Imaging of Select Multisystem Disorders

Editor

SRINIVASA R. PRASAD

RADIOLOGIC CLINICS
OF NORTH AMERICA

www.radiologic.theclinics.com

Consulting Editor
FRANK H. MILLER

May 2016 • Volume 54 • Number 3

ELSEVIER

1600 John F. Kennedy Boulevard • Suite 1800 • Philadelphia, Pennsylvania, 19103-2899

http://www.theclinics.com

RADIOLOGIC CLINICS OF NORTH AMERICA Volume 54, Number 3
May 2016 ISSN 0033-8389, ISBN 13: 978-0-323-44479-8

Editor: John Vassallo (j.vassallo@elsevier.com)
Developmental Editor: Donald Mumford

Radiologic Clinics of North America (ISSN 0033-8389) is published bimonthly by Elsevier Inc., 360 Park Avenue South, New York, NY 10010-1710. Months of issue are January, March, May, July, September, and November. Periodicals postage paid at New York, NY and additional mailing offices. Subscription prices are USD 460 per year for US individuals, USD 784 per year for US institutions, USD 100 per year for US students and residents, USD 535 per year for Canadian individuals, USD 1002 per year for Canadian institutions, USD 660 per year for international individuals, USD 1002 per year for international institutions, and USD 315 per year for Canadian and foreign students/residents. To receive student and resident rate, orders must be accompanied by name of affiliated institution, date of term and the signature of program/residency coordinatior on institution letterhead. Orders will be billed at individual rate until proof of status is received. Foreign air speed delivery is included in all *Clinics* subscription prices. All prices are subject to change without notice. **POSTMASTER:** Send address changes to *Radiologic Clinics of North America*, Elsevier Health Sciences Division, Subscription Customer Service, 3251 Riverport Lane, Maryland Heights, MO63043. **Customer Service: Telephone: 1-800-654-2452** (U.S. and Canada); **1-314-447-8871** (outside U.S. and Canada). **Fax: 1-314-447-8029.** E-mail: journalscustomerservice-usa@elsevier.com **(for print support);** journalsonlinesupport-usa@elsevier.com **(for online support).**

Reprints. For copies of 100 or more of articles in this publication, please contact the Commercial Reprints Department, Elsevier Inc., 360 Park Avenue South, New York, New York 10010-1710. Tel.: +1-212-633-3874; Fax: +1-212-633-3820; E-mail: reprints@elsevier.com.

Radiologic Clinics of North America also published in Greek Paschalidis Medical Publications, Athens, Greece.

Radiologic Clinics of North America is covered in *MEDLINE/PubMed (Index Medicus), EMBASE/Excerpta Medica, Current Contents/Life Sciences, Current Contents/Clinical Medicine, RSNA Index to Imaging Literature, BIOSIS, Science Citation Index,* and *ISI/BIOMED.*

Printed in the United States of America.

Contributors

CONSULTING EDITOR

FRANK H. MILLER, MD
Chief, Body Imaging Section and Fellowship
Program; Medical Director of MRI; Professor,
Department of Radiology, Northwestern
University Feinberg School of Medicine,
Chicago, Illinois

EDITOR

SRINIVASA R. PRASAD, MD
Professor, Department of Radiology, The
University of Texas MD Anderson Cancer
Center, Houston, Texas

AUTHORS

BEHRANG AMINI, MD, PhD
Assistant Professor, Musculoskeletal Imaging,
Diagnostic Radiology, The University of Texas
MD Anderson Cancer Center, Houston, Texas

BRICE ANDRING, MD
Department of Radiology, University of Texas
Southwestern Medical Center, Dallas, Texas

BENJAMIN ATCHIE, MD
Department of Radiology, University of Texas
Southwestern Medical Center, Dallas, Texas

HERSH CHANDARANA, MD
Associate Professor, Department of Radiology,
NYU Langone Medical Center, New York,
New York

**ESHWAR N. CHANDRA, MD, DNB, FRCR,
FICR**
Professor and Head, Department of Radiology,
Kamineni Academy of Medical Sciences and
Research Centre, Hyderabad, Telangana, India

STEVEN CHUA, MD
Department of Diagnostic and Interventional
Imaging, The University of Texas Health
Science Center at Houston, Houston, Texas

GIRISH FATTERPAKER, MD
Associate Professor, Department of Radiology,
NYU Langone Medical Center, New York,
New York

ROBERT GAINES FRICKE, MD
Department of Diagnostic Radiology,
University of Arkansas for Medical Sciences,
Little Rock, Arkansas

JAMES GLOCKNER, MD, PhD
Department of Radiology, Mayo Clinic,
Rochester, Minnesota

JOSEPH R. GRAJO, MD
Director of Body MRI; Assistant Professor,
Division of Abdominal Imaging, Department of
Radiology, Shands Medical Center, University
of Florida College of Medicine, Gainesville,
Florida

CAREY GUIDRY, MD
Department of Diagnostic Radiology,
University of Arkansas for Medical Sciences,
Little Rock, Arkansas

ROBERT P. HARTMAN, MD
Department of Radiology, Mayo Clinic,
Rochester, Minnesota

MICHAEL HOCH, MD
Department of Radiology, NYU Langone
Medical Center, New York, New York

BENJAMIN M. HOWE, MD
Department of Radiology, Mayo Clinic,
Rochester, Minnesota

KEDAR JAMBHEKAR, MD
Department of Diagnostic Radiology,
University of Arkansas for Medical Sciences,
Little Rock, Arkansas

SANJEEVA P. KALVA, MD
Department of Radiology, University of Texas
Southwestern Medical Center; Chief,
Interventional Radiology, UT Southwestern
Medical Center, Dallas, Texas

AVINASH KAMBADAKONE, MD
Medical Director of Martha's Vineyard Hospital
Imaging; Assistant Professor, Division of
Abdominal Imaging, Department of Radiology,
Massachusetts General Hospital, Harvard
Medical School, Boston, Massachusetts

VENKATA S. KATABATHINA, MD
Department of Radiology, University of Texas
Health Science Center at San Antonio, San
Antonio, Texas

RASHMI KATRE, MD
Assistant Professor, Department of Radiology,
The University of Texas Health Science Center
at San Antonio, San Antonio, Texas

AKIRA KAWASHIMA, MD, PhD
Department of Radiology, Mayo Clinic,
Rochester, Minnesota

RAVI K. KAZA, MD
Associate Professor, Department of Radiology,
University of Michigan Hospitals, Ann Arbor,
Michigan

ABHISHEK R. KERALIYA, MD
Department of Imaging, Dana Farber Cancer
Institute; Department of Radiology, Brigham
and Women's Hospital, Harvard Medical
School, Boston, Massachusetts

SUHARE KHALIL, MD
Department of Radiology, University of Texas
Health Science Center at San Antonio, San
Antonio, Texas

**NIRANJAN KHANDELWAL, MD, Dip NBE,
FICR, FAMS**
Professor and Head, Department of
Radiodiagnosis, Post Graduate Institute of
Medical Education and Research, Chandigarh,
India

ANKAJ KHOSLA, MD
Department of Radiology, University of Texas
Southwestern Medical Center, Dallas, Texas

ANANT KRISHNAN, MD
Associate Professor of Radiology, Department
of Diagnostic Radiology, The Oakland
University William Beaumont School of
Medicine and Beaumont Hospital, Royal Oak,
Michigan

NEERAJ LALWANI, MD
Department of Radiology, University of
Washington, Seattle, Washington

NARAYAN LATH, MD
Department of Radiology, Singapore General
Hospital, Singapore, Singapore

JARROD MACFARLANE, MD
Department of Radiology, University of Texas
Southwestern Medical Center, Dallas, Texas

CHRISTINE O. MENIAS, MD
Department of Radiology, Mayo Clinic,
Scottsdale, Arizona

AMY MUMBOWER, MD
Assistant Professor, Department of Radiology,
The University of Texas Health Science Center
at San Antonio, San Antonio, Texas

PRASHANT S. NAPHADE, MD, DNB
Fellow in Neuroradiology; Consultant
Radiologist, CT/MRI Department, ESIC
Hospital, Mumbai, India

TARUN PANDEY, MD, FRCR
Department of Diagnostic Radiology,
University of Arkansas for Medical Sciences,
Little Rock, Arkansas

RAJ MOHAN PASPULATI, MD
Director of Medical Student Education;
Associate Professor, Department of Radiology,
University Hospitals Case Medical Center,
Case Western Reserve University, Cleveland,
Ohio

RAJAN P. PATEL, MD
Department of Diagnostic and Interventional Imaging, The University of Texas Health Science Center at Houston, Houston, Texas

SRINIVASA R. PRASAD, MD
Professor, Department of Radiology, The University of Texas MD Anderson Cancer Center, Houston, Texas

ROOPA RAM, MD
Department of Diagnostic Radiology, University of Arkansas for Medical Sciences, Little Rock, Arkansas

NIKHIL H. RAMAIYA, MD
Department of Imaging, Dana Farber Cancer Institute; Department of Radiology, Brigham and Women's Hospital, Harvard Medical School, Boston, Massachusetts

RAVI RAMAKANTAN, MD
Consultant Radiologist and Head of Department, Department of Radiology, Kokilaben Dhirubhai Ambani Hospital, Mumbai, Maharashtra, India

ABHIJIT A. RAUT, MD
Consultant Radiologist, Department of Radiology, Kokilaben Dhirubhai Ambani Hospital, Mumbai, Maharashtra, India

JYOTHI G. REDDY, DNB
Senior Resident, Department of Radiology, Kamineni Academy of Medical Sciences and Research Centre, Hyderabad, Telangana, India

CARLOS SANTIAGO RESTREPO, MD
Director, Cardio-Thoracic Radiology; Professor, Department of Radiology, The University of Texas Health Science Center at San Antonio, San Antonio, Texas

ERIC ROHREN, MD, PhD
Professor, Nuclear Medicine, The University of Texas MD Anderson Cancer Center, Houston, Texas

DUSHYANT V. SAHANI, MD
Director of CT; Associate Professor, Division of Abdominal Imaging, Department of Radiology, Massachusetts General Hospital, Harvard Medical School, Boston, Massachusetts

SHETAL SHAH, MD
Associate Professor, Diagnostic Radiology, Cleveland Clinic, Cleveland, Ohio

KRISHNA PRASAD SHANBHOGUE, MD
Assistant Professor, Department of Radiology, NYU Langone Medical Center, New York, New York

SOOYOUNG SHIN, MD
Department of Radiology, The University of Texas MD Anderson Cancer Center, Houston, Texas

ATUL B. SHINAGARE, MD
Department of Imaging, Dana Farber Cancer Institute; Department of Radiology, Brigham and Women's Hospital, Harvard Medical School, Boston, Massachusetts

ANINDITA SINHA, MD
Assistant Professor, Department of Radiodiagnosis, Post Graduate Institute of Medical Education and Research, Chandigarh, India

KUSHALJIT SINGH SODHI, MD, PhD, MAMS, FICR
Additional Professor, Department of Radiodiagnosis, Post Graduate Institute of Medical Education and Research, Chandigarh, India

VENKATESWAR R. SURABHI, MD
Department of Diagnostic and Interventional Imaging, The University of Texas Health Science Center at Houston, Houston, Texas

NAOKI TAKAHASHI, MD
Department of Radiology, Mayo Clinic, Rochester, Minnesota

SREE HARSHA TIRUMANI, MD
Department of Imaging, Dana Farber Cancer Institute; Department of Radiology, Brigham and Women's Hospital, Harvard Medical School, Boston, Massachusetts

RAGHUNANDAN VIKRAM, MD
Associate Professor, Abdominal Imaging, Diagnostic Radiology, The University of Texas MD Anderson Cancer Center, Houston, Texas

DHARSHAN R. VUMMIDI, MD
Clinical Lecturer, Department of Radiology,
University of Michigan Hospitals, Ann Arbor,
Michigan

BENJAMIN WHITE, MD
Department of Radiology, University of Texas
Southwestern Medical Center, Dallas, Texas

SARVARI YELLAPRAGADA, MD
Assistant Professor, Medicine-Hematology
and Oncology, Baylor College of Medicine;

Staff Physician, Michael E DeBakey VA
Medical Center, Houston, Texas

ATIF ZAHEER, MD
The Russell H. Morgan Department of
Radiology and Radiological Science, Johns
Hopkins Medical Institutions, Baltimore,
Maryland

JOSEPH ZERR, MD
Department of Radiology, University of Texas
Southwestern Medical Center, Dallas, Texas

Contents

von Hippel-Lindau (VHL) disease is an autosomal-dominant, hereditary, multisystem neoplasia syndrome with increased susceptibility to several benign and malignant tumors. VHL occurs in about 1 in 36,000 live births and is associated with germline mutation of the VHL tumor suppressor gene on the short arm of chromosome 3. VHL disease exhibits diverse genotype and phenotype correlations, exhibits variable intrafamilial and interfamilial expressivity, and can manifest with benign and malignant tumors of the central nervous system, kidneys, adrenals, pancreas, and reproductive organs. Imaging and management of this entity are therefore multidisciplinary. An overview of VHL disease is presented.

Tuberous sclerosis complex (TSC) is a multisystem, genetic disorder characterized by development of hamartomas in the brain, abdomen, and thorax. It results from a mutation in one of 2 tumor suppressor genes that activates the mammalian target of rapamycin pathway. This article discusses the origins of the disorder, the recently updated criteria for the diagnosis of TSC, and the cross-sectional imaging findings and recommendations for surveillance. Familiarity with the diverse radiological features facilitates diagnosis and helps in treatment planning and monitoring response to treatment of this multisystem disorder.

MEN1, MEN2, and MEN4 comprise a series of familial disorders involving the simultaneous occurrence of tumors in more than one endocrine organ, collectively known as multiple endocrine neoplasia. Patients with this family of disorders develop tumors of the parathyroid gland, pancreas, pituitary gland, adrenal gland, and thyroid gland, along with miscellaneous neuroendocrine tumors of the respiratory and gastrointestinal tracts. Although some patients undergo early prophylactic surgical management, particularly in the setting of familial medullary thyroid carcinoma, many develop tumors later in life. These tumors are often discovered at imaging for screening purposes. Recognition of the imaging features of the known tumors is important for appropriate patient management.

Despite significant improvements in the diagnosis and treatment of tuberculosis achieved during the last 3 decades, tuberculosis still remains one of the deadliest communicable diseases worldwide. Tuberculosis is still present in all regions of the world, with a more significant impact in developing countries. This article reviews the most common imaging manifestations of primary and postprimary tuberculosis, their complications, and the critical role of imaging in the diagnosis and follow-up of affected patients.

Imaging Spectrum of Extrathoracic Tuberculosis

Abhijit A. Raut, Prashant S. Naphade, and Ravi Ramakantan

The incidence of extrathoracic tuberculosis (ETB) continues to increase slowly, especially in immunocompromised and multidrug-resistant tuberculosis (TB) patients. ETB manifests with nonspecific clinical symptoms, and being less frequent, is less familiar to most physicians. Imaging modalities of choice are computed tomography (lymphadenopathy and abdominal TB) and MR imaging (central nervous system and musculoskeletal system TB). ETB commonly involves multiple organ systems with characteristic imaging findings that permit accurate diagnosis and timely management.

Multidetector Computed Tomography and MR Imaging Findings in Mycotic Infections

Niranjan Khandelwal, Kushaljit Singh Sodhi, Anindita Sinha, Jyothi G. Reddy, and Eshwar N. Chandra

Fungal infections constitute a diverse spectrum of infections with variable clinical and imaging features. They are commonly opportunistic infections that affect immunocompromised individuals secondary to inherited or acquired disorders. Fungal infections may affect multiple organ systems and contribute to significant morbidity and mortality. Although the imaging features of some fungal infections are characteristic and permit their diagnosis, many mycotic infections manifest nonspecific findings. Definitive diagnosis often depends on histopathological analysis. Early diagnosis requires both clinical suspicion and supporting radiological evidence. Early treatment results in reduced morbidity and mortality. This article reviews the imaging findings in opportunistic and endemic fungal infections.

Imaging of Sarcoidosis: A Contemporary Review

Carey Guidry, R. Gaines Fricke, Roopa Ram, Tarun Pandey, and Kedar Jambhekar

Sarcoidosis is a systemic granulomatous disorder with a variety of clinical presentations and radiological appearances. Although it primarily affects the lungs and lymphatics, sarcoidosis potentially involves essentially every organ system. On imaging, sarcoidosis can mimic different disease entities, including primary and metastatic neoplasms, vasculitis, and other granulomatous infections. Definitive diagnosis often requires a combination of clinical, radiological, and histologic information. Imaging plays a crucial role in diagnosis and evaluating response to therapy. This review covers imaging findings in sarcoidosis within each organ system, with an emphasis on the use of imaging in the diagnosis and management of this condition.

Immunoglobulin G4–Related Disease: Recent Advances in Pathogenesis and Imaging Findings

Venkata S. Katabathina, Suhare Khalil, Sooyoung Shin, Narayan Lath, Christine O. Menias, and Srinivasa R. Prasad

Immunoglobulin G4–related disease (IgG4-RD) is a novel, immune-mediated, multisystem disease characterized by the development of tumefactive lesions in multiple organs. IgG4-RD encompasses many fibroinflammatory diseases that had been thought to be confined to single organs. Delayed diagnosis or misdiagnosis as malignancies leading to aggressive treatment may be averted by identification of the multisystem nature of IgG4-RD. Most cases show exquisite response to steroid therapy; steroid-resistant cases are being treated by novel therapeutic agents, including B-cell depleting agents such as rituximab. Cross-sectional imaging studies play a pivotal role in the initial diagnosis, assessing response to therapy and long-term surveillance.

Inflammatory myofibroblastic tumor (IMT) is a mesenchymal neoplasm of intermediate biological potential with a predilection for the lung and abdominopelvic region. IMT represents the neoplastic subset of the family of inflammatory pseudotumors, an umbrella term for spindle cell proliferations of uncertain histogenesis with a variable inflammatory component. IMTs show characteristic fasciitis-like, compact spindle cell and hypocellular fibrous histologic patterns and distinctive molecular features. Imaging findings reflect pathologic features and vary from an ill-defined, infiltrating lesion to a well circumscribed, soft tissue mass owing to variable inflammatory, stromal, and myofibroblastic components.

Optimal management of solitary fibrous tumor requires a multidisciplinary approach with proper histopathological mapping and use of various imaging modalities for exact delineation of primary tumor and metastatic disease if present. In this article, the authors present a comprehensive review of the spectrum of imaging findings of solitary fibrous tumors involving various organ systems and discuss the role of molecular targeted therapies in the management of metastatic disease.

Monoclonal gammopathy of unknown significance (MGUS) is a clinically asymptomatic premalignant clonal plasma cell or lymphoplasmacytic proliferative disorder. Smoldering multiple myeloma, also called asymptomatic multiple myeloma, is an intermediate stage between MGUS and symptomatic multiple myeloma. As the name implies, extraosseous or extramedullary myeloma refers to the presence of myeloma deposits outside the skeletal system. Waldenström macroglobulinemia is a distinct subtype of plasma cell dyscrasia characterized by lymphoplasmacytic lymphoma in the bone marrow with an associated IgM monoclonal gammopathy. Amyloidosis is a condition characterized by extracellular deposition of fibrils composed of a variety of normal serum proteins.

Amyloidosis is a heterogeneous group of disorders that are characterized by extracellular deposition of misfolded and aggregated autologous proteins leading to organ dysfunction. Amyloid deposits produce diverse clinical syndromes depending on their type, location, and the amount of deposition. Clinical and imaging features of amyloidosis in various organ systems are described.

Systemic vasculopathies represent a wide spectrum of heterogeneous vascular disorders characterized by variable target vessel involvement, vascular abnormalities, and end organ damage. The revised 2012 Chapel Hill Consensus Conference scheme classifies systemic vasculitis syndromes into primary systemic, secondary systemic, single-vessel, and variable-vessel vasculitis categories with associated management implications. Multimodality imaging not only allows diagnosis, characterization, and localization of vascular abnormalities but also permits evaluation of natural history and complications, thus, facilitating optimal patient management. This article discusses epidemiologic and radiologic characteristics of several common systemic vasculopathies with an emphasis on the role of endovascular therapy for management of select disorders.

PROGRAM OBJECTIVE

The objective of the *Radiologic Clinics of North America* is to keep practicing radiologists and radiology residents up to date with current clinical practice in radiology by providing timely articles reviewing the state of the art in patient care.

TARGET AUDIENCE

Practicing radiologists, radiology residents, and other health care professionals who provide patient care utilizing radiologic findings.

LEARNING OBJECTIVES

Upon completion of this activity, participants will be able to:
1. Review updates in imaging of myofibroblastic and solitary fibrous tumors.
2. Discuss the imaging spectrum and manifestation of thoracic and extra-thoracic tuberculosis.
3. Recognize updates in the imaging of multi-system disorders.

ACCREDITATION

The Elsevier Office of Continuing Medical Education (EOCME) is accredited by the Accreditation Council for Continuing Medical Education (ACCME) to provide continuing medical education for physicians.

The EOCME designates this enduring material for a maximum of 15 *AMA PRA Category 1 Credit*(s)™. Physicians should claim only the credit commensurate with the extent of their participation in the activity.

All other health care professionals requesting continuing education credit for this enduring material will be issued a certificate of participation.

DISCLOSURE OF CONFLICTS OF INTEREST

The EOCME assesses conflict of interest with its instructors, faculty, planners, and other individuals who are in a position to control the content of CME activities. All relevant conflicts of interest that are identified are thoroughly vetted by EOCME for fair balance, scientific objectivity, and patient care recommendations. EOCME is committed to providing its learners with CME activities that promote improvements or quality in healthcare and not a specific proprietary business or a commercial interest.

The planning committee, staff, authors and editors listed below have identified no financial relationships or relationships to products or devices they or their spouse/life partner have with commercial interest related to the content of this CME activity:

Behrang Amini, MD, PhD; Brice Andring, MD; Benjamin Atchie, MD; Hersh Chandarana, MD; Eshwar N Chandra, MD, DNB, FRCR, FICR; Steven Chua, MD; Girish Fatterpaker, MD; Anjali Fortna; R. Gaines Fricke, MD; James Glockner, MD, PhD; Joseph R. Grajo, MD; Carey Guidry, MD; Robert P. Hartman, MD; Michael Hoch, MD; Benjamin M. Howe, MD; Kedar Jambhekar, MD; Sanjeeva P. Kalva, MD; Avinash Kambadakone, MD; Venkata S. Katabathina, MD; Rashmi Katre, MD; Akira Kawashima, MD, PhD; Abhishek R. Keraliya, MD; Suhare Khalil, MD; Niranjan Khandelwal, MD, Dip NBE, FICR, FAMS; Ankaj Khosla, MD; Anant Krishnan, MD; Neeraj Lalwani, MD; Narayan Lath, MD; Jarrod MacFarlane, MD; Christine O. Menias, MD; Frank H. Miller, MD; Amy Mumbower, MD; Prashant S. Naphade, MD, DNB; Tarun Pandey, MD, FRCR; Raj Mohan Paspulati, MD; Rajan P. Patel, MD; Srinivasa R. Prasad, MD; Roopa Ram, MD; Nikhil H. Ramaiya, MD; Ravi Ramakantan, MD; Abhijit A. Raut, MD; Jyothi G. Reddy, DNB; Carlos Santiago Restrepo, MD; Eric Rohren, MD, PhD; Dushyant V. Sahani, MD; Erin Scheckenbach; Shetal Shah, MD; Krishna Prasad Shanbhogue, MD; Sooyoung Shin, MD; Atul B. Shinagare, MD; Kushaljit Singh Sodhi, MD, PhD, MAMS, FICR; Anindita Sinja, MD; Karthik Subramaniam; Venkateswar R. Surabhi, MD; Naoki Takahashi, MD; Sree Harsha Tirumani, MD; John Vassallo; Raghunandan Vikram, MD; Benjamin White, MD; Sarvari Yellapragada, MD; Atif Zaheer, MD; Joseph Zerr, MD.

UNAPPROVED/OFF-LABEL USE DISCLOSURE

The EOCME requires CME faculty to disclose to the participants:
1. When products or procedures being discussed are off-label, unlabelled, experimental, and/or investigational (not US Food and Drug Administration [FDA] approved); and
2. Any limitations on the information presented, such as data that are preliminary or that represent ongoing research, interim analyses, and/or unsupported opinions. Faculty may discuss information about pharmaceutical agents that is outside of FDA-approved labelling. This information is intended solely for CME and is not intended to promote off-label use of these medications. If you have any questions, contact the medical affairs department of the manufacturer for the most recent prescribing information.

TO ENROLL

To enroll in the *Radiologic Clinics of North America* Continuing Medical Education program, call customer service at 1-800-654-2452 or sign up online at http://www.theclinics.com/home/cme. The CME program is available to subscribers for an additional annual fee of USD 315.

METHOD OF PARTICIPATION

In order to claim credit, participants must complete the following:

1. Complete enrolment as indicated above.
2. Read the activity.
3. Complete the CME Test and Evaluation. Participants must achieve a score of 70% on the test. All CME Tests and Evaluations must be completed online.

CME INQUIRIES/SPECIAL NEEDS

For all CME inquiries or special needs, please contact elsevierCME@elsevier.com.

RADIOLOGIC CLINICS OF NORTH AMERICA

ISSUE OF RELATED INTEREST

Neuroimaging Clinics, February 2016 (Vol. 24, Issue 1)
Plaque Imaging
J. Kevin DeMarco, *Editor*
Available at: http://www.neuroimaging.theclinics.com

THE CLINICS ARE AVAILABLE ONLINE!
Access your subscription at:
www.theclinics.com

Preface
Imaging of Select Multisystem Disorders

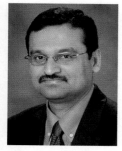

Srinivasa R. Prasad, MD
Editor

Recent advances in pathology and genetics have thrown fresh light on the pathogenesis of many "old diseases," clarified the nosology of some entities such as solitary fibrous tumors, and facilitated the diagnosis and management of some recently described disorders such as "IgG4-related disease." A comprehensive understanding of epidemiology and pathogenesis permits radiologists to make sense of the protean manifestations of many multisystem disorders as well as to allow accurate diagnosis based on pathognomic imaging features of select entities. This issue of the *Radiologic Clinics of North America* titled, "Imaging of Select Multisystem Disorders," aims to provide state-of-the-art, yet practical information for practicing radiologists, clinicians, trainees, and academicians albeit in "bite-size" format to enable optimal patient care. In this subspecialized world, I am fortunate to get the support of esteemed "multi-system" experts from reputed institutions, who agreed to share their "cutting-edge" insights and expertise with us all.

As the editor of this issue, I selected a wide variety of distinctive, multisystem disorders to include hereditary, infectious, inflammatory, proliferative, and neoplastic entities. The covered topics include von Hippel-Lindau syndrome, tuberous sclerosis, MEN syndromes, tuberculosis, fungal infections, sarcoidosis, inflammatory myofibroblastic tumor, IgG4-related disease, solitary fibrous tumor, multiple myeloma/plasmacytoma, amyloidosis, and systemic vasculopathy syndromes.

As the saying goes, "it takes a village to raise a child"; this issue would not have been possible without the combined efforts and expert contributions of all the authors who willingly shared their "phenomenal" cases with us. It has been a distinct privilege and pleasure to work with the authors, some of whom I consider as my "Gurus." I am indebted to Frank Miller, MD (Consulting Editor) for giving me this opportunity to edit this issue. I am thankful to John Vassallo (Acquisitions Editor) and the staff at Elsevier for making this a pleasurable experience. I am blessed to have the enthusiastic support of my family, including my wife, Raji, and the boys, Aditya and Rohan.

Today's radiologists are forced to not only manage "image overload" but also learn to deal with "information overload." I hope that this issue provides the readers with a contemporary and comprehensive imaging update on a variety of uncommon, yet fascinating spectrum of disorders that affect multiple organ systems. I am confident that this will serve as a valuable and practical resource to all who care for their patients in the upcoming years.

Srinivasa R. Prasad, MD
Department of Radiology
The University of Texas
MD Anderson Cancer Center
1515 Holcombe Boulevard
Houston, TX 77030, USA

E-mail address:
sprasad2@mdanderson.org

Radiol Clin N Am 54 (2016) xv
http://dx.doi.org/10.1016/j.rcl.2016.02.001
0033-8389/16/$ – see front matter © 2016 Published by Elsevier Inc.

radiologic.theclinics.com

Erratum

In the March 2016 issue (Volume 54, number 2), in the article, "Surgical Techniques and Imaging Complications of Liver Transplant," authored by Akshay D. Baheti, Rupan Sanyal, Matthew T. Heller, and Puneet Bhargava, Figure 13(B) on page 209 is incorrect. The correct figure and caption is below.

Figure 13(B). HIDA scan performed subsequently shows complete leakage of the radiotracer into the peritoneal cavity.

http://dx.doi.org/10.1016/j.rcl.2016.04.003
0033-8389/16/$ – see front matter

radiologic.theclinics.com

von Hippel-Lindau Disease
Review of Genetics and Imaging

Krishna Prasad Shanbhogue, MD*, Michael Hoch, MD,
Girish Fatterpaker, MD, Hersh Chandarana, MD

KEYWORDS

- von Hippel-Lindau disease • Hemangioblastoma • Serous cystadenoma
- Clear cell renal cell carcinoma • Pheochromocytoma

KEY POINTS

- von Hippel-Lindau (VHL) disease is an autosomal-dominant, familial cancer syndrome that genetically predisposes affected individuals to characteristic tumors in multiple organs.
- The natural history of VHL disease, including the development of tumors and disease severity, is highly variable.
- Given the highly variable penetrance of disease, imaging study might be the first to raise suspicion of VHL disease when characteristic lesions are seen, such as multifocal renal cell carcinomas, bilateral pheochromocytomas or multiple pancreatic cysts, and serous cystadenomas.
- Renal cell carcinoma and central nervous system hemangioblastoma are major causes of death in VHL patients. With improved surveillance, early diagnosis of lesions by modern imaging studies, and advances in treatment, prognosis of VHL has improved.

INTRODUCTION

von Hippel-Lindau (VHL) disease is a rare, multisystem familial neoplasia syndrome that genetically predisposes affected individuals to tumor formation in multiple organ systems. VHL disease is inherited in an autosomal-dominant fashion with high penetrance and variable expression.[1,2] In the central nervous system (CNS), characteristic hemangioblastomas (HBs) are seen in the retina, brain, and spine with additional tumors of the endolymphatic sac (ELS). Outside of the CNS, VHL disease presents with tumors of the pancreas, kidneys, adrenals, and reproductive organs. Therefore, it is essential that radiologists be familiar with their imaging appearance. Collins, an English ophthalmologist, first described a case of 2 siblings with retinal HBs in 1894.[3] von Hippel, a German ophthalmologist, first recognized the familial nature of retinal HBs in 1904, and a Swedish ophthalmologist, Arvid Lindau, first described the association of retinal and cerebellar lesions.[4,5] The term "von Hippel-Lindau Disease" was coined by Melmon and Rosen,[6] who studied a large family with the disorder in 1964. In 1993, the VHL tumor suppressor gene was isolated to the short arm of chromosome 3 (3p25.5).[7]

Criteria have been established for clinical diagnosis of VHL disease. VHL disease is clinically diagnosed in patients with a family history, and a CNS HB (including retinal HBs), pheochromocytoma (PCC), or clear cell renal carcinoma (RCC). In patients without family history, the presence of 2 or more CNS HBs, or one CNS HB and a visceral tumor (with the exception of epididymal and renal cysts, which are frequent in the general population), meet the diagnostic criteria.[6,8]

Disclosure Statement: The authors have nothing to disclose.
Department of Radiology, NYU Langone Medical Center, 660 First Avenue, 3rd Floor, New York, NY 10016, USA
* Corresponding author.
E-mail address: Alampady.Shanbhogue@nyumc.org

Radiol Clin N Am 54 (2016) 409–422
http://dx.doi.org/10.1016/j.rcl.2015.12.004

The natural history of VHL disease, including the manifestation of tumors and its severity, is highly variable, both within and between families. Mean age of first manifestation of VHL disease is 24 to 26 years.[9,10] It is rare for the diagnosis to be made after the age of 60, but there is no age at which lesions cease to occur. The average age of death is 49 years old, usually from complications of cerebellar tumor or metastatic clear cell RCC.[1] However, morbidity and mortality have decreased in recent history because of genetic testing, improved screening techniques, and surgical and chemotherapy advances.[11]

GENETICS AND PATHOLOGY

The inheritance of VHL disease is autosomal-dominant; therefore, there is a 50% chance of inheriting the *VHL* gene from a carrier. Because there is variable gene expression, a wide spectrum of manifestations results with most patients with *VHL* gene mutation presenting with disease-related symptoms by the age of 65 years.[1] The *VHL* gene, located on the short arm of chromosome 3 (3p25.5), is a tumor suppressor gene. Inactivation of its gene product, VHL protein, results in unregulated cell growth.[7]

VHL is a relatively small gene encoding 854 nucleotides on 3 exons and encodes the VHL protein.[7] Under normal tissue oxygen levels, the VHL protein forms a complex with elongin B, elongin C, Cul 2, and Rbx1, which in turn initiates ubiquitin-mediated degradation of hypoxia-inducible factors (HIFs), HIF-1α and HIF-2α.[12–14] HIF regulates expression of several genes, including vascular endothelial growth factor, platelet-derived growth factor, epidermal growth factor receptor, transforming growth factor -α, and glucose transporter -1 genes. VHL gene mutations lead to stabilization of HIF-1 and HIF-2, and activation of these HIF-dependent genes are implicated in angiogenesis, proliferation, and metabolism.[15,16]

More than 300 germline mutations have been identified in families with VHL disease.[17] About 20% of VHL cases are due to sporadic mutations and present later than people with inherited VHL disease.[18] Although sporadic cases require a "2-hit" model of gene inactivation, familial cases require only a single "hit" because one allele is already affected at the time of conception.[19] VHL gene deletions, frameshifts, and missense mutations have been implicated in the development of VHL disease. VHL disease has been classified into distinct clinical subtypes (type 1/2A/2B/2C) based on clustering of tumors (**Table 1**). It appears that missense mutations predominate in VHL disease with PCC; germline deletion or truncating mutation implies a low risk of PCC.[20] VHL gene mutations lead to impaired apoptosis of sympathoadrenal precursor cells during embryogenesis, thereby increasing the risk of developing into PCCs in the later life.[21,22] RCCs are more frequently seen in patients with truncating mutations compared with missense mutations.[23,24] Individuals with deletion of VHL gene (VHL type 1B) have also been found to have reduced risk for RCC, in addition to PCC.[25–27] Acquired somatic mutations in VHL have been found to be associated with sporadic VHL-type tumors such as clear cell RCCs and HBs.[28,29] Missense mutations carry an overall high risk for tumor development, although predicting the actual risk is more complex due to considerable allelic heterogeneity.[27,30] However, proposed type 1/2A/2B/2C classification of VHL disease can be accurately used only in large scale and is primarily based on clinical phenotype.[31]

Table 1
von Hippel-Lindau disease subtypes: genotype-phenotype correlation

Subtype	Phenotype	Genotype
VHL type 1 (low risk for PCC)	Retinal angioma, CNS HB, renal cell carcinoma, pancreatic cysts, and neuroendocrine tumors	Truncating mutations or missense mutations that grossly disrupt the folding of the VHL protein
VHL type 2 (high risk for PCC)		
Type 2A (low risk for renal cell carcinoma)	PCC, retinal angiomas, and CNS HB	Missense mutation
Type 2B (high risk for renal cell carcinoma)	PCC, renal cell carcinoma, retinal angioma, CNS HBs, pancreatic cysts, and neuroendocrine tumors	
Type 2C	Risk for PCC only; some individuals within families with apparent type 2C disease have developed HBs	

Central Nervous System Manifestations

CNS tumors seen in VHL disease include retinal HB, CNS HB, and endolymphatic sac tumors (ELSTs).

HB is a benign vascular lesion that contains channels lined by cuboidal endothelium, is interspersed with nests of foamy stromal cells and pericytes, and is supported by collagenous tissue of varying thickness. Mast cells are also found and may be responsible for the production of erythropoietin-causing polycythemia.[32] At gross inspection, HBs are well circumscribed but without a true capsule. They may be purely solid or partially cystic with most of the cystic lesions having yellow- or amber-colored proteinaceous fluid. HBs are very vascular with the solid reddish nodule generally close to the pial surface. Microscopic examination shows a rich capillary network and large vacuolated stromal cells that have a clear cytoplasm.[19,32] HBs have no well-defined histologic origin. There is no agreeable explanation for most of these tumors to be located posteriorly within the brain around the fourth ventricle. Lindau suggested that a segment of the primitive choroid plexus likely becomes incorporated within the developing cerebellum. HBs were thought to develop from these choroid remnants. This theory would seem plausible in light of the observation that one of the functions of the primordial choroid plexus is hematopoiesis, but it does not account for the occurrence of HBs elsewhere in the CNS.

RETINAL HEMANGIOBLASTOMAS

Retinal HBs generally are the first CNS lesions in VHL to come to clinical attention with lesions occurring at 25 years of age.[9] They also occur frequently with 45% to 60% of VHL cases having a retinal lesion, and 50% are bilateral.[9,33] They have historically been called retinal angiomas or hemangiomas, but should be characterized as HBs because they are pathologically identical to other CNS HBs. They are histologically composed of significant vascular channels lined by cuboidal endothelial cells, foamy stromal cells, and pericytes.[34] Symptoms vary by location. About 85% are located in the peripheral retina and are commonly asymptomatic, but when large or involving the optic disc, they can cause vision loss. Leaky capillaries with exudate and arteriovenous (AV) shunting cause complications, such as retinal detachment, macular edema, glaucoma, cataracts, uveitis, and ophthalmitis.[6,9]

Ophthalmoscopy shows small lesions (<3 mm) as a red hue and large lesions as nodular and exudative lesions. On fluorescein angiography, dilated feeding arteries and veins may be seen with microaneurysms.[32,35,36] On MR imaging, the visible lesions appear hyperintense on T1-weighted images (T1WI) when compared with the surrounding vitreous and show significant enhancement. The lesions may show calcifications when detected late.[6] However, only large lesions may be seen with MR imaging, and by then, it is usually too late because large lesions cause profound vision loss.[32,37] This finding heightens the need for aggressive screening ophthalmoscopy that some argue should begin in infancy of familial cases to identify lesions at their smallest and most easily treatable. Treatment of small lesions usually consists of laser photocoagulation. Larger and complicated lesions may be treated by cryotherapy, radiotherapy, or vitreoretinal surgery. Enucleation is a possible treatment for lesions causing intractable pain or glaucoma.[9,33,38]

CENTRAL NERVOUS SYSTEM HEMANGIOBLASTOMAS

HBs of the CNS are classified as World Health Organization grade I tumors. Sixty percent to 80% of VHL patients will have a CNS HB. The cerebellum is the most common site (44%–72%), followed by spinal cord (13%–50%), brainstem, dorsal medulla and pons (10%–25%), and rarely, supratentorial structures, such as the optic pathways, choroid plexus, anterior pituitary, and infundibulum (1%).[32,39,40] HBs tend to occur around the age of 30 years in VHL disease but can be seen earlier.[9] The National Institutes of Health recommends contrast-enhanced MR imaging of the brain and spine in VHL cases from age 11, every 2 years, along with annual physical and neurologic examinations. When an unsuspected isolated CNS HB is found on imaging, a complete CNS contrast-enhanced MR imaging should be performed.

Cerebellar HBs represent 2% of all brain tumors and 7% to 10% of all posterior fossa tumors. Only 5% to 30% of HBs are due to VHL disease. HBs in patients with VHL disease tend to be multiple, present sooner, and have a worse prognosis.[32] Patients usually present with headache (75%) and posterior fossa symptoms, such as ataxia (55%), dysmetria (29%), and obstructive hydrocephalus (28%).[41] Surgical resection of symptomatic cerebellar and spine HBs is the standard treatment.[41,42] Stereotactic radiosurgery for control of smaller and noncystic lesions, deep lesions, and multiple lesions that would require multiple surgeries has gained increased use. However, lesions tend to recur because of residual tumor.[43,44]

HBs may vary in size from a tiny lesion to a large mass with an even larger cystic component. Some authorities think that the lesions begin as small nodules that become cystic, enlarge, and cause symptoms and that small solid nodules can be observed with routine imaging.[45,46] This theory is supported by 75% of symptomatic tumors having an associated cyst and peritumoral edema.[32] Multiple periods of tumor growth (usually associated with increasing cyst size) separated by periods of growth arrest termed "stuttering growth rate" have been described.[39,42] However, none of the lesions ever diminish in size.

Angiography shows an intensely vascular mass with a prolonged homogenous contrast blush. AV shunting is easily seen when the lesions are large, and early draining veins may be common.[32,47] On computed tomography (CT), most lesions will have a well-defined cerebellar cystic mass with an enhancing mural nodule that typically abuts the pial surface. About 33% will not have an associated cyst.[32,47] On MR imaging, T1WI, the nodule will appear isointense to hypointense with the cyst slightly hyperintense to cerebrospinal fluid due to protein and blood products. T2-weighted image (T2WI) demonstrates the nodule and cyst both to be hyperintense; prominent flow voids may be seen. Fluid attenuated inversion recovery (FLAIR) will show a hyperintense cyst with variable surrounding edema. Hemorrhage within the cyst appears as a blooming artifact on susceptibility-weighted sequences. The nodule enhances avidly with gadolinium; the cyst wall typically does not enhance. One should take care to evaluate for other tiny asymptomatic enhancing nodules as well[32,47] (Fig. 1).

Unlike the posterior fossa, most (80%) spinal cord HBs are associated with VHL disease. Patients may present with progressive myelopathy, localizing pain, paraparesis, and muscle wasting.[32,47] The lesions can occur anywhere in the cord and even along the cauda equine; however, they usually are seen more frequently at the craniocervical junction and conus medullaris.[48] Spinal cord HBs may be intramedullary, both intramedullary and extramedullary, or entirely extramedullary. The CT and MR imaging characteristics of spinal cord HBs are similar to that of posterior fossa

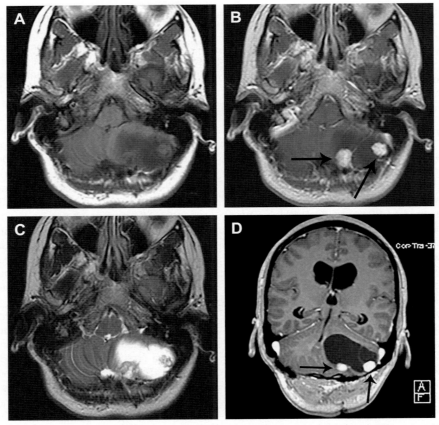

Fig. 1. HBs of the posterior fossa. Axial (A) T1 precontrast, (B) T1 postcontrast, (C) T2, and (D) coronal T1-weighted postcontrast MR images show 2 adjacent cystic lesions each with avidly enhancing nodules (*black arrows*) abutting the pial surface of the left cerebellum. Note the lack of edema and invasion of adjacent tissue.

HBs. HBs may appear as cystic lesions with enhancing nodules or as small multiple enhancing nodules along the posterior (more frequent than anterior) pial surface of the cord (**Fig. 2**). Enlargement of the cord secondary to edema may be seen when there are large, multiple, lesions with significant AV shunting.[32,47] A variable (25%–95%) proportion of cord lesions may be associated with a syrinx.[39,49,50] If no gadolinium contrast is administered, this could serve as a potential pitfall, and one could miss a small enhancing mural nodule and the correct diagnosis. Another possible pitfall is mistaking a prominent draining vein of a HB for a dural AV fistula. Angiography and embolization may be required before surgery for extensive spinal cord tumors. Drainage of an associated syrinx or posterior fossa cyst without removal of the nodule is ineffective.[38,51]

ENDOLYMPHATIC SAC TUMOR

The ELS is located at the end of the endolymphatic duct, at the aperture of the vestibular aqueduct, and lies within the dura of the posterior fossa. The ELS plays a role in the production and resorption of endolymph, which is found within the cochlea and semicircular canals. The ELSTs can grow outward into the cerebellopontine angle and mimic other tumors more commonly found at this site. They generally occur around 31 years of age.[9] They are pathologically distinct from HBs and resemble papillary cystadenomas (PCAs) of the epididymis, which are also seen in VHL disease.[52] Bilateral ELSTs should prompt further workup for VHL in previously undiagnosed cases.

ELSTs are benign tumors that do not metastasize, but are locally aggressive.[53] Patients may manifest disequilibrium, aural fullness, and hearing loss. The onset of hearing loss can be sudden and profound.[54] Large lesions (>3 cm) can erode into the facial nerve canal and cause ipsilateral facial nerve paralysis.[48] Prompt surgical intervention is required to prevent progression of symptoms and deafness.[54]

On CT, the ELSTs typically show destructive changes in the petrous bone, with a "moth-eaten"

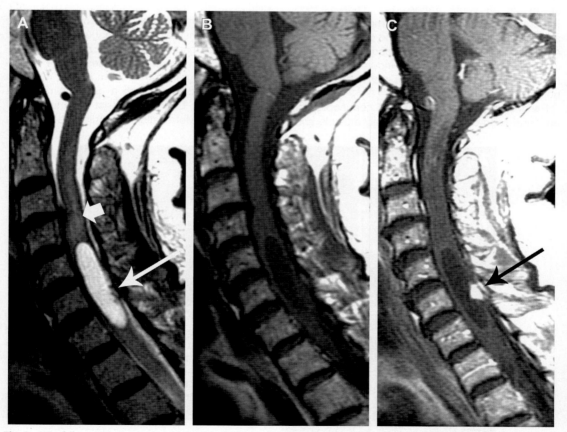

Fig. 2. HB of the cervical spinal cord. (*A*) T2, (*B*) T1 precontrast, and (*C*) T1 postcontrast sagittal MR images show a focal cystic intramedullary mass with prominent feeding vessels (*long white arrow*), cord expansion, and edema (*short white arrow*). There is an enhancing nodule posteriorly (*black arrow*).

appearance. The intratumoral bone may show spiculated or reticular pattern.[55] Direct extension and erosion of the vestibular aqueduct, vestibular-semicircular canal complex, and cochlea may be seen. On T1WI MR imaging, the lesion is heterogeneously hyperintense owing to protein and hemorrhage.[55] T2WI and FLAIR show a hyperintense mass. The lesion has a "stippled" or "paintbrush" pattern of heterogeneous contrast enhancement.[32,47,55]

Abdominal Manifestations

Tumors of the pancreas, kidney, adrenal glands, and reproductive organs occur in VHL disease.

Pancreas

An estimated 35% to 70% of patients with VHL present with pancreatic findings. Pancreatic manifestations of VHL include simple pancreatic cysts, serous cystadenomas, and neuroendocrine tumors (PNETs). Overall prevalence of pancreatic cysts and serous cystadenomas (SCAs) is about 20% to 56% and prevalence of PNETs is 8% to 20%.[56–62] Mean age at diagnosis of pancreatic lesions is 36 years (range: 1–7 decades).[62,63] Pancreatic lesions in VHL often remain asymptomatic, are incidentally detected, and can be the only manifestation of disease.[64] Endocrine or exocrine insufficiency is rare even with innumerable cysts replacing the pancreas. PNETs in VHL are usually not hormonally active.

Pancreatic cysts in VHL are nonneoplastic, epithelial-lined cysts that are usually multiple and distributed throughout the pancreas. PNETs in VHL are slow-growing, but malignant behavior has been observed, particularly in tumors greater than 3 cm in size.[65,66] On CT, pancreatic cysts are seen as simple cysts without enhancing septations, solid components, ductal communication, or ductal dilatation. MR imaging is better in delineating and characterizing pancreatic cystic lesions. SCAs appear as multiseptated, complex cystic lesions with multiple (>6) small cystic components with each component measuring less than 2 cm in size (microcystic adenoma). A central scar with calcification is characteristic (**Fig. 3**). PNETs frequently appear as solid, hypervascular lesions with arterial enhancement (**Fig. 4**); cystic tumors are uncommon.

Management of pancreatic lesions in VHL primarily involves surveillance of cysts. The SCAs are almost exclusively benign, and hence, do not warrant surgical resection. Large, symptomatic SCAs are resected, however. PNETs in VHL are often hormonally inactive and slow-growing; however, they can present with distant metastases. Surgical resection is therefore performed for PNETs greater than 3 cm in size in the pancreatic body or tail, and greater than 2 cm in size in the head.[59,67] Blansfield and colleagues[68] proposed additional prognostic criteria for resection in patients with high risk of metastases. These criteria include tumor greater than 3 cm in size, mutation in exon 3, and tumor with a doubling rate less than 500 days. Liver is the most common site of metastases. Metastatic liver disease can be

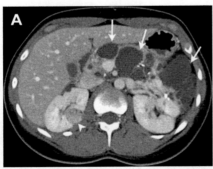
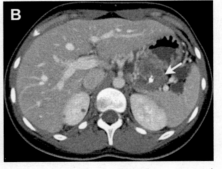
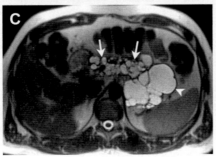

Fig. 3. Multiple pancreatic cysts and SCA. Axial contrast-enhanced CT images (*A*, *B*) and axial T2WIMR image (*C*) demonstrate multiple simple cysts scattered throughout the pancreas (*arrows*). SCA in the pancreatic tail demonstrates a characteristic multicystic appearance with a central scar that shows calcification (*arrowhead* in *C*).

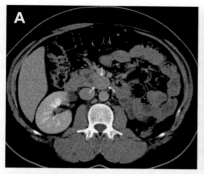
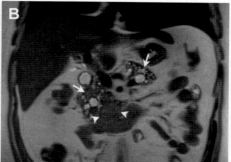
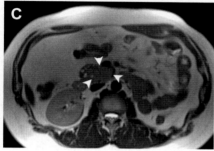

Fig. 4. Pancreatic neuroendocrine tumor. Axial contrast-enhanced CT (*A*), axial T2WIMR (*B*), and coronal T2WI (*C*) show a solid enhancing mass in the head/uncinate process (*arrows* in *A*; *arrowheads* in *B* and *C*) compatible with neuroendocrine tumor. Multiple pancreatic cystic lesions are also seen (*arrows* in *B*). Surgical resection (pancreaticoduodenectomy) revealed this to be a well-differentiated neuroendocrine tumor with innumerable additional smaller neuroendocrine tumors, cysts, and cystadenomas in the pancreatic head.

treated by a combination of locoregional therapy (including ablation) and hepatic arterial chemotherapeutic infusion.

Kidney

Renal manifestations of VHL disease include multiple benign renal cysts and clear cell carcinomas. Multiple bilateral renal cysts are common in VHL disease and are found on screening in approximately 50% to 70% of patients with VHL disease.[60,69] Renal cysts are asymptomatic, and unlike autosomal-dominant polycystic kidney disease, chronic renal failure is infrequent even in patients with innumerable bilateral renal cysts.[70] Although these are considered to be precursors to malignancy, malignant transformation is uncommon.[60,69] Renal cysts have not been associated with any specific genotype.

VHL patients are predisposed to development of clear cell RCCs in up to 45% of affected individuals by age 60 years; RCCs are a leading cause of mortality in VHL disease.[1,9] RCCs in VHL disease tend to be multiple and bilateral. Small renal lesions in VHL are low-grade and minimally invasive. However, an estimated 30% to 50% of symptomatic RCCs in VHL present with metastases with resultant poor prognosis.[71] Mean age of diagnosis of RCC in VHL disease is 39 years (range: 16–67 years).[10] Mutations in VHL are the most common cause of both inheritable and sporadic RCCs.[50,70,72–75]

VHL gene alteration affecting both the alpha domain (which binds elongin) and the beta subunit (which targets HIF for breakdown) with resultant increased expression of HIF-regulated genes is the primary molecular pathogenesis in clear cell RCC. Specifically, sustained activation of pathways for cellular proliferation and neovascularization is seen in patients with VHL mutations.[76,77] Most systemic agents used to treat metastatic clear cell RCC (including sunitinib, sorafenib, temsirolimus, and everolimus) target VHL transcription products.[78,79] Two distinct subgroups of VHL mutated tumors have been identified: one expressing both HIF-1α and HIF-2α (H1H2) and the other expressing only HIF-2α (H2).[79,80] Overproduction of HIF-2α activated c-myc and promotes cell proliferation; overproduction of HIF-1α antagonizes c-myc activity and suppresses tumor formation.[79,80] Overexpression of HIF-1α also downregulates HIF-2α. Hence, it is the HIF-2α, rather than HIF-1α, that promotes renal carcinogenesis.[81–83] Attempts have been made to elucidate potential molecular biomarkers along the VHL/HIF pathway, including VHL gene status, HIF1/HIF2 protein expression, and HIF-1 gene signature to predict response to therapy and guide treatment decision in clear cell RCCs.[77]

Renal cysts in VHL are asymptomatic and do not warrant treatment. Many VHL-associated RCCs often remain asymptomatic; advanced cases may present with hematuria, flank pain, or mass. Occurrence of up to 600 microscopic tumors and more than 1100 cysts per kidney has been described in VHL patients.[13,24] On gross pathology, RCCs are encapsulated solid or solid-cystic masses, which are yellow or orange on the cut surface. Histologically, clear-cell subtype predominates, and small carcinomas tend to be low grade.[73]

On imaging, simple cysts appear as homogeneous low-attenuation (<20 HU) masses with well-defined wall, and without enhancement. Clear cell RCCs present as solid or complex cystic enhancing renal masses (**Fig. 5**). Multiplicity and bilaterality are characteristic and should raise suspicion for VHL disease in adult patients. Given that these lesions tend to be asymptomatic, serial imaging surveillance is necessary for early detection of low-grade tumors. Surveillance is also adopted for asymptomatic incidentally discovered complex cysts because these may harbor RCCs. Although contrast-enhanced CT is the usual imaging modality used for screening/surveillance, MR imaging is being increasingly used to reduce radiation burden in young individuals and in those with impaired renal function.

Early surgery is the best option for renal cell carcinoma, and often a nephron-sparing or partial nephrectomy is performed in tumors greater than 3 cm in size.[84] The primary goal of early surgery is to preserve the renal function and decrease the risk of metastases. With this approach, no evidence of metastases or need for dialysis/kidney transplantation was found in a series of 52 patients

followed up for 60 months.[85] Percutaneous radiofrequency ablation or cryoablation is being increasingly used for small lesions (<3 cm) or in individuals who are likely to require multiple surgical procedures.[86] Cryoablation has also been used to treat patients with tumors as large as 5 cm. Total nephrectomy may be required in large tumors with advanced stage.[86,87] Renal transplantation has been successful in individuals in whom bilateral nephrectomy has been necessary. It is imperative to evaluate any living related potential donor for VHL disease and to exclude those found to have VHL disease.

Adrenal pheochromocytoma

PCC occurs in up to 20% of patients with VHL.[8,9] In comparison to sporadic PCC, VHL-associated PCCs tend to occur in younger patients and are frequently multifocal and bilateral. Extra-adrenal paragangliomas, including glomus jugulare, carotid body, and periaortic tumors, have also been reported. Mean age at diagnosis of PCC in VHL disease is 30 years (range: 5–58 years).[10] Approximately 20% of all PCCs are secondary to VHL.[88–90]

PCC can be the sole manifestation of VHL, and unusual clustering of PCCs in a subset of families has been reported. Clinically, PCC may present with sustained or episodic hypertension, sweating,

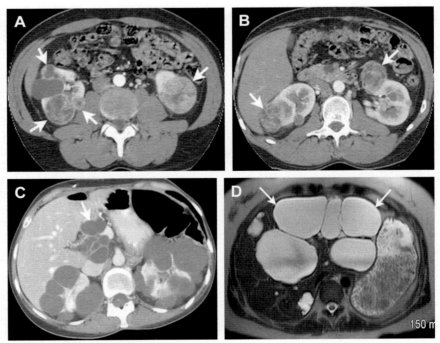

Fig. 5. Multiple renal cell carcinomas in VHL. Axial contrast-enhanced CT images demonstrate multifocal solid and complex cystic enhancing renal masses bilaterally consistent with multifocal RCC (*arrows* in A, B). Multiple simple cysts are also seen (*arrow* in C, D).

pallor, palpitations, headache, or nausea. PCC manifesting before the age of 10 years, and presenting with hypertensive crisis in young children, has been reported in VHL disease. Biochemical tests also remain unremarkable in a subset of patients; however, their biological behavior is variable with rapid progression reported in some cases.[91] Given the early onset of tumors and

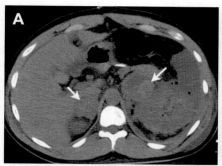

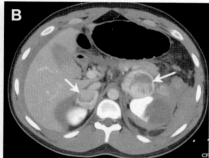

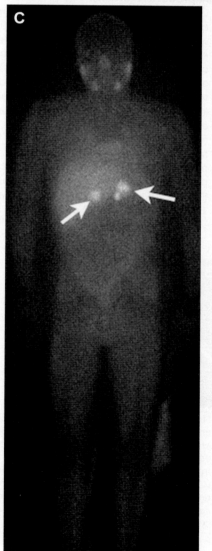

Fig. 6. Bilateral adrenal PCC incidentally detected in a 25-year-old patient presenting with motor vehicle accident. Axial unenhanced (A) and contrast-enhanced (B) CT image demonstrates intensely enhancing bilateral adrenal masses (arrows). Hypodensity in the upper pole of the left kidney is also seen compatible with laceration. (C) Whole-body I-123 metaiodobenzylguanidine scan reveals intense uptake in bilateral adrenal lesions (arrows). Surgical resection was performed. Genetic analysis revealed VHL mutation.

frequent absence of signs and symptoms, biochemical screening for PCC is routinely performed in individuals with known VHL mutation, beginning at about the age of 2 years. Measurements of plasma-free metanephrines and 24-hour urinary catecholamines are the commonly used biochemical tests for screening for PCC. On gross pathology, PCC appears as a red or orange encapsulated mass with foci of hemorrhage and necrosis. Histologically, these are composed of well-defined clusters of chromaffin cells containing eosinophilic cytoplasm and a fibrovascular stroma.

On imaging, PCCs demonstrate varied manifestations. Small tumors tend to be solid and hypervascular (**Fig. 6**). Larger tumors may show varying degrees of cystic change or necrosis. T2 hyperintense signal is classical but only seen in a small subset of patients with PCCs. Atypical imaging manifestations of PCCs include predominantly cystic appearance, presence of microscopic/macroscopic fat, and delayed washout on adrenal protocol CT. VHL disease can be first suspected in young patients with bilateral PCCs incidentally detected on imaging. Other syndromes that result in bilateral PCCs include neurofibromatosis type 1, MEN 2A/2B, and hereditary paraganglioma-PCC syndrome.[92] VHL disease can also be suspected in patients with solitary PCC with concomitant RCCs or pancreatic lesions (**Fig. 7**).

Surgical resection is usually performed for PCC with abnormal function, meta-iodobenzylguanidine uptake, and tumors greater than 3·5 cm in size.[85] Early intervention with cortical-sparing adrenal surgery is preferred to decrease recurrence rates and long-term corticosteroid dependence.[93] Treatment of choice for symptomatic PCCs is surgical excision, which can be often done via laparoscopic approach. Adrenal-sparing surgery is performed in bilateral PCCs to preserve adrenal function.[94] Preoperative treatment with α-adrenergic blockade (± β-adrenergic blockade) for 7 to 10 days before surgery is usually performed even in individuals without hypertension. PCCs in VHL disease are usually benign; malignant behavior has been reported to occur in up to 5% of cases.[95] A long-term follow-up study (9.25 years) in 36 individuals with VHL-related PCC showed local recurrence (partial adrenalectomy) in up to 11% cases and no evidence of metastatic disease in any individual.[96]

Reproductive organs

Cysts and PCAs of the epididymis are relatively common and are seen in 25% to 60% of men with VHL disease. They can be multiple and bilateral.[32] These cysts and PCAs are benign and typically appear during teenage years. Epididymal cysts are often asymptomatic and incidentally detected; bilateral disease has been associated with infertility.[97] Pathologically, these arise from the epididymal duct derived from the embryonic mesonephric duct. Epididymal cysts have been rarely reported as the first clinical manifestation of VHL.[98,99] Sonographic criteria have been proposed for diagnosis of PCAs, which include (1) predominantly solid tumor greater than 14 × 10 mm in size, (2) occurrence in a man with VHL disease, and (3) slow growth[100] (**Fig. 8**).

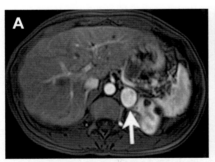
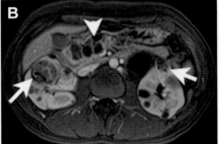
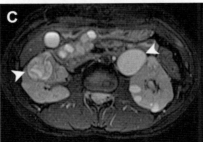

Fig. 7. Multifocal renal cell carcinoma, left adrenal PCC, and multiple pancreatic cysts in VHL. (*A*) Axial contrast-enhanced T1WIMR image demonstrates intensely enhancing left adrenal mass consistent with PCC (*arrow* in *A*). (*B*) Axial contrast-enhanced T1WIMR image and (*C*) Axial T2WIMR image demonstrates multiple bilateral enhancing solid as well as complex cystic renal masses consistent with RCC (*arrows* in *B*). Multiple pancreatic cysts are also noted (*arrowhead* in *B*).

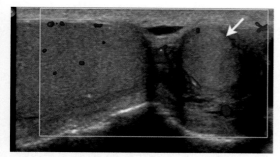

Fig. 8. PCA of the epididymis in a 35-year-old patient with VHL. Ultrasound image through the epididymal head reveals a solid isoechoic to mildly hyperechoic lesion (*arrow*).

Although epididymal PCAs appear solid on imaging, they are histologically composed of multiple cysts lined by epithelium with clear cell features and papillary fronds with a fibrovascular core. PCA of the broad ligament is the analogous lesion that occurs in female patients with VHL disease, but is less commonly encountered. Mean age of onset is 20 to 40 years, although it has been reported to occur at 16 years of age.[101,102] On imaging, PCAs manifest as cystic lesions (**Fig. 9**). Although asymptomatic cases are conservatively managed, symptomatic patients with secondary infertility benefit from surgical excision.

In summary, VHL disease is an autosomal-dominant, rare inherited neoplasia syndrome characterized by development of characteristic tumors such as CNS HBs, ELSTs, and clear cell RCCs. Given the variable penetrance of disease, the radiologist may be the first physician to raise the suspicion of VHL disease. Molecular genetic testing is performed in all individuals suspected of having VHL disease based on clinical or imaging manifestations.[103] Treatment of VHL disease primarily relies on early detection and removal of tumors to prevent/minimize secondary deficits. Specific surveillance guidelines exist for early detection of tumors in patients with VHL disease, those with a *VHL* disease-causing mutation, and at-risk relatives of unknown genetic status. Annual abdominal ultrasound and biannual MR imaging of the abdomen is performed in patients older than 16 years of age. MR imaging of the brain and spine is also performed every 2 years in these patients. RCCs and CNS HBs are the major causes of death in VHL disease. With improved surveillance, early diagnosis of lesions by imaging studies, and advances in treatment, the prognosis of patients with VHL has improved.[60]

REFERENCES

1. Maher ER, Iselius L, Yates JR, et al. von Hippel-Lindau disease: a genetic study. J Med Genet 1991;28(7):443–7.
2. Neumann HP, Wiestler OD. Clustering of features and genetics of von Hippel-Lindau syndrome. Lancet 1991;338(8761):258.
3. Collins ET. Two cases, brother and sister, with peculiar vascular new growth, probably primarily retinal, affecting both eyes. Trans Am Ophthalmol Soc 1894;14:141–7.
4. von Hippel E. Uber eine sehr self seltene erkrankung der netzhaut. Klinische Beobachtungen Arch Ophthalmol 1904;59:83–106.
5. Lindau A. Studien ber kleinbirncysten bau: pathogenese und beziehungen zur angiomatosis rentinae. Acta Path Microbiol Scandinavica 1926;1(suppl):1–128.
6. Melmon KL, Rosen SW. Lindau's disease. review of the literature and study of a large kindred. Am J Med 1964;36:595–617.
7. Latif F, Tory K, Gnarra J, et al. Identification of the von Hippel-Lindau disease tumor suppressor gene. Science 1993;260(5112):1317–20.
8. Lamiell JM, Salazar FG, Hsia YE. von Hippel-Lindau disease affecting 43 members of a single kindred. Medicine (Baltimore) 1989;68(1):1–29.
9. Maher ER, Yates JR, Harries R, et al. Clinical features and natural history of von Hippel-Lindau disease. Q J Med 1990;77(283):1151–63.
10. Ong KR, Woodward ER, Killick P, et al. Genotype-phenotype correlations in von Hippel-Lindau disease. Hum Mutat 2007;28(2):143–9.
11. Hes FJ, Feldberg MA. Von Hippel-Lindau disease: strategies in early detection (renal-, adrenal-, pancreatic masses). Eur Radiol 1999;9(4):598–610.

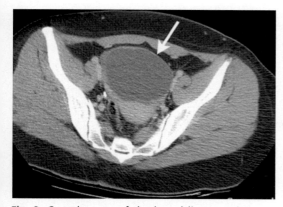

Fig. 9. Cystadenoma of the broad ligament in a patient with VHL. Axial contrast-enhanced CT image demonstrates a large hypodense lesion in the pelvis adjacent to the uterus in a patient with VHL (*arrow*). Surgical resection confirmed the diagnosis of broad ligament cystadenoma.

12. Duan DR, Pause A, Burgess WH, et al. Inhibition of transcription elongation by the VHL tumor suppressor protein. Science 1995;269(5229):1402–6.

13. Kibel A, Iliopoulos O, DeCaprio JA, et al. Binding of the von Hippel-Lindau tumor suppressor protein to Elongin B and C. Science 1995;269(5229):1444–6.

14. Pause A, Lee S, Worrell RA, et al. The von Hippel-Lindau tumor-suppressor gene product forms a stable complex with human CUL-2, a member of the Cdc53 family of proteins. Proc Natl Acad Sci U S A 1997;94(6):2156–61.

15. Rosner I, Bratslavsky G, Pinto PA, et al. The clinical implications of the genetics of renal cell carcinoma. Urol Oncol 2009;27(2):131–6.

16. Singer EA, Bratslavsky G, Middelton L, et al. Impact of genetics on the diagnosis and treatment of renal cancer. Curr Urol Rep 2011;12(1):47–55.

17. Beroud C, Joly D, Gallou C, et al. Software and database for the analysis of mutations in the VHL gene. Nucleic Acids Res 1998;26(1):256–8.

18. Conway JE, Chou D, Clatterbuck RE, et al. Hemangioblastomas of the central nervous system in von Hippel-Lindau syndrome and sporadic disease. Neurosurgery 2001;48(1):55–62 [discussion: 53].

19. Wizigmann-Voos S, Plate KH. Pathology, genetics and cell biology of hemangioblastomas. Histol Histopathol 1996;11(4):1049–61.

20. Nordstrom-O'Brien M, van der Luijt RB, van Rooijen E, et al. Genetic analysis of von Hippel-Lindau disease. Hum Mutat 2010;31(5):521–37.

21. Kaelin WG. von Hippel-Lindau disease. Annu Rev Pathol 2007;2:145–73.

22. Lee S, Nakamura E, Yang H, et al. Neuronal apoptosis linked to EgIN3 prolyl hydroxylase and familial pheochromocytoma genes: developmental culling and cancer. Cancer Cell 2005;8(2):155–67.

23. Gallou C, Chauveau D, Richard S, et al. Genotype-phenotype correlation in von Hippel-Lindau families with renal lesions. Hum Mutat 2004;24(3):215–24.

24. Maranchie JK, Afonso A, Albert PS, et al. Solid renal tumor severity in von Hippel Lindau disease is related to germline deletion length and location. Hum Mutat 2004;23(1):40–6.

25. Chen F, Kishida T, Yao M, et al. Germline mutations in the von Hippel-Lindau disease tumor suppressor gene: correlations with phenotype. Hum Mutat 1995;5(1):66–75.

26. Neumann HP, Bender BU. Genotype-phenotype correlations in von Hippel-Lindau disease. J Intern Med 1998;243(6):541–5.

27. Zbar B, Kishida T, Chen F, et al. Germline mutations in the von Hippel-Lindau disease (VHL) gene in families from North America, Europe, and Japan. Hum Mutat 1996;8(4):348–57.

28. Iliopoulos O. von Hippel-Lindau disease: genetic and clinical observations. Front Horm Res 2001; 28:131–66.

29. Kim M, Yan Y, Lee K, et al. Ectopic expression of von Hippel-Lindau tumor suppressor induces apoptosis in 786-O renal cell carcinoma cells and regresses tumor growth of 786-O cells in nude mouse. Biochem Biophys Res Commun 2004; 320(3):945–50.

30. Maher ER, Webster AR, Richards FM, et al. Phenotypic expression in von Hippel-Lindau disease: correlations with germline VHL gene mutations. J Med Genet 1996;33(4):328–32.

31. McNeill A, Rattenberry E, Barber R, et al. Genotype-phenotype correlations in VHL exon deletions. Am J Med Genet A 2009;149A(10):2147–51.

32. Choyke PL, Glenn GM, Walther MM, et al. von Hippel-Lindau disease: genetic, clinical, and imaging features. Radiology 1995;194(3):629–42.

33. Martz CH. von Hippel-Lindau disease: a genetic condition predisposing tumor formation. Oncol Nurs Forum 1991;18(3):545–51.

34. Grossniklaus HE, Thomas JW, Vigneswaran N, et al. Retinal hemangioblastoma. A histologic, immunohistochemical, and ultrastructural evaluation. Ophthalmology 1992;99(1):140–5.

35. Karsdorp N, Elderson A, Wittebol-Post D, et al. von Hippel-Lindau disease: new strategies in early detection and treatment. Am J Med 1994;97(2): 158–68.

36. Moore AT, Maher ER, Rosen P, et al. Ophthalmological screening for von Hippel-Lindau disease. Eye (Lond) 1991;5(Pt 6):723–8.

37. Filling-Katz MR, Choyke PL, Patronas NJ, et al. Radiologic screening for von Hippel-Lindau disease: the role of Gd-DTPA enhanced MR imaging of the CNS. J Comput Assist Tomogr 1989;13(5): 743–55.

38. Goodman J, Kleinholz E, Peck FC Jr. Lindau's disease–in the Hudson Valley. J Neurosurg 1964;21: 97–103.

39. Wanebo JE, Lonser RR, Glenn GM, et al. The natural history of hemangioblastomas of the central nervous system in patients with von Hippel-Lindau disease. J Neurosurg 2003;98(1):82–94.

40. Weil RJ, Lonser RR, DeVroom HL, et al. Surgical management of brainstem hemangioblastomas in patients with von Hippel-Lindau disease. J Neurosurg 2003;98(1):95–105.

41. Jagannathan J, Lonser RR, Smith R, et al. Surgical management of cerebellar hemangioblastomas in patients with von Hippel-Lindau disease. J Neurosurg 2008;108(2):210–22.

42. Ammerman JM, Lonser RR, Dambrosia J, et al. Long-term natural history of hemangioblastomas in patients with von Hippel-Lindau disease: implications for treatment. J Neurosurg 2006;105(2): 248–55.

43. Chang SD, Meisel JA, Hancock SL, et al. Treatment of hemangioblastomas in von Hippel-Lindau

disease with linear accelerator-based radiosurgery. Neurosurgery 1998;43(1):28–34 [discussion: 25].

44. Wang EM, Pan L, Wang BJ, et al. The long-term results of gamma knife radiosurgery for hemangioblastomas of the brain. J Neurosurg 2005; 102(Suppl):225–9.

45. Kurosaki Y, Tanaka YO, Itai Y. Solid cerebellar hemangioblastoma with an evolving large cystic component. Eur Radiol 1997;7(6):910–2.

46. Slater A, Moore NR, Huson SM. The natural history of cerebellar hemangioblastomas in von Hippel-Lindau disease. AJNR Am J Neuroradiol 2003; 24(8):1570–4.

47. Leung RS, Biswas SV, Duncan M, et al. Imaging features of von Hippel-Lindau disease. Radiographics 2008;28(1):65–79 [quiz: 323].

48. Filling-Katz MR, Choyke PL, Oldfield E, et al. Central nervous system involvement in von Hippel-Lindau disease. Neurology 1991;41(1):41–6.

49. Fill WL, Lamiell JM, Polk NO. The radiographic manifestations of von Hippel-Lindau disease. Radiology 1979;133(2):289–95.

50. Horton WA, Wong V, Eldridge R. Von Hippel-Lindau disease: clinical and pathological manifestations in nine families with 50 affected members. Arch Intern Med 1976;136(7):769–77.

51. Bonebrake RA, Siquerira EB. The familial occurrence of solitary hemangioblastoma of the cerebellum. Neurology 1964;14:733–43.

52. Price EB Jr. Papillary cystadenoma of the epididymis. A clinicopathologic analysis of 20 cases. Arch Pathol 1971;91(5):456–70.

53. Lo WW, Applegate LJ, Carberry JN, et al. Endolymphatic sac tumors: radiologic appearance. Radiology 1993;189(1):199–204.

54. Choo D, Shotland L, Mastroianni M, et al. Endolymphatic sac tumors in von Hippel-Lindau disease. J Neurosurg 2004;100(3):480–7.

55. Ayadi K, Mahfoudh KB, Khannous M, et al. Endolymphatic sac tumor and von Hippel-Lindau disease: imaging features. AJR Am J Roentgenol 2000;175(3):925–6.

56. Binkovitz LA, Johnson CD, Stephens DH. Islet cell tumors in von Hippel-Lindau disease: increased prevalence and relationship to the multiple endocrine neoplasias. AJR Am J Roentgenol 1990; 155(3):501–5.

57. Hammel PR, Vilgrain V, Terris B, et al. Pancreatic involvement in von Hippel-Lindau disease. The Groupe Francophone d'Etude de la Maladie de von Hippel-Lindau. Gastroenterology 2000;119(4): 1087–95.

58. Hough DM, Stephens DH, Johnson CD, et al. Pancreatic lesions in von Hippel-Lindau disease: prevalence, clinical significance, and CT findings. AJR Am J Roentgenol 1994;162(5): 1091–4.

59. Libutti SK, Choyke PL, Bartlett DL, et al. Pancreatic neuroendocrine tumors associated with von Hippel Lindau disease: diagnostic and management recommendations. Surgery 1998;124(6):1153–9.

60. Lonser RR, Glenn GM, Walther M, et al. von Hippel-Lindau disease. Lancet 2003;361(9374): 2059–67.

61. Lubensky IA, Pack S, Ault D, et al. Multiple neuroendocrine tumors of the pancreas in von Hippel-Lindau disease patients: histopathological and molecular genetic analysis. Am J Pathol 1998; 153(1):223–31.

62. Neumann HP, Dinkel E, Brambs H, et al. Pancreatic lesions in the von Hippel-Lindau syndrome. Gastroenterology 1991;101(2):465–71.

63. Bickler S, Wile AG, Melicharek M, et al. Pancreatic involvement in Hippel-Lindau disease. West J Med 1984;140(2):280–2.

64. Charlesworth M, Verbeke CS, Falk GA, et al. Pancreatic lesions in von Hippel-Lindau disease? A systematic review and meta-synthesis of the literature. J Gastrointest Surg 2012;16(7):1422–8.

65. Corcos O, Couvelard A, Giraud S, et al. Endocrine pancreatic tumors in von Hippel-Lindau disease: clinical, histological, and genetic features. Pancreas 2008;37(1):85–93.

66. Marcos HB, Libutti SK, Alexander HR, et al. Neuroendocrine tumors of the pancreas in von Hippel-Lindau disease: spectrum of appearances at CT and MR imaging with histopathologic comparison. Radiology 2002;225(3):751–8.

67. Libutti SK, Choyke PL, Alexander HR, et al. Clinical and genetic analysis of patients with pancreatic neuroendocrine tumors associated with von Hippel-Lindau disease. Surgery 2000;128(6):1022–7 [discussion: 1027–8].

68. Blansfield JA, Choyke L, Morita SY, et al. Clinical, genetic and radiographic analysis of 108 patients with von Hippel-Lindau disease (VHL) manifested by pancreatic neuroendocrine neoplasms (PNETs). Surgery 2007;142(6):814–8 [discussion: 818.e1–2].

69. Choyke PL, Glenn GM, Walther MM, et al. The natural history of renal lesions in von Hippel-Lindau disease: a serial CT study in 28 patients. AJR Am J Roentgenol 1992;159(6):1229–34.

70. Frimodt-Moller PC, Nissen HM, Dyreborg U. Polycystic kidneys as the renal lesion in Lindau's disease. J Urol 1981;125(6):868–70.

71. Neumann HP, Lips CJ, Hsia YE, et al. von Hippel-Lindau syndrome. Brain Pathol 1995;5(2):181–93.

72. Malek RS, Omess PJ, Benson RC Jr, et al. Renal cell carcinoma in von Hippel-Lindau syndrome. Am J Med 1987;82(2):236–8.

73. Poston CD, Jaffe GS, Lubensky IA, et al. Characterization of the renal pathology of a familial form of renal cell carcinoma associated with von Hippel-

Lindau disease: clinical and molecular genetic implications. J Urol 1995;153(1):22–6.

74. Richard S, Chauveau D, Chretien Y, et al. Renal lesions and pheochromocytoma in von Hippel-Lindau disease. Adv Nephrol Necker Hosp 1994;23:1–27.

75. Solomon D, Schwartz A. Renal pathology in von Hippel-Lindau disease. Hum Pathol 1988;19(9): 1072–9.

76. Kaelin WG Jr. The von Hippel-Lindau tumor suppressor protein and clear cell renal carcinoma. Clin Cancer Res 2007;13(2 Pt 2):680s–4s.

77. Linehan WM, Vasselli J, Srinivasan R, et al. Genetic basis of cancer of the kidney: disease-specific approaches to therapy. Clin Cancer Res 2004;10(18 Pt 2):6282S–9S.

78. Linehan WM. Editorial: kidney cancer–a unique opportunity for the development of disease specific therapy. J Urol 2002;168(6):2411–2.

79. Singer EA, Bratslavsky G, Linehan WM, et al. Targeted therapies for non-clear renal cell carcinoma. Target Oncol 2010;5(2):119–29.

80. Nelson EC, Evans CP, Lara PN Jr. Renal cell carcinoma: current status and emerging therapies. Cancer Treat Rev 2007;33(3):299–313.

81. Linehan WM, Zbar B. Focus on kidney cancer. Cancer Cell 2004;6(3):223–8.

82. Rini BI. Metastatic renal cell carcinoma: many treatment options, one patient. J Clin Oncol 2009; 27(19):3225–34.

83. Singer EA, Gupta GN, Srinivasan R. Update on targeted therapies for clear cell renal cell carcinoma. Curr Opin Oncol 2011;23(3):283–9.

84. Grubb RL 3rd, Choyke PL, Pinto PA, et al. Management of von Hippel-Lindau-associated kidney cancer. Nat Clin Pract Urol 2005;2(5):248–55.

85. Walther MM, Choyke PL, Glenn G, et al. Renal cancer in families with hereditary renal cancer: prospective analysis of a tumor size threshold for renal parenchymal sparing surgery. J Urol 1999;161(5):1475–9.

86. Shingleton WB, Sewell PE Jr. Percutaneous renal cryoablation of renal tumors in patients with von Hippel-Lindau disease. J Urol 2002;167(3):1268–70.

87. Pavlovich CP, Walther M, Choyke PL, et al. Percutaneous radio frequency ablation of small renal tumors: initial results. J Urol 2002;167(1):10–5.

88. Atuk NO, McDonald T, Wood T, et al. Familial pheochromocytoma, hypercalcemia, and von Hippel-Lindau disease. A ten year study of a large family. Medicine (Baltimore) 1979;58(3):209–18.

89. Neumann HP, Berger DP, Sigmund G, et al. Pheochromocytomas, multiple endocrine neoplasia type 2, and von Hippel-Lindau disease. N Engl J Med 1993;329(21):1531–8.

90. Sato Y, Waziri M, Smith W, et al. Hippel-Lindau disease: MR imaging. Radiology 1988;166(1 Pt 1):241–6.

91. Cryer PE. Phaeochromocytoma. Clin Endocrinol Metab 1985;14(1):203–20.

92. Neumann HP, Bausch B, McWhinney SR, et al. Germ-line mutations in nonsyndromic pheochromocytoma. N Engl J Med 2002;346(19):1459–66.

93. Baghai M, Thompson GB, Young WF Jr, et al. Pheochromocytomas and paragangliomas in von Hippel-Lindau disease: a role for laparoscopic and cortical-sparing surgery. Arch Surg 2002; 137(6):682–8 [discussion: 688–9].

94. Pavlovich CP, Linehan WM, Walther MM. Partial adrenalectomy in patients with multiple adrenal tumors. Curr Urol Rep 2001;2(1):19–23.

95. Walther MM, Reiter R, Keiser HR, et al. Clinical and genetic characterization of pheochromocytoma in von Hippel-Lindau families: comparison with sporadic pheochromocytoma gives insight into natural history of pheochromocytoma. J Urol 1999;162(3 Pt 1):659–64.

96. Benhammou JN, Boris RS, Pacak K, et al. Functional and oncologic outcomes of partial adrenalectomy for pheochromocytoma in patients with von Hippel-Lindau syndrome after at least 5 years of followup. J Urol 2010;184(5):1855–9.

97. Witten FR, O'Brien DP 3rd, Sewell CW, et al. Bilateral clear cell papillary cystadenoma of the epididymides presenting as infertility: an early manifestation of von Hippel-Lindau's syndrome. J Urol 1985; 133(6):1062–4.

98. Kroes HY, Sijmons RH, Van Den Berg A, et al. Early-onset renal cell cancer and bilateral epididymal cysts as presenting symptoms of von Hippel-Lindau disease. Br J Urol 1998;81(6):915.

99. Nicolaij D, Vogel-Kerebyn C, van den Bergh R, et al. Bilateral epididymal cysts as the first clinical manifestation of von Hippel-Lindau-disease. A case report. Andrologia 1979;11(3):234–5.

100. Choyke PL, Glenn GM, Wagner JP, et al. Epididymal cystadenomas in von Hippel-Lindau disease. Urology 1997;49(6):926–31.

101. Funk KC, Heiken JP. Papillary cystadenoma of the broad ligament in a patient with von Hippel-Lindau disease. AJR Am J Roentgenol 1989; 153(3):527–8.

102. Gersell DJ, King TC. Papillary cystadenoma of the mesosalpinx in von Hippel-Lindau disease. Am J Surg Pathol 1988;12(2):145–9.

103. Rasmussen A, Nava-Salazar S, Yescas P, et al. Von Hippel-Lindau disease germline mutations in Mexican patients with cerebellar hemangioblastoma. J Neurosurg 2006;104(3):389–94.

Cross-sectional Imaging Review of Tuberous Sclerosis

Anant Krishnan, MD[a],*, Ravi K. Kaza, MD[b], Dharshan R. Vummidi, MD[c]

KEYWORDS

- Tuberous sclerosis • MR imaging • Tuber • Subependymal giant cell astrocytoma (SEGA) • mTOR
- Angiomyolipoma • Lymphangioleiomyomatosis

KEY POINTS

- Tuberous sclerosis results from uninhibited activation of the mammalian target of rapamycin pathway secondary to inactivating mutations of tuberous sclerosis complex (TSC) 1 or *TSC2* genes (prototype tumor suppressor genes).
- Neurologic manifestations are the primary cause of morbidity and mortality in TSC. Pathologic findings include cortical and cerebellar tubers, radial migration lines, subependymal nodules, and subependymal giant cell astrocytomas (SEGAs).
- Imaging of neuropathological abnormalities depends on the age of the patient; most lesions under 6 months of age appear hyperintense on T1-weighted imaging. Serial growth of an enhancing nodule near the foramen of Monro suggests a SEGA.
- Renal angiomyolipomas (AMLs) are the second most common cause of morbidly and mortality in TSC. The risk of hemorrhage is higher in AMLs larger than 4 cm or AMLs with aneurysms larger than 5 mm.

INTRODUCTION

Tuberous sclerosis complex (TSC) is an autosomal dominant, neurocutaneous disorder that is characterized by development of hamartomatous tumors in multiple organs and neuronal migration abnormalities.[1] Although TSC was first described by von Recklinghausen in 1862,[2] it was recognized as a distinct disease by Bourneville in 1880 (thus also referred to as Bourneville disease). TSC affects 1 million people worldwide, and occurs in 1 in 6000 to 1 in 10,000 live births, with a population prevalence of around 1 in 20,000.[2] TSC is marked by high penetrance, albeit with variable phenotypic manifestations.

This article begins with a brief discussion on the advances in the genetics and etiopathogenesis of the condition as well as the recently updated criteria for the diagnosis of TSC. Cross-sectional imaging spectrum of the neurologic, abdominal, and thoracic manifestations of this protean disorder are discussed subsequently.

Disclosure: The authors have nothing to disclose.
[a] Department of Diagnostic Radiology, The Oakland University William Beaumont School of Medicine and Beaumont Hospital, 3601 West 13 Mile Road, Royal Oak, MI 48073, USA; [b] Department of Radiology, University of Michigan Hospitals, 1500 East Medical Center Drive, UH B1 502 E, Ann Arbor, MI 48109, USA; [c] Department of Radiology, University of Michigan Hospitals, 1500 East Medical Center Drive, CVC5581, Ann Arbor, MI 48109, USA
* Corresponding author.
E-mail address: akrishnan@beaumont.edu

Radiol Clin N Am 54 (2016) 423–440
http://dx.doi.org/10.1016/j.rcl.2015.12.003

CAUSE AND GENETICS

Tuberous sclerosis results from a mutation in one of 2 tumor suppressor genes: TSC1 (located on 9q34 and encoding hamartin) or TSC2 (located on 16p13 and encoding tuberin),[1] with TSC2 mutations 3 times more common and associated with more severe disease manifestations.[3] The protein products of TSC1 (hamartin) and TSC2 (tuberin) form a heterodimer that functions as a master switch to primarily inhibit the mammalian target of rapamycin (mTOR) complex 1 (mTORC1).[4] mTOR is a key protein kinase that senses a variety of environmental signals, such as growth factors and metabolic milieu, while regulating many critical cellular processes, including protein/lipid synthesis, cell cycle progression, proliferation, cytoskeleton organization, and cell survival. In TSC, the inactivating mutations of the TSC1 or TSC2 genes result in uninhibited activation of the mTOR pathway.[5]

Although approximately one-third of patients have inherited mutations from their parents, most seem to be mutations that arose sporadically in very early somatic cells and may not equally affect all organ systems.[5] Some studies also suggest that a second hit (based on Knudson's two-hit hypothesis) may account for brain lesions.[6] Such genetic complexity may explain the considerable phenotypic diversity observed in patients with TSC. In addition, improved knowledge of the genetics of TSC and mTOR complex has led to the development of targeted therapeutics for management of patients with TSC.[5]

REVISED DIAGNOSTIC CRITERIA

In 2012, the second International Tuberous Sclerosis Complex Consensus Conference was held in Washington, DC, with the major goal to revisit the diagnostic criteria[2] (**Box 1**). One of the major changes was the inclusion of genetic testing for the identification of a pathogenic mutation in TSC1 and TSC2. Because approximately 10% to 25% of patients with TSC do not have a genetic mutation by conventional genetic testing, a normal result does not exclude the diagnosis.

Pertinent changes include:

- Combination of radial migration lines (RMLs; previously minor criteria) and cortical tubers into one major criteria called cortical dysplasia
- The word renal removed from "renal angiomyolipoma" to accommodate liver angiomyolipoma (AML)
- To separate sporadic lymphangioleiomyomatosis (LAM) from tuberous sclerosis-related LAM; when both are present, together constitute only one major criterion

Because 2 major criteria constitute a definite diagnosis of TSC, it follows that the detection of these findings on an imaging study of the brain is conclusive in making a diagnosis of TSC even in the absence of other typical clinical signs and symptoms.

NEUROLOGIC MANIFESTATIONS OF TUBEROUS SCLEROSIS COMPLEX

Neurologic manifestations are present in approximately 85% of patients with TSC and are the primary cause of morbidity and mortality.[7,8] Seizures are present in most of these patients and often begin in the first year of life as intractable infantile spasms.[5] Certain neuroradiological features, such as greater than 7 tubers,[9] large tuber size,[10] and increased tuber/brain ratio, favor a more severe epilepsy or early onset of epilepsy as well as intellectual impairment. Other manifestations include cognitive impairment (>50% of patients), challenging behavioral problems, and autism.[5,11] There is a higher risk of severe cognitive and behavioral difficulties in patients with involvement of the temporal or occipital lobes, particularly the left temporal lobe in right-handed patients.[12] A recently coined term, TSC-associated neuropsychiatric disorders, refers to the constellation of behavioral, psychiatric, intellectual, and psychosocial difficulties than can affect more than 90% of patients with TSC.[13]

These clinical manifestations arise from underlying neuropathological abnormalities, including cerebral and cerebellar tubers, white matter RMLs, subependymal nodules (SENs), subependymal giant cell astrocytomas (SEGAs), and rarely vascular abnormalities such as intracranial aneurysms.

IMAGING TECHNIQUES

MR imaging is the primary imaging modality in the diagnosis, characterization, and monitoring of the intracranial lesions of TSC.[7,8] Although the classic subependymal calcifications are best seen by computed tomography (CT) (**Fig. 1**), MR imaging techniques such as gradient T2* and three-dimensional susceptibility-weighted imaging[14] may be an alternative to avoid ionizing radiation. Ultrasonography is most valuable in the prenatal period, although its main contribution is in the detection of cardiac rhabdomyomas.[7] Prenatal ultrasonography can detect subependymal nodules and tubers, although fetal MR imaging is more sensitive[15] (**Fig. 2**). Similarly, in the neonatal period, although transfontanelle ultrasonography can be used, MR imaging is still the preferred test.

Box 1
Updated diagnostic criteria for tuberous sclerosis complex 2012

A. Genetic diagnostic criteria

The identification of either a *TSC1* or *TSC2* pathogenic mutation in DNA from normal tissue is sufficient to make a definite diagnosis of TSC. Note that 10% to 25% of patients with TSC have no mutation identified by conventional genetic testing, and a normal result does not exclude TSC, or have any effect on the use of clinical diagnostic criteria to diagnose TSC.

B. Clinical diagnostic criteria

Major features

1. Hypomelanotic macules ($\geq$3, at least 5 mm in diameter)
2. Angiofibromas ($\geq$3) or fibrous cephalic plaque
3. Ungual fibromas ($\geq$2)
4. Shagreen patch
5. Multiple retinal hamartomas
6. Cortical dysplasias[a]
7. Subependymal nodules
8. Subependymal giant cell astrocytoma
9. Cardiac rhabdomyoma
10. Lymphangioleiomyomatosis (LAM)[b]
11. Angiomyolipomas ($\geq$2)[b]

Minor features

1. Confetti skin lesions
2. Dental enamel pits (>3)
3. Intraoral fibromas ($\geq$2)
4. Retinal achromic patch
5. Multiple renal cysts
6. Nonrenal hamartomas

Definite diagnosis: 2 major features or 1 major feature with 2 or more minor features.

Possible diagnosis: either 1 major feature or 2 or more minor features.

[a] Includes tubers and cerebral white matter radial migration lines.
[b] A combination of the 2 major clinical features (LAM and angiomyolipomas) without other features does not meet criteria for a definite diagnosis.
Data from Northrup H, Krueger DA, International Tuberous Sclerosis Complex Consensus Group. Tuberous sclerosis complex diagnostic criteria update: recommendations of the 2012 International Tuberous Sclerosis Complex Consensus Conference. Pediatr Neurol 2013;49(4):243–54.

Detection of TSC lesions depends on the age of the patient. In a child less than 6 months old, T1-weighted sequences are most helpful in the detection of lesions because most lesions are hyperintense (**Fig. 3**) on T1-weighted images (T1WIs).[16] The lesions in this age group can be harder to detect on T2-weighted images (T2WIs) or fluid-attenuated inversion recovery (FLAIR) sequences as a result of the native high T2 signal of the unmyelinated white matter. In older children (>12 months) and adults, FLAIR sequences are the most sensitive in detection of lesions.[7] Postcontrast sequences are required for identifying enhancing lesions such as SEGA. Some investigators have suggested improved sensitivity in detection of cortical tubers and RMLs with the use of magnetization transfer T1-weighted sequences.[17,18]

NEUROPATHOLOGICAL MANIFESTATIONS OF TUBEROUS SCLEROSIS
Cerebral Tubers

Tubers (grossly akin to potato tubers), after which the disease tuberous sclerosis is named, are

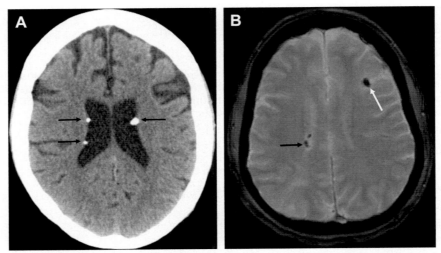

Fig. 1. Head CT. (*A*) Multiple calcified subependymal nodules (*arrows*). Gradient T2* sequence (*B*) in a different patient shows calcified subependymal nodules (*black arrow*) and tuber (*white arrow*).

glioneuronal hamartomas composed of enlarged atypical and disorganized neuronal and glial elements with astrocytosis.[7,19,20] They are present in more than 90% of patients, and are often multiple and bilateral (65%–92%).[21] They are most commonly located in the frontal lobes.[7,21]

Tubers have been historically classified based on their gross pathology and related radiology appearance into the smooth surfaced type 1 and the dimpled cystic type 2.[22,23] More recently, 3 types of tubers (**Figs. 4** and **5**) have been described based on their imaging appearance on MR imaging. Type A tubers are mildly hyperintense on T2WI/FLAIR, isointense on T1WI, and hence

harder to detect. Type B tubers are hyperintense on T2WI and hypointense on T1WI. Type C (cystic) tubers are prominently hyperintense on T2WI, centrally suppress on FLAIR, and are hypointense on T1WI.[22] Patients with type C tuber predominance have more severe manifestations, have a higher incidence of SEGA, and have been associated with *TSC2* gene mutations.[4]

On CT, tubers appear hypodense, show enhancement in only 3% to 4% of cases, but can be calcified in as many as 50% of patients[24,25] (see **Fig. 1**B). In adults, tubers are T2 hyperintense and T1 hypointense, whereas in infants they are often hyperintense on T1WI (some cases have

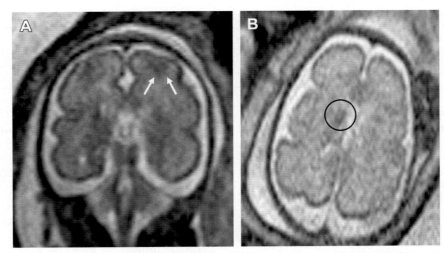

Fig. 2. Coronal (*A*), and axial (*B*) HASTE T2-weighted fetal MR images show cortical tuber (*white arrows in A*), and subependymal nodule (*circled*). HASTE, half-fourier acquisition single-shot turbo spin echo imaging. (*Courtesy of Dr Hemant Parmar, University of Michigan, Ann Arbor, MI.*)

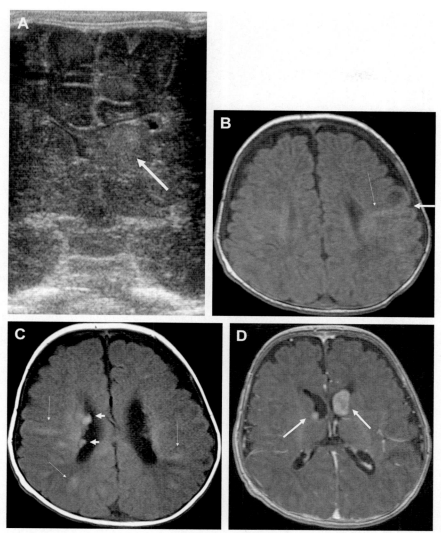

Fig. 3. Transfontanelle coronal ultrasonography (*A*) in a 10-day-old shows a large left subependymal mass (*arrow*). Axial MPRAGE T1 images (*B, C*) show multiple hyperintense SENs (*arrowheads*), RMLs (*arrows*), and cortical dysplasia (*short arrow*) in this 2-month-old patient with TSC. Postcontrast image (*D*) confirms large left and smaller right enhancing nodules (*arrows*); focus on left suspicious for SEGA. MPRAGE, magnetization prepared rapid gradient echo.

mixed signal) and hypointense on T2WI.[16] Less than half the tubers in one study[16] could be seen on T2WIs in children less than 6 month of age. Large transmantle dysplasias can also be seen in infants (**Fig. 6**). Less than 10% of cortical tubers enhance by MR imaging. Calcified lesions can cause blooming or hypointense signal on T2*-weighted sequences.

Box 2 shows the imaging findings of tubers.

On MR spectroscopy, tubers show decreased N-acetyl aspartate (NAA), presumably from loss of neurons, and increased myoinositol from gliosis or immature neurons.[26] On diffusion tensor imaging, tubers have decreased fractional anisotropy

(FA) and increased apparent diffusion coefficients (ADCs).[24] Tubers with significantly higher ADCs and lower FA have increased epileptogenic potential compared with other lesions.[8] Fluorodeoxyglucose (FDG)-PET is also helpful in separating epileptogenic from nonepileptogenic tubers by showing larger volumes of hypometabolism relative to MR imaging size in epileptogenic lesions.[27]

Cerebellar Tubers

Cerebellar tubers are reported in 10% to 40% of patients with TSC, with recent reports suggesting they occur in a third of pediatric patients.[28–30]

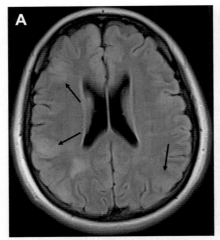

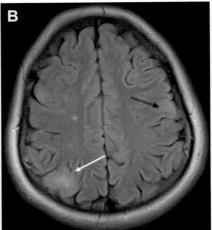

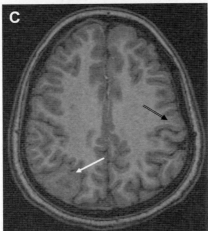

Fig. 4. Axial FLAIR images (*A, B*) in a 20-year-old with TSC show multiple cortical tubers (*black arrows*). The tuber in the right high parietal lobe (*white arrow in B*) is more distinct than the focus on the left (*double arrow*). Axial MPRAGE T1 sequence (*C*) shows the corresponding subtle nature of the left frontal type A tuber (*double arrow*) versus the more defined cortical thickening with subcortical hypointensity in the right parietal type B tuber (*white arrow*).

They always occur in association with cortical tubers. Additionally, patients who have both cerebral and cerebellar tubers have significantly more global cortical lesions than patients without cerebellar tubers.[31] Cerebellar tubers are thus a marker for severity of disease.

Cerebellar tubers are wedge-shaped lesions (presumably from the inward migration of the granule cell neurons from the surface) that are hyperintense on T2WI and hypointense to isointense on T1WI (**Fig. 7**). These lesions are more likely to enhance (30.7%[28]–51%[30]) than supratentorial tubers (10% enhance). A zebralike pattern of enhancement has been described, presumably reflecting the cerebellar anatomy, with interposed cerebrospinal fluid–filled sulci. Cerebellar tubers commonly calcify (29%–54%), and even more commonly undergo retraction (74%–85%).[28,30] Other infratentorial abnormalities seen in TSC include linear and gyriform cerebellar folia calcifications, vermis and cerebellar hemispheric

hypoplasia, and agenesis.[7] Some lesions (20%–52%) increase in size, enhancement, and calcification and this occurs in the first 8 years of life.[28] Similarly, some tubers can also decrease in size in early adulthood.

Cerebellar atrophy occurs in 4% to 13% of patients with TSC[29,31] but it is unclear whether this is from the presence of cerebellar tubers, or a primary aberrant neuronal developmental process, or a sequela of seizures and treatment of the same. Cerebellar tubers have been associated with more severe clinical disease. Patients have more severe communication and social disturbances when these tubers are located in the right cerebellar hemisphere.[32]

Radial Migration Lines

RMLs represent arrested migratory neurons and glial cells.[7,25] They extend outward from the ependymal ventricular surface toward the cortex. They

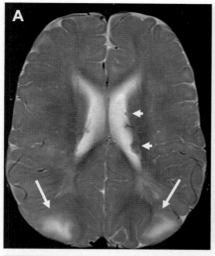

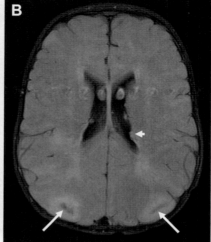

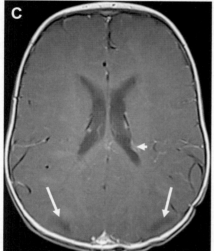

Fig. 5. Axial T2WI (*A*), axial FLAIR (*B*), and postcontrast T1WI (*C*) from a 9-month-old child with numerous lesions show the cystic type C cortical tubers (*white arrows*) that centrally suppress on FLAIR and are markedly centrally hypointense on T1. Also seen are subependymal nodules (*arrowheads*).

are thus most commonly identified in the subcortical white matter and are the most common lesions in TSC (**Fig. 8**). The strong correlation between RML, tubers, and subependymal nodules suggests that these lesions originate from a common biological dysfunction in the periventricular zone.[33]

RMLs are harder to identify by CT. On MR imaging, on which they are well seen, they appear as curvilinear or band-shaped T2/FLAIR hyperintense lesions traversing the deep white matter. These lines do not typically enhance. In addition to RML, some patients also show small cysts (see **Fig. 8**A) in the white matter that resemble perivascular spaces.[24] In a study on RML,[33] the investigators found a strong association between the frequency of RMLs and age of seizure onset and history of seizures. Additionally, the RML

frequency was also strongly associated with the level of intelligence and rate of autistic features. They suggested that, in TSC, neurocognitive deficits are caused by focal migration and proliferation abnormalities.

Subependymal Nodules

SENs are hamartomatous lesions that are scattered along the ependymal surface of the lateral ventricles.[24] Although they can occur anywhere along the lateral ventricle, they are most common at the caudothalamic groove in the region of the foramen of Monro.[25] They are hyperintense on T1WI at all ages (thus lacking the inverse signal abnormalities described earlier in tubers and RML between infants and adults) and are isointense/hypointense on T2WI. The T2 signal depends on

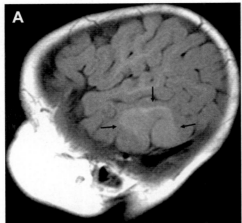

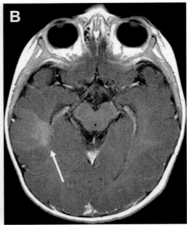

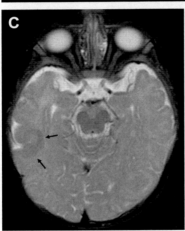

Fig. 6. Sagittal T1WI (*A*) in a 7-month-old shows a T1 hyperintense tuber (*small arrows*) bridging 2 gyri in the right temporal lobe. Axial postcontrast T1WI (*B*) shows an even more hyperintense T1 curvilinear abnormality (*arrow*) deep to the tuber extending to the ventricle, compatible with a transmantle dysplasia. Axial T2WI (*C*) shows the hypointense signal of the tuber (*small arrows*).

whether they are calcified. Most SENs (>90%) calcify (see **Fig. 1**) and calcifications can be seen by the end of the first year. Cranial CT in children detects more than 80% of calcified SENs and around 30% of noncalcified tubers.[34] It is important to remember that SENs can enhance and enhancement does not imply that a nodule is going to transform into a SEGA or that surgical intervention is necessary.[25]

Subependymal Giant Cell Astrocytoma

SEGAs are low-grade tumors (World Health Organization [WHO] grade I), and the most common brain tumors in TSC.[11,25] They occur in approximately 10% to 15% of patients with TSC. Although the name may suggest that they are astrocytomas (and they are included under the astrocytoma category in

Box 2 Imaging findings of tubers	
CT	Hypodense subcortical lesions, rarely enhance
MR imaging <6 mo	Hyperintense on T1, hypointense on T2 but difficult to detect as a result of unmyelinated white matter signal
MR imaging 6–12 mo	Variable appearance as signal characteristics on T1, T2 reverse from neonatal to adult (>12 mo)
MR imaging >12 mo or adults	Hypointense on T1, hyperintense on T2 and FLAIR
	If cystic, lesions may suppress centrally on FLAIR
	May enhance

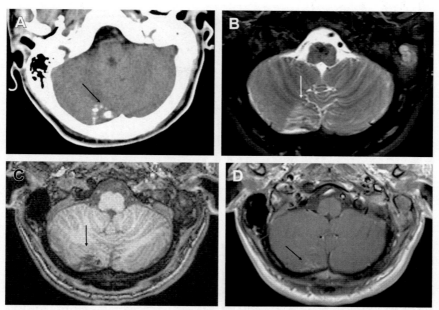

Fig. 7. Axial CT (*A*), axial T2WI (*B*), T1WI (*C*), and postcontrast T1WI (*D*) show a calcified, wedge-shaped, and mildly enhancing right cerebellar tuber (*arrow*).

the current WHO classification), they are now thought to be of glioneuronal origin.[35] As a result, a better term may be subependymal giant cell tumor.

SEGAs are slow growing but vascular tumors. They are believed to arise from SENs, and are also most commonly located near the foramen of Monro, and frequently bilateral. The biggest concern with SEGAs is the possibility of obstructing the ventricle and causing potentially fatal hydrocephalus, and this is proportional to the volume of the tumor.[35] SEGAs most commonly occur between 8 and 14 years of age[7] but may occur in the first few months of life or even prenatally.[36]

Subependymal nodule versus subependymal giant cell astrocytoma

Historically, features used in separating SEGAs from SENs include location near the foramen of Monro, size (>1 cm favoring SEGA), enhancement, and growth.[16,23] In a study by Nabout and colleagues,[37] nodules more than 0.5 cm in diameter that were incompletely calcified and enhanced by gadolinium were at higher risk of growth, particularly in children with a familial history of TSC. Recently, a panel of European experts suggested that a SEGA should be considered if a lesion near the foramen of Monro is more than 0.5 cm in diameter, with any documented growth, and gadolinium enhancement.[38]

SEGAs are isodense or hyperdense on CT and frequently show calcifications (**Fig. 9**). On MR

imaging, they are hypointense/isointense on T1WI and hyperintense on T2WI. Intense enhancement is seen, particularly in noncalcified lesions. SEGAs are believed to develop from SENs, but, unlike SENs, show growth, with a growth rate of less than 0.5 cm/y in longest dimension.[39] However, rapid growth may occur, with transformation from a SEN to an obstructive SEGA in as little as 18 months.[23] Because early detection and treatment is critical, periodic surveillance with imaging every 1 to 3 years is recommended until the age of 25 years.[40] Monitoring also depends on size, with some investigators suggesting 6-monthly screening in lesions greater than 1 cm.[38] Treatment options include surgical resection, gamma knife radiosurgery, and pharmacotherapy with mTOR inhibitors.[39,41]

- Surgical resection is the standard therapy for SEGAs with documented growth or if associated with obstructive hydrocephalus.
- mTOR inhibitors such as everolimus may be used in patients aged 3 years and older for asymptomatic SEGAs, when surgery is contraindicated, or in recurrent lesions when scarring and distorted anatomy may increase morbidity and mortality from surgery.

Other Less Common Associations with Tuberous Sclerosis Complex

Hemimegalencephaly

There are scattered reports of uncommon association of TSC with hemimegalencephaly.[42] Most

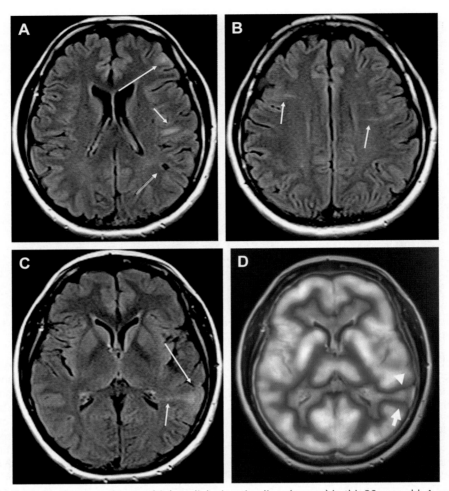

Fig. 8. Axial FLAIR (*A–C*) images show multiple radial migration lines (*arrows*) in this 36-year-old. A cystic lesion is also seen in the left inferior parietal lobe (*double arrow* in Fig. 9A). Tubers (*long arrows*) are also seen. (*D*) Inter-ictal FDG-PET fused onto MR imaging shows a corresponding focus of hypometabolism in the left temporal lobe (*arrowheads*). (*Courtesy of* [*D*] Dr Oliver Wong, Beaumont Hospital, Royal Oak, MI.)

interestingly, there may be a common abnormality, namely an alteration in the mTOR signaling pathway and upregulation of an abnormal phosphorylated tau protein.[43] This possibility led the investigators[43] to suggest that conditions such as hemimegalencephaly, TSC, and focal cortical dysplasia may be referred to as infantile tauopathies. Clinically, all entities produce highly epileptogenic foci in the cerebral cortex.

Aneurysms

Intracranial arteriopathy, including aneurysms, may be part of the clinical spectrum of TSC and is probably caused by a dysfunction of smooth muscle cells, again potentially mediated by the mTOR pathway.[44,45] Baronat and colleagues[45] reported intracranial aneurysms in 3 of 404 patients with definite TSC. Intracranial aneurysms in TSC seem to affect mainly the internal carotid artery and are more frequently fusiform. They may be multiple, giant (>2.5 cm), and may occur at an early age, particularly in male patients.

Chordomas

Chordomas have been reported in patients with TSC, ranging from the sacrococcygeal region to the clivus and the cervical spine.[46,47] Chordomas are distinctly uncommon in children and adolescents, but almost all the chordomas described in TSC were seen in individuals aged 16 years of age or younger and in many less than 5 years of age. In a recent review comparing 10 patients with chordomas and TSC versus chordomas in the general pediatric population,[46] chordomas occurred at a younger age in TSC (median age of 6.2 months vs 12 years in general pediatric

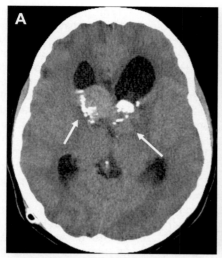

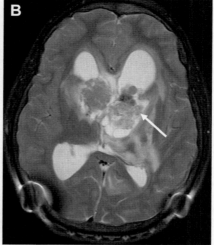

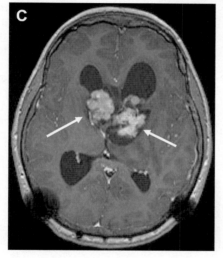

Fig. 9. SEGA. Head CT (*A*) shows bilateral partially calcified large masses (*arrows*) at the foramen of Monro, with hydrocephalus. The masses are heterogeneous on the T2WI (*B*) and show intense enhancement on the postcontrast image (*C*).

population), more commonly involved the sacrum (40% vs 9.4%), and had better survival. The investigators also suggested that chordomas may be a rare pediatric manifestation of TSC and that future studies were necessary to assess whether even the typical adult chordomas were somehow related to TSC.

ABDOMINAL MANIFESTATIONS
Renal Manifestations

Kidneys are the most common abdominal organs to be involved in TSC. Renal manifestation in TSC is most commonly in the form of AMLs, with renal cysts and renal cell carcinomas noted infrequently.[24,48,49]

Angiomyolipomas

AMLs are the most common benign renal neoplasms, composed of varying amounts of blood vessels, smooth muscle, and fat. Although AMLs are present in 80% of patients with TSC, only 20% of patients with AML have TSC.[50] AMLs in patients with TSC are more commonly seen in younger patients and are multiple, involving both kidneys, as opposed to incidental AMLs in patients without TSC, which are usually seen in middle-aged women and are solitary.[50] The radiological hallmark of AML is the presence of macroscopic fat within it. Smaller AMLs are usually homogeneous and may be seen as an entirely fat-containing lesion, whereas larger lesions tend to be more heterogeneous with varying degrees of enhancement and soft tissue component within the lesions. On ultrasonography, AMLs are seen as uniformly hyperechoic lesions (**Fig. 10**) that may be homogeneous or heterogeneous depending on the size of the lesions; associated speed-propagation artifact, when present, is diagnostic of AMLs. Vascular flow may be seen with color

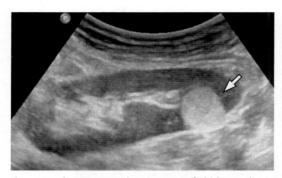

Fig. 10. Ultrasonography image of kidney shows a well-defined, homogeneously hyperechoic lesion in the lower pole (*arrow*) representing an angiomyolipoma.

Doppler in classic, triphasic AMLs containing fat, blood vessels, and smooth muscle. However, 10% of renal cell carcinomas may also present as homogeneously hyperechoic masses and distinguishing them from AML based on ultrasonography may be difficult, necessitating further evaluation with CT scan or MR imaging for definitive diagnosis.[48]

CT and MR imaging enable a specific diagnosis of AML to be made by detection of macroscopic fat within most (approximately 95%) of the lesions.

A thin-slice CT scan (**Fig. 11**) performed before intravenous contrast administration is needed to detect small amounts of fat within AML, which are seen as areas with attenuation of less than -10 Hounsfield units.[51] CT scan done after intravenous contrast administration shows heterogeneous areas of soft tissue and enhancement within larger AMLs and could potentially obscure small areas of fat within the lesions. Fat in AML is seen as areas of increased signal on T1WI and T2WI with corresponding areas of decreased signal on the fat-suppressed T1WI and T2WI. On T1-weighted opposed-phase images, AMLs show a characteristic linear area of signal loss along the periphery of the lesion, at fat-parenchymal interfaces, termed India ink etching artifact.[52] About 5% of AMLs do not contain macroscopic fat and are termed minimal fat AML.[53] These minimal fat AMLs are seen as homogeneously enhancing renal masses that are radiologically indistinguishable from renal cell carcinoma and often require a biopsy to establish a diagnosis.[54]

Renal AMLs are usually asymptomatic at presentation. The major clinical concern with renal AML is the risk of hemorrhage (**Fig. 12**) caused by the rupture of small renal artery aneurysms (**Fig. 13**) within them. The risk of hemorrhage is

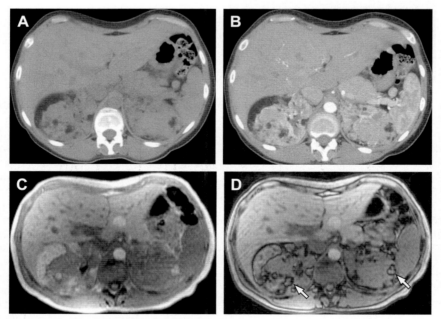

Fig. 11. Axial CT scan of abdomen done before (*A*) and following (*B*) administration of intravenous contrast in a patient with known TSC shows multiple fat density lesions in both kidneys, representing angiomyolipomas. There is heterogeneous enhancement of the soft tissue components of the angiomyolipomas following contrast administration. Axial T1-weighted in-phase (*C*) and opposed-phase (*D*) images at the same level show multiple T1 hyperintense lesions with India ink etching artifact (*arrows*) seen on the opposed-phase gradient recalled echo images.

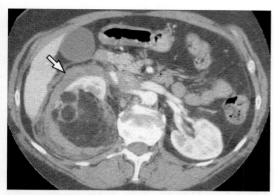

Fig. 12. Axial contrast-enhanced CT of abdomen shows a large fat-containing AML in the right kidney with high-density hemorrhage in the perinephric region (*arrow*) representing an AML that has bled.

higher in AMLs larger than 4 cm or AMLs with aneurysms larger than 5 mm.[55] Embolization is recommended for AMLs with higher risk of hemorrhage.

Renal Cysts

Simple renal cysts can be seen in up to 53% of patients with tuberous sclerosis. Although renal cysts

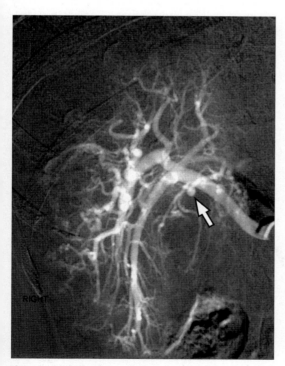

Fig. 13. Digital subtraction angiography in a patient with known tuberous sclerosis and multiple renal AMLs shows diffuse irregularity and tortuosity of renal parenchymal vessels and a 6-mm aneurysm (*arrow*) arising from a renal artery branch.

tend to occur in younger patients with TSC, they are usually asymptomatic. Approximately 2% to 3% of patients with TSC who have a contiguous mutation involving the *TSC2* gene and the polycystic kidney disease-1 (*PKD1*) gene on chromosome 16, present with features similar to adult polycystic kidney disease, with enlarged lobulated kidneys containing multiple cysts causing hypertension or renal failure.[56]

Renal Cell Carcinoma

Tuberous sclerosis does not seem to increase the risk of developing renal cell carcinoma, with a 2% to 3% lifetime risk of developing renal cell carcinoma (RCC) being similar in patients with TSC and in the general population.[57] However, RCC tends to occur at a younger age in patients with TSC (mean age of 28 years), compared with the general population (mean age of 53 years) and tends to show slower rate of growth.[58] A variety of distinct histologic subtypes of renal epithelial tumors occur more commonly in patients with TSC and include RCCs with (angio)leiomyomatous stroma, chromophobe and hybrid oncocytic tumors, and papillary tumors with clear cell morphology.[59,60] They are seen as enhancing solid renal masses, with degree of enhancement and heterogeneity depending on individual subtypes of cancers. Characteristic features of TSC-associated RCCs include predilection to affect young women and development of bilateral, multiple tumors that have an indolent course.[60]

Other Abdominal Manifestations

Hepatic AMLs may be seen in 16% to 24% of patients with TSC. However, most hepatic AMLs are sporadic and only 5.8% are associated with TSC.[61] Imaging features are similar to renal AMLs, with the lesions seen as fat-containing lesions in hepatic parenchyma. Hepatic AMLs are predominantly asymptomatic with a potential risk of hemorrhage in larger AMLs. Other rare reported abdominal manifestations of TSC in abdominal organs include splenic hamartomas, pancreatic neuroendocrine tumors, and intestinal polyps.[24,48,49] LAM, which frequently involves the lungs in patients with TSC, may also involve the retroperitoneum.[62] The obstructed lymphatic ducts are distended and are seen as multiple cystic lesions in the retroperitoneum.

CARDIOTHORACIC MANIFESTATIONS
Cardiac Manifestations

Cardiac rhabdomyoma is a common manifestation of TSC with a frequency of 50% to 65%, commonly manifesting before the age of 1 year.[63] Approximately 40% to 80% of patients who have this benign striated muscle–containing tumor have TSC.[64] It may also be diagnosed on antenatal ultrasonography or fetal MR imaging (**Fig. 14**). Cardiac rhabdomyomas are seen as solitary or multiple hypoechoic ventricular septal masses on echocardiography.[65] On cardiac MR imaging (**Fig. 15**), these lesions are isointense to myocardium on T1WIs and hyperintense on T2WIs.[66]

Frequently asymptomatic, 80% of these tumors regress before birth.[67] There is spontaneous regression of these tumors before the age of 4 years in 70% of the children. Symptoms are rare but can include heart failure, arrhythmias, and outflow obstruction,[68] with outflow obstruction sometimes necessitating surgery. Echocardiography has been recommended every 1 to 3 years to monitor the regression or stability of these tumors.[48]

Thoracic Manifestations

Thoracic manifestations include LAM and multifocal micronodular pneumocyte hyperplasia.

Lymphangioleiomyomatosis

LAM consists of smooth muscle proliferations in the lymphatics associated with cystic change in the lung parenchyma. Almost exclusively occurring in women, 1% to 3 % of patients with TSC (TSC-LAM) have LAM in contradistinction to the rarer sporadicvariant.[11] Clinical symptoms include

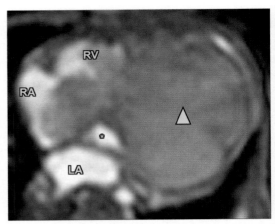

Fig. 15. A 3-day-old infant with masses noted on echocardiography underwent cardiac MR imaging. Axial b-TFE image shows the large hypointense mass (*arrowhead*) centered on the interventricular septum-balanced turbo field-echo (b-TFE) with extension into the right atrium (RA) and right ventricle (RV), and narrowing the left ventricular outflow tract (*asterisk*). Subsequent diagnosis of TSC was confirmed with characteristic findings on MR imaging brain. LA, left atrium.

dyspnea and hemoptysis with spirometry showing evidence of obstruction. LAM is characterized by recurrent pneumothoraces, chylothoraces, enlarged lymph nodes, and renal AMLs.[69]

The characteristic finding (**Fig. 16**) of LAM on high-resolution CT (HRCT) is diffuse, thin-walled, well-circumscribed lung cysts surrounded by normal lung parenchyma and presenting with either pneumothorax (up to 50%) or chylothorax (<15% of the cases).[62] These cysts are of varying size and uniformly distributed throughout the lungs. Communication between bronchioles and cysts may cause a decrease in cyst size on expiration. Reticular opacities are also recognized because of lymphatic obstruction. Presence of these characteristic features is sufficient for diagnosis without biopsy.

LAM is slowly progressive, eventually requiring lung transplant. In a study of 69 patients published by Urban and colleagues,[70] the 10-year survival rate was 79%. LAM is a low-grade metastasizing tumor classified as a mesenchymal tumor by the WHO.[71] The TSC consensus group recommends HRCT surveillance every 5 to 10 years in women at risk for LAM and annual pulmonary function testing in those with cysts on HRCT.[40]

Multifocal Micronodular Pneumocyte Hyperplasia

Multifocal micronodular pneumocyte hyperplasia (MMPH) is a rare disorder; it still constitutes the

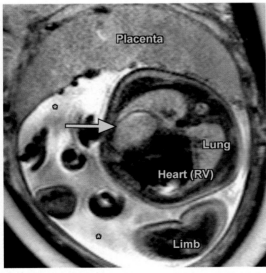

Fig. 14. Fetal MR imaging at 26 gestational weeks shows a hyperintense 3.5-cm mass (*arrow*) arising from the left ventricle, suggestive of a rhabdomyoma. The asterisk indicates amniotic fluid. RV, right ventricle.

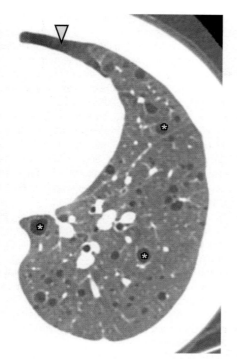

Fig. 16. A 30-year-old woman with TSC-LAM manifested as multiple thin-walled lung cysts (*asterisks*) and normal intervening lung presenting with a small spontaneous left pneumothorax (*arrowhead*).

second most common pulmonary manifestation of TSC.[48] As suggested by the name, this disorder is characterized by the multifocal nodular proliferation of type II pneumocytes along the alveolar septae. On imaging, this nonprogressive condition is manifest as multiple discrete solid or ground-glass lung nodules varying in size between 2 and 8 mm. Differential considerations include other causes for miliary or random lung nodules; however, the association with TSC should prompt the diagnosis of MMPH.[72]

SURVEILLANCE AND MONITORING OF PATIENTS WITH TUBEROUS SCLEROSIS COMPLEX

Recommendations from the 2012 TSC consensus conference[40] are presented here.

At Initial Diagnosis

- All individuals should undergo MR imaging brain with and without contrast.
- MR imaging abdomen may be performed following diagnosis or in concert with brain MR imaging in young children, to avoid repeat anesthesia administration.

- To evaluate for LAM, high-resolution chest CT with low-dose protocol was suggested in women 18 years of age or older. Adult men, if symptomatic, should also undergo testing.

Follow-up Recommendations

- Brain: MR imaging of the brain is to be obtained every 1 to 3 years in asymptomatic patients with TSC younger than 25 years of age to monitor for new occurrence of SEGA. After the age of 25 years, in patients without evidence of SEGA, no additional imaging is warranted. In contrast, patients with SEGAs need periodic imaging after 25 years, the exact interval of which was not defined, and depends on location (near foramen of Monro), size, and recent discovery.
- Renal: MR imaging abdomen to assess for the progression of AML and renal cystic disease every 1 to 3 years throughout the lifetime of the patient.
- Lungs: HRCT every 5 to 10 years in asymptomatic individuals at risk of LAM if there is no evidence of lung cysts on their baseline HRCT imaging. Individuals with lung cysts detected on HRCT should have the HRCT interval reduced to every 2 to 3 years.

TREATMENT

- Seizure control: in addition to standard antiepileptic drugs, Vigabatrin and corticotropin are used in the management of infantile spasms.[40,73] Vigabatrin can cause toxicity and abnormalities in the brain.
- Surgical resection of refractory epileptogenic tubers and growing SEGAs, or if associated with hydrocephalus.
- mTOR inhibitors are now approved and used for treatment of SEGA,[74] and AMLs (asymptomatic growing AMLs >3 cm in diameter).

SUMMARY

TSC is a multisystem genetic disorder with specific intracranial manifestations such as cortical and cerebellar tubers, subependymal nodules, and SEGAs, as well as abdominal and thoracic manifestations such as AMLs and LAM. TSC results from a mutation in the *TSC1* or *TSC2* genes, with approximately one-third of cases being inherited. The common underlying biochemical pathways have also been identified. It is important for radiologists involved in the interpretation and care of these children and adults to be abreast of this rapidly changing field.

REFERENCES

1. Crino PB, Nathanson KL, Henske EP. The tuberous sclerosis complex. N Engl J Med 2006;355(13): 1345–56.

2. Northrup H, Krueger DA, International Tuberous Sclerosis Complex Consensus Group. Tuberous sclerosis complex diagnostic criteria update: recommendations of the 2012 International Tuberous Sclerosis Complex Consensus Conference. Pediatr Neurol 2013;49(4):243–54.

3. Dabora SL, Jozwiak S, Franz DN, et al. Mutational analysis in a cohort of 224 tuberous sclerosis patients indicates increased severity of TSC2, compared with TSC1, disease in multiple organs. Am J Hum Genet 2001;68(1):64–80.

4. Chu-Shore CJ, Major P, Montenegro M, et al. Cyst-like tubers are associated with TSC2 and epilepsy in tuberous sclerosis complex. Neurology 2009; 72(13):1165–9.

5. Feliciano DM, Lin TV, Hartman NW, et al. A circuitry and biochemical basis for tuberous sclerosis symptoms: From epilepsy to neurocognitive deficits. Int J Dev Neurosci 2013;31(7):667–78.

6. Jozwiak S, Kwiatkowski D, Kotulska K, et al. Tuberin and hamartin expression is reduced in the majority of subependymal giant cell astrocytomas in tuberous sclerosis complex consistent with a two-hit model of pathogenesis. J Child Neurol 2004;19(2):102–6.

7. Rovira A, Ruiz-Falco ML, Garcia-Esparza E, et al. Recommendations for the radiological diagnosis and follow-up of neuropathological abnormalities associated with tuberous sclerosis complex. J Neurooncol 2014;118(2):205–23.

8. Luat AF, Makki M, Chugani HT. Neuroimaging in tuberous sclerosis complex. Curr Opin Neurol 2007; 20(2):142–50.

9. Goodman M, Lamm SH, Engel A, et al. Cortical tuber count: a biomarker indicating neurologic severity of tuberous sclerosis complex. J Child Neurol 1997;12(2):85–90.

10. Pascual-Castroviejo I, Hernandez-Moneo JL, Pascual-Pascual SI, et al. Significance of tuber size for complications of tuberous sclerosis complex. Neurologia 2013;28(9):550–7.

11. Curatolo P, Bombardieri R, Jozwiak S. Tuberous sclerosis. Lancet 2008;372(9639):657–68.

12. Chou IJ, Lin KL, Wong AM, et al. Neuroimaging correlation with neurological severity in tuberous sclerosis complex. Eur J Paediatr Neurol 2008;12(2): 108–12.

13. de Vries PJ, Whittemore VH, Leclezio L, et al. Tuberous sclerosis associated neuropsychiatric disorders (TAND) and the TAND checklist. Pediatr Neurol 2015;52(1):25–35.

14. Gumus K, Koc G, Doganay S, et al. Susceptibility-based differentiation of intracranial calcification and hemorrhage in pediatric patients. J Child Neurol 2015;30(8):1029–36.

15. Chen CP, Liu YP, Huang JK, et al. Contribution of ultrafast magnetic resonance imaging in prenatal diagnosis of sonographically undetected cerebral tuberous sclerosis associated with cardiac rhabdomyomas. Prenat Diagn 2005;25(6):523–4.

16. Baron Y, Barkovich AJ. MR imaging of tuberous sclerosis in neonates and young infants. AJNR Am J Neuroradiol 1999;20(5):907–16.

17. Girard N, Zimmerman RA, Schnur RE, et al. Magnetization transfer in the investigation of patients with tuberous sclerosis. Neuroradiology 1997;39(7): 523–8.

18. Pinto Gama HP, da Rocha AJ, Braga FT, et al. Comparative analysis of MR sequences to detect structural brain lesions in tuberous sclerosis. Pediatr Radiol 2006;36(2):119–25.

19. Trombley IK, Mirra SS. Ultrastructure of tuberous sclerosis: Cortical tuber and subependymal tumor. Ann Neurol 1981;9(2):174–81.

20. Sosunov AA, Wu X, Weiner HL, et al. Tuberous sclerosis: a primary pathology of astrocytes? Epilepsia 2008;49(Suppl 2):53–62.

21. Ridler K, Suckling J, Higgins N, et al. Standardized whole brain mapping of tubers and subependymal nodules in tuberous sclerosis complex. J Child Neurol 2004;19(9):658–65.

22. Gallagher A, Grant EP, Madan N, et al. MRI findings reveal three different types of tubers in patients with tuberous sclerosis complex. J Neurol 2010;257(8): 1373–81.

23. Braffman BH, Bilaniuk LT, Naidich TP, et al. MR imaging of tuberous sclerosis: Pathogenesis of this phakomatosis, use of gadopentetate dimeglumine, and literature review. Radiology 1992; 183(1):227–38.

24. Baskin HJ Jr. The pathogenesis and imaging of the tuberous sclerosis complex. Pediatr Radiol 2008; 38(9):936–52.

25. Kalantari BN, Salamon N. Neuroimaging of tuberous sclerosis: spectrum of pathologic findings and frontiers in imaging. AJR Am J Roentgenol 2008;190(5): W304–9.

26. Mukonoweshuro W, Wilkinson ID, Griffiths PD. Proton MR spectroscopy of cortical tubers in adults with tuberous sclerosis complex. AJNR Am J Neuroradiol 2001;22(10):1920–5.

27. Chandra PS, Salamon N, Huang J, et al. FDG-PET/MRI coregistration and diffusion-tensor imaging distinguish epileptogenic tubers and cortex in patients with tuberous sclerosis complex: a preliminary report. Epilepsia 2006;47(9):1543–9.

28. Daghistani R, Rutka J, Widjaja E. MRI characteristics of cerebellar tubers and their longitudinal changes in children with tuberous sclerosis complex. Childs Nerv Syst 2015;31(1):109–13.

29. Ertan G, Arulrajah S, Tekes A, et al. Cerebellar abnormality in children and young adults with tuberous sclerosis complex: MR and diffusion weighted imaging findings. J Neuroradiol 2010; 37(4):231–8.

30. Vaughn J, Hagiwara M, Katz J, et al. MRI characterization and longitudinal study of focal cerebellar lesions in a young tuberous sclerosis cohort. AJNR Am J Neuroradiol 2013;34(3):655–9.

31. Marti-Bonmati L, Menor F, Dosda R. Tuberous sclerosis: Differences between cerebral and cerebellar cortical tubers in a pediatric population. AJNR Am J Neuroradiol 2000;21(3):557–60.

32. Eluvathingal TJ, Behen ME, Chugani HT, et al. Cerebellar lesions in tuberous sclerosis complex: Neurobehavioral and neuroimaging correlates. J Child Neurol 2006;21(10):846–51.

33. van Eeghen AM, Ortiz-Teran L, Johnson J, et al. The neuroanatomical phenotype of tuberous sclerosis complex: Focus on radial migration lines. Neuroradiology 2013;55(8):1007–14.

34. Jozwiak S, Schwartz RA, Janniger CK, et al. Usefulness of diagnostic criteria of tuberous sclerosis complex in pediatric patients. J Child Neurol 2000; 15(10):652–9.

35. Goh S, Butler W, Thiele EA. Subependymal giant cell tumors in tuberous sclerosis complex. Neurology 2004;63(8):1457–61.

36. Hussain N, Curran A, Pilling D, et al. Congenital subependymal giant cell astrocytoma diagnosed on fetal MRI. Arch Dis Child 2006;91(6):520.

37. Nabbout R, Santos M, Rolland Y, et al. Early diagnosis of subependymal giant cell astrocytoma in children with tuberous sclerosis. J Neurol Neurosurg Psychiatry 1999;66(3):370–5.

38. Jozwiak S, Nabbout R, Curatolo P, Participants of the TSC Consensus Meeting for SEGA and Epilepsy Management. Management of subependymal giant cell astrocytoma (SEGA) associated with tuberous sclerosis complex (TSC): Clinical recommendations. Eur J Paediatr Neurol 2013; 17(4):348–52.

39. Cuccia V, Zuccaro G, Sosa F, et al. Subependymal giant cell astrocytoma in children with tuberous sclerosis. Childs Nerv Syst 2003;19(4):232–43.

40. Krueger DA, Northrup H, International Tuberous Sclerosis Complex Consensus Group. Tuberous sclerosis complex surveillance and management: Recommendations of the 2012 International Tuberous Sclerosis Complex Consensus Conference. Pediatr Neurol 2013;49(4):255–65.

41. Beaumont TL, Limbrick DD, Smyth MD. Advances in the management of subependymal giant cell astrocytoma. Childs Nerv Syst 2012;28(7):963–8.

42. Parmar H, Patkar D, Shah J, et al. Hemimegalencephaly with tuberous sclerosis: a longitudinal imaging study. Australas Radiol 2003;47(4):438–42.

43. Sarnat HB, Flores-Sarnat L. Infantile tauopathies: Hemimegalencephaly; tuberous sclerosis complex; focal cortical dysplasia 2; ganglioglioma. Brain Dev 2015;37(6):553–62.

44. Beltramello A, Puppini G, Bricolo A, et al. Does the tuberous sclerosis complex include intracranial aneurysms? A case report with a review of the literature. Pediatr Radiol 1999;29(3):206–11.

45. Boronat S, Shaaya EA, Auladell M, et al. Intracranial arteriopathy in tuberous sclerosis complex. J Child Neurol 2014;29(7):912–9.

46. McMaster ML, Goldstein AM, Parry DM. Clinical features distinguish childhood chordoma associated with tuberous sclerosis complex (TSC) from chordoma in the general paediatric population. J Med Genet 2011;48(7):444–9.

47. Lee-Jones L, Aligianis I, Davies PA, et al. Sacrococcygeal chordomas in patients with tuberous sclerosis complex show somatic loss of TSC1 or TSC2. Genes Chromosomes Cancer 2004;41(1): 80–5.

48. Manoukian SB, Kowal DJ. Comprehensive imaging manifestations of tuberous sclerosis. Am J Roentgenol 2015;204(5):933–43.

49. Umeoka S, Koyama T, Miki Y, et al. Pictorial review of tuberous sclerosis in various organs. Radiographics 2008;28(7):e32.

50. Ewalt DH, Sheffield E, Sparagana SP, et al. Renal lesion growth in children with tuberous sclerosis complex. J Urol 1998;160(1):141–5.

51. Davenport MS, Neville AM, Ellis JH, et al. Diagnosis of renal angiomyolipoma with Hounsfield unit thresholds: Effect of size of region of interest and nephrographic phase imaging. Radiology 2011;260(1): 158–65.

52. Israel GM, Hindman N, Hecht E, et al. The use of opposed-phase chemical shift MRI in the diagnosis of renal angiomyolipomas. Am J Roentgenol 2005; 184(6):1868–72.

53. Jinzaki M, Tanimoto A, Narimatsu Y, et al. Angiomyolipoma: Imaging findings in lesions with minimal fat. Radiology 1997;205(2):497–502.

54. Chaudhry HS, Davenport MS, Nieman CM, et al. Histogram analysis of small solid renal masses: Differentiating minimal fat angiomyolipoma from renal cell carcinoma. Am J Roentgenol 2012; 198(2):377–83.

55. Yamakado K, Tanaka N, Nakagawa T, et al. Renal angiomyolipoma: Relationships between tumor size, aneurysm formation, and rupture. Radiology 2002;225(1):78–82.

56. Brook-Carter PT, Peral B, Ward CJ, et al. Deletion of the TSC2 and PKD1 genes associated with severe infantile polycystic kidney disease–a contiguous gene syndrome. Nat Genet 1994;8(4):328–32.

57. Tello R, Blickman JG, Buonomo C, et al. Meta analysis of the relationship between tuberous sclerosis

complex and renal cell carcinoma. Eur J Radiol 1998;27(2):131–8.

58. Washecka R, Hanna M. Malignant renal tumors in tuberous sclerosis. Urology 1991;37(4):340–3.

59. Delahunt B, Srigley JR. The evolving classification of renal cell neoplasia. Semin Diagn Pathol 2015;32(2): 90–102.

60. Guo J, Tretiakova MS, Troxell ML, et al. Tuberous sclerosis-associated renal cell carcinoma: A clinicopathologic study of 57 separate carcinomas in 18 patients. Am J Surg Pathol 2014;38(11):1457–67.

61. Fricke BL, Donnelly LF, Casper KA, et al. Frequency and imaging appearance of hepatic angiomyolipomas in pediatric and adult patients with tuberous sclerosis. AJR Am J Roentgenol 2004; 182(4):1027–30.

62. Pallisa E, Sanz P, Roman A, et al. Lymphangioleiomyomatosis: pulmonary and abdominal findings with pathologic correlation. Radiographics 2002;22 Spec No:S185–98.

63. Gibbs JL. The heart and tuberous sclerosis. an echocardiographic and electrocardiographic study. Br Heart J 1985;54(6):596–9.

64. Webb DW, Thomas RD, Osborne JP. Cardiac rhabdomyomas and their association with tuberous sclerosis. Arch Dis Child 1993;68(3):367–70.

65. Bader RS, Chitayat D, Kelly E, et al. Fetal rhabdomyoma: Prenatal diagnosis, clinical outcome, and incidence of associated tuberous sclerosis complex. J Pediatr 2003;143(5):620–4.

66. Christophe C, Bartholome J, Blum D, et al. Neonatal tuberous sclerosis. US, CT, and MR diagnosis of brain and cardiac lesions. Pediatr Radiol 1989; 19(6–7):446–8.

67. Nir A, Tajik AJ, Freeman WK, et al. Tuberous sclerosis and cardiac rhabdomyoma. Am J Cardiol 1995;76(5):419–21.

68. Smythe JF, Dyck JD, Smallhorn JF, et al. Natural history of cardiac rhabdomyoma in infancy and childhood. Am J Cardiol 1990;66(17):1247–9.

69. Xu KF, Lo BH. Lymphangioleiomyomatosis: Differential diagnosis and optimal management. Ther Clin Risk Manag 2014;10:691–700.

70. Urban T, Lazor R, Lacronique J, et al. Pulmonary lymphangioleiomyomatosis. A study of 69 patients. Groupe d'etudes et de recherche sur les maladies "orphelines" pulmonaires (GERM"O"P). Medicine (Baltimore) 1999;78(5):321–37.

71. McCormack FX, Travis WD, Colby TV, et al. Lymphangioleiomyomatosis: Calling it what it is: A low-grade, destructive, metastasizing neoplasm. Am J Respir Crit Care Med 2012;186(12):1210–2.

72. Ristagno RL, Biddinger PW, Pina EM, et al. Multifocal micronodular pneumocyte hyperplasia in tuberous sclerosis. AJR Am J Roentgenol 2005; 184(3 Suppl):S37–9.

73. Camposano SE, Major P, Halpern E, et al. Vigabatrin in the treatment of childhood epilepsy: A retrospective chart review of efficacy and safety profile. Epilepsia 2008;49(7):1186–91.

74. Franz DN, Belousova E, Sparagana S, et al. Efficacy and safety of everolimus for subependymal giant cell astrocytomas associated with tuberous sclerosis complex (EXIST-1): A multicentre, randomised, placebo-controlled phase 3 trial. Lancet 2013; 381(9861):125–32.

Multiple Endocrine Neoplasia Syndromes
A Comprehensive Imaging Review

Joseph R. Grajo, MD[a],*, Raj Mohan Paspulati, MD[b],
Dushyant V. Sahani, MD[c], Avinash Kambadakone, MD[c]

KEYWORDS

- Multiple endocrine neoplasia • MEN1 • MEN2 • MEN4 • Neuroendocrine tumor

KEY POINTS

- Multiple endocrine neoplasia is composed of a series of genetically inherited disorders involving concomitant tumors within two or more endocrine organs.
- Patients with MEN1 develop tumors of the parathyroid gland, pancreas, and pituitary gland and adrenal cortical tumors and neuroendocrine tumors of the thymus, bronchi, and stomach.
- MEN2 is comprised of three subtypes (MEN2A, MEN2B, and familial medullary thyroid carcinoma), the hallmark of which is medullary thyroid cancer, adrenal pheochromocytoma, and parathyroid tumor.
- MEN4 represents a newly described group of patients who develop parathyroid and pituitary tumors.

INTRODUCTION

Multiple endocrine neoplasia (MEN) encompasses a series of familial, genetically inherited conditions in which tumors simultaneously occur in two or more endocrine organs. MEN syndromes are autosomal-dominant disorders categorized into three main patterns: (1) MEN1 (Wermer syndrome), (2) MEN2 (including MEN2A or Sipple syndrome, MEN2B or Wagenmann-Froboese syndrome, and familial medullary thyroid cancer [FMTC]), and (3) MEN4. Although MEN1 and MEN2 are most common and usually manifest as distinct syndromes, other presentations do occur, including hyperparathyroidism–jaw tumor syndrome and "overlap syndromes," in which tumors typically associated with one syndrome develop in combination. This article outlines the imaging characteristics of the endocrine tumors that occur in patients with MEN syndromes.

MEN1 SYNDROME

Patients with MEN1 (or Wermer) syndrome develop germline-inactivating mutations of the MEN1 tumor suppressor gene, resulting in tumors of the parathyroid gland (95%), pancreas (40%), and pituitary gland (30%).[1] Other tumors occurring with MEN1 include angiofibromas (88%), collagenomas (72%), adrenal cortical tumors (35%), and facial ependymomas (<5%).[1] Clinical symptoms of MEN1 syndrome almost uniformly present by the fifth decade and are seen in children at 5 years of age.[2–4]

Disclosures: None.
a Division of Abdominal Imaging, Department of Radiology, Shands Medical Center, University of Florida College of Medicine, PO Box 100374, Gainesville, FL 32610, USA; b Department of Radiology, University Hospitals Case Medical Center, Case Western Reserve University, 11100 Euclid Avenue, Cleveland, OH 44106, USA; c Division of Abdominal Imaging, Department of Radiology, Massachusetts General Hospital, Harvard Medical School, 55 Fruit Street, White 270, Boston, MA 02114, USA
* Corresponding author.
E-mail address: grajjr@radiology.ufl.edu

radiologic.theclinics.com

Table 1	
Imaging features of parathyroid adenomas	
Echogenicity on ultrasound	• Typically uniformly hypoechoic relative to the thyroid gland on gray-scale imaging (perhaps caused by compact cellularity) • Commonly detected on gray-scale alone when >1 cm in size
Shape	• Usually oval or bean-shaped • Larger adenomas can be multilobulated
Vascularity on ultrasound	• Classic extrathyroidal feeding vessel supplying the upper or lower pole of the parathyroid glad (usually a branch of the inferior thyroidal artery) • Characteristic rim of vascularity (resulting from branching of the feeding vessel around the periphery of the gland before diving deeper) (**Fig. 1**) • Color Doppler imaging of the overlying thyroid gland may show focal asymmetric hypervascularity, which may help direct identification of an underlying parathyroid adenoma
99mTc-sestamibi uptake	• Initial planar images shortly after radiotracer administration: uptake in thyroid gland and normal parathyroid tissue • Early dynamic images: asymmetric focal activity within the abnormal parathyroid gland (adenoma or hyperplasia) superimposed on normal thyroid uptake • Delayed images: retained radiotracer activity within hyperfunctioning parathyroid tissue (typically at 2-hour delay) (**Fig. 2**)

Data from Johnson NA, Tublin ME, Ogilvie JB. Parathyroid imaging: technique and role in the preoperative evaluation of primary hyperparathyroidism. AJR Am J Roentgenol 2007;188(6):1706–15.

MEN1 Tumors

Parathyroid tumors

Parathyroid adenomas are the most common tumors associated with MEN1. They typically present as the initial manifestation of the syndrome, usually occurring in the third decade of life.[1] Patients with primary hyperparathyroidism can be asymptomatic with biochemical abnormalities or demonstrate the classic symptoms of abdominal pain/constipation/peptic ulceration, nephrolithiasis/polyuria/polydipsia, confusion/dementia/depression, and fatigue/aching/fractures (commonly referred to as moans, stones, groans, and bones).

Cross-sectional investigation for a parathyroid adenoma usually begins with high-resolution ultrasound, which has a sensitivity of up to 82% when performed by experienced sonographers.[5] Computed tomography (CT) does not add additional information other than localizing ectopic parathyroid glands within the superior mediastinum. Parathyroid glands are typically T1 hypointense and T2 hyperintense on MR imaging. Although MR imaging is slightly more sensitive than CT in the detection of parathyroid adenomas, it is also not frequently used for this purpose. Planar and single-photon emission CT sestamibi imaging has a high sensitivity for detection of parathyroid adenomas, particularly when used in conjunction with ultrasound. Adenomas demonstrate asymmetric focal radiotracer uptake with retention on delayed imaging (**Table 1**).

Pancreatic neuroendocrine tumors

Pancreatic neuroendocrine tumors (NETs) are the second most common neoplasm associated with MEN1, occurring in up to 80% of patients.[4] NETs are functioning or nonfunctioning, and present with biochemical abnormalities or screening imaging of patients with known MEN syndromes.[3] More than half of pancreatic NETs are gastrinomas; one-third are insulinomas; and less than 5% are glucagonomas, vasoactive intestinal

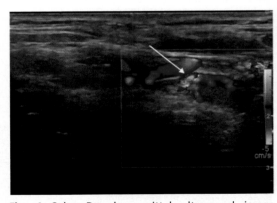

Fig. 1. Color Doppler sagittal ultrasound image demonstrating an ovoid soft tissue nodule, which is slightly hypoechoic to the adjacent thyroid gland (not shown). The peripheral flow emanating from a feeding vessel at the superior pole of this nodule (*arrow*) is the typical sonographic appearance of a parathyroid gland.

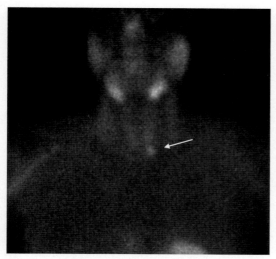

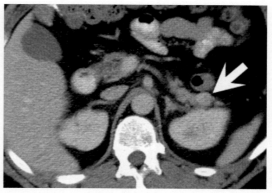

Fig. 3. Axial contrast-enhanced CT image demonstrating an arterially enhancing mass (*arrow*) in the pancreatic tail. Surgical pathology revealed the lesion to be an insulinoma.

Fig. 2. Delayed planar ^{99m}Tc-sestamibi scan demonstrating focal radiotracer uptake at the lower pole of the left thyroid lobe (*arrow*), corresponding to the parathyroid adenoma seen sonographically in Fig. 1.

peptide-omas, and pancreatic polypeptide-omas.[1] When they occur in the setting of MEN1, pancreatic NETs cause the most morbidity and mortality. NETs can be multiple, occur anywhere in the pancreas, and range from indolent mircoadenomas to aggressive invasive and even metastatic adenocarcinomas. NETs associated with MEN1 also develop in the duodenum, most commonly microgastrinomas.[5]

Ultrasound is not an effective method for investigating pancreaticoduodenal NETs, unless used with endoscopic or intraoperative approach. CT is the most commonly used method to evaluate for evaluating pancreatic NETs, with a sensitivity of 70% to 80%.[5] On CT, NETs are often small, multiple, and isodense to the pancreas on unenhanced imaging. Pancreatic protocol CT demonstrates hyperenhancement of the tumor, particularly on the arterial phase (**Fig. 3**). High-quality pancreatic CT

imaging is important because NETs may be visualized only on the arterial phase (25–30 seconds after intravenous contrast administration) and not on the pancreatic phase (35–40 seconds) or portal venous phase (60–70 seconds). Conspicuity of NETs, especially small tumors, is increased with narrowed windows and thin-section imaging (1.25–2.5 mm slices rather than 5 mm) (**Fig. 4**).[5] CT is also first-line for identifying metastatic disease, most commonly to the liver. MR imaging offers increased sensitivity in the detection of pancreatic NET compared with CT,[6,7] with a sensitivity ranging from 65% to 85%[7,8] and a positive predictive value approaching 96%.[9] NETs are typically T1 hypointense and T2 hyperintense but can demonstrate variable T2-signal intensity depending on the degree of underlying collage content. Liver metastases classically demonstrate T2 hyperintensity (**Fig. 5**), early arterial ringlike enhancement (**Fig. 6**), and restricted diffusion (**Fig. 7**). The sensitivity for detection of NET liver metastases with T2-weighted imaging and dynamic contrast-enhanced T1-weighted images is approximately 48% to 56% but is 72% for diffusion-weighted imaging. When

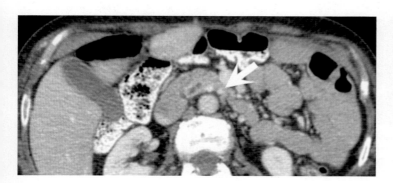

Fig. 4. Thin-section axial contrast-enhanced CT image showing a small subcentimeter hyperenhancing mass at the junction of the pancreatic body and tail (*arrow*), which was later discovered to represent a somatostatinoma.

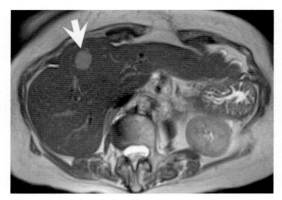

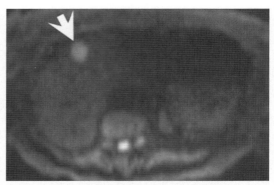

Fig. 7. Axial diffusion-weighted image demonstrating restricted diffusion (*arrow*) within the same glucagonoma metastasis depicted in **Figs. 5** and **6**.

Fig. 5. Axial T2-weighted MR image demonstrating a hyperintense mass within hepatic segment IV (*arrow*). This mass represented a metastasis from a known primary glucagonoma within the pancreas (not shown).

using all three MR imaging parameters, the sensitivity approaches 100% with a specificity of 89% to 100% for each sequence.[10]

Somatostatin receptor imaging with ^{111}In-octreotide is a whole-body nuclear medicine imaging technique helpful for detecting NETs and distant metastases, with a sensitivity of 70% to 90% for gastrinomas and 50% for insulinomas (**Fig. 8**).[5] Unfortunately, not all NETs have somatostatin receptors, which can result in false-negative results. Aggressive NETs, which are less likely to have somatostatin receptors, may demonstrate hypermetabolic activity on ^{18}F-FDG PET imaging (**Fig. 9**). Radionuclide imaging is helpful for evaluating disease response in patients with NETs demonstrating radiotracer uptake either on ^{111}In-octreotide or ^{18}F-FDG PET imaging (**Table 2**).

Pituitary tumors
Pituitary tumors in MEN1 occur in the anterior pituitary gland (or adenohypophysis). As in the

pancreas, these anterior pituitary tumors are neuroendocrine in etiology. Anterior pituitary NETs occur in 30% to 50% of patients with MEN1, with a higher incidence in women.[11] Clinical symptoms occur as a result of hypersecretion of hormones or compression of adjacent structures by the mass. Two-thirds of the tumors are prolactinomas, one-quarter are somatotrophinomas,

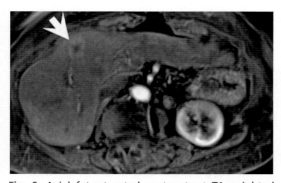

Fig. 6. Axial fat-saturated postcontrast T1-weighted image in the arterial phase shows that the glucagonoma metastasis (same lesion as in **Fig. 5**) demonstrates peripheral arterial hyperenhancement (*arrow*).

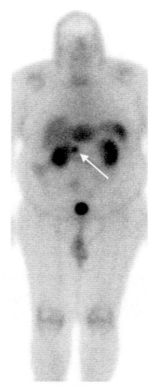

Fig. 8. Whole-body [111]In Octreoscan demonstrating focal radiotracer uptake (*arrow*) within a neuroendocrine tumor in the pancreatic head in this patient with MEN1 syndrome.

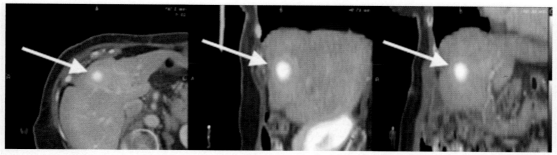

Fig. 9. Fused PET-CT image showing focal hypermetabolic activity (*arrows*) within the same segment IV glucagonoma metastasis depicted in **Figs. 5–7**.

about 5% are adrenocorticotrophinomas, and about 5% are nonfunctioning adenomas.[1] Prolactinomas (secreting prolactin) are the most common anterior pituitary NET, resulting in secondary amenorrhea, galactorrhea, and infertility (in women), and impotence (in men). Somatotrophinomas (secreting growth hormone) result in acromegaly, whereas adrenocorticotrophinomas (secreting ACTH) result in Cushing disease.

Small field of view MR imaging with precontrast and postcontrast imaging of the sella is the modality of choice for detection of pituitary tumors. Adenomas are typically hypointense to the normal pituitary gland on precontrast and postcontrast T1 weighted. Microadenomas (measuring <10 mm)

are not always visualized on imaging. In these cases, secondary signs, such as focal convexity of the superior pituitary gland or erosion of the sellar floor, can be used to suggest the diagnosis. Macroadenomas (measuring >10 mm) may cause mass effect on adjacent structures (**Table 3**).

Adrenal cortical tumors

As in the general population, most adrenal cortical tumors are benign and nonfunctioning. They occur in 10% to 30% of patients with MEN1 syndrome.[12] Although tumors less than 4 cm generally do not require surgical resection, functioning cortical adenomas in patients with MEN1 resulting in Cushing

---

Table 2
Imaging features of pancreatic neuroendocrine tumors on CT and MR imaging

Margins	• Well-circumscribed round or oval masses • Tend to displace, rather than invade surrounding structures
Composition	• Usually solid • Can be cystic, may demonstrate hypervascular rim
Signal characteristics on MR imaging	• Hypointense on T1 weighted relative to the normally T1 hyperintense pancreas (on both fat saturation and non–fat saturation sequences) • Hyperintense on T2 weighted compared with background parenchyma • Can also be T2 intermediate or hypointense (because of presence of collagen)
Enhancement	• Typically avidly enhancing in the arterial and venous phases (because of rich capillary networks) • May demonstrate homogeneous, ring, or heterogeneous enhancement (depending on the degree of cystic degeneration and/or necrosis in larger tumors)
Homogeneity	• Smaller lesions are usually more homogeneous • Larger lesions may demonstrate heterogeneity (because of cystic degeneration, necrosis, calcification)

Metastases	• Liver metastases
	  ○ Hypervascular, often with ringlike arterial enhancement
	  ○ T1 hypointense and T2 hyperintense, often more conspicuous on fat-suppressed T2 weighted
	• Lymph node metastases
	  ○ Also hypervascular (best seen on arterial phase)

Data from Lewis RB, Lattin GE Jr, Paal E. Pancreatic endocrine tumors: radiologic-clinicopathologic correlation. Radiographics 2010;30(6):1445–64.

Table 3 Imaging features of pituitary adenomas on MR imaging	
Size	• Microadenomas: <10 mm in size; may not be clearly visualized even with thin-section MR imaging; focal convexity of the superior margin of the pituitary gland or erosion of the sellar floor may suggest the presence of an underlying microadenoma • Macroadenomas: >10 mm in size, may compress adjacent structures (eg, the optic chiasm)
Signal characteristics on MR imaging	Hypointense on T1 weighted relative to the normal pituitary gland
Enhancement	Typically hypointense to the normal pituitary gland on postcontrast images (may be more conspicuous on sagittal and coronal imaging planes)

Data from Scarsbrook AF, Thakker RV, Wass JA, et al. Multiple endocrine neoplasia: spectrum of radiologic appearances and discussion of a multitechnique imaging approach. Radiographics 2006;26(2):433–51.

syndrome (hypercortisolemia) and Conn syndrome (hyperaldosteronism) warrant adrenelectomy.[13]

Adrenal adenomas are typically diagnosed on either CT or MR imaging. Approximately 70% to 80% of adenomas are lipid-rich, whereas up to 30% of adenomas are lipid-poor. Lipid-rich adenomas are identified when these lesions contain intracellular fat, which is characterized on unenhanced CT (density <10 HU) or adrenal protocol CT using unenhanced, portal venous phase, and 15-minute delayed images (relative washout exceeding 40% or absolute washout exceeding 60%). Alternatively, signal drop-out on opposed-phase T1-weighted gradient recalled echo imaging can identify intracellular fat on chemical shift MR imaging. Lipid-poor adenomas are difficult to characterize because of density values exceeding 10 HU on unenhanced CT and lack of chemical shift artifact on opposed-phased T1-weighted MR imaging. However, washout values and T2 signal that mirrors that of normal adrenal cortex are imaging features that suggest a lipid-poor adenoma.[14] Adrenal cortical carcinomas are extremely rare. These aggressive malignant tumors are frequently large, show necrosis/hemorrhage, and have a tendency to invade locally and into the blood vessels (into adrenal/renal veins and inferior vena cava) and distant metastasis (Table 4).

Other neuroendocrine tumors
Patients with MEN1 may also develop NETs of the thymus, respiratory tract, and upper gastrointestinal tract (Fig. 10). The presentation of these NETs ranges from asymptomatic disease to metastatic carcinoma. Patients with metastatic NETs may manifest features of carcinoid syndrome, including facial flushing, bronchospasm, and diarrhea.[1]

Early detection of NETs may be attempted with endoscopy or cross-sectional imaging (CT or MR imaging). Whole-body functional imaging with Octreoscan (Mallinckrodt, Inc, St. Louis, MO) or PET scan is also a consideration, although false-negatives may occur in poorly differentiated NETs[5] (Table 5).

MEN2 SYNDROME

MEN2 syndrome is comprised of three disease groups: (1) MEN2A (55% of patients), (2) MEN2B (10%), and (3) FMTC (35%).[15] The hallmark tumors of MEN2 include medullary thyroid carcinoma (MTC), pheochromocytomas of the adrenal glands, and parathyroid tumors (Table 6).

Table 4 Adrenal cortical tumors	
Adenomas	• Present in up to 40% of MEN1 (rarely functional) • Typically diagnosed on CT (ie, density of <10 HU, or relative washout >40%/absolute washout >60%) or MR imaging (ie, signal dropout on opposed-phase T1-weighted gradient recalled echo images)
Adrenal cortical carcinoma	• Typically large (>5 cm) • May demonstrate central necrosis, hemorrhage, or calcification • May present with local invasion, nodal spread, and distant metastases

Data from Scarsbrook AF, Thakker RV, Wass JA, et al. Multiple endocrine neoplasia: spectrum of radiologic appearances and discussion of a multitechnique imaging approach. Radiographics 2006;26(2):433–51.

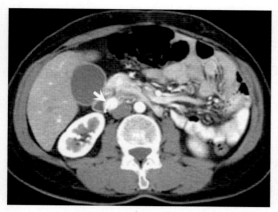

Fig. 10. Axial contrast-enhanced CT image demonstrating a hyperenhancing mass within the second portion of the duodenum (*arrow*), which represents a gastrinoma in this patient with MEN1 syndrome.

MEN2 Tumors

Medullary thyroid carcinoma

MTC is multicentric and bilateral in patients with MEN2, requiring total thyroidectomy and central lymph node dissection in patients with symptomatic thyroid nodules.[1] It is characterized by increased levels of calcitonin and carcinoembryonic antigen, which are secreted by parafollicular C cells of the thyroid gland. MTC is an aggressive cancer that can metastasize to the liver, lungs, bone, and brain. Early prophylactic total thyroidectomy is recommended between ages 5 and 10 for patients with MEN2A or FMTC and

by 6 months of age in children with MEN2B.[16] Early detection by calcitonin screening and *RET* mutational analysis in MEN2 families is required for prompt operative planning.[1]

MTC presents as a solid mass with possible calcifications on ultrasound, CT, or MR imaging. Local invasion, nodal disease, and distant metastases can be characterized with these modalities. However, whole-body radionuclide imaging with ^{123}I-MIGH, pentavalent ^{99m}Tc-dimer-captosuccinic acid, and ^{111}In-octreotide permit accurate staging and restaging for treatment planning, although no single imaging technique provides complete diagnostic confidence[5] (**Table 7**).

Pheochromocytoma

Pheochromocytomas are benign adrenal tumors in patients with MEN2 that often develop bilaterally in the fourth decade of life. They are characterized clinically by labile or refractory hypertension. Pheochromocytomas increase the perioperative morbidity and mortality of patients with MEN2. Therefore, laboratory screening with urinary metanephrines and radiologic screening with MR imaging or MIBG scan is required before thyroid surgery in patients with FMTC.[1] Screening for pheochromocytomas is recommended starting at the age of 20 years for patients with MEN2A and FMTC and at the age of 8 years for children with MEN2B.[15,16]

On contrast-enhanced CT, pheochromocytomas demonstrate avid enhancement and may contain calcifications and/or necrosis (**Fig. 11**).

Table 5 Imaging features of MEN1-associated carcinoids	
Thymic carcinoid	• Typically seen in males • Manifests in middle age • Commonly asymptomatic and hormonally inactive • May be large at the time of diagnosis • On cross-sectional imaging, may be locally invasive and indistinguishable from a thymoma
Bronchial carcinoid	• More common in females • Usually benign low-grade tumors • Can be more aggressive when occurring in males • On cross-sectional imaging, typically a well-circumscribed spherical or ovoid nodule associated with central bronchi; atypical bronchial carcinoids are typically larger and more peripheral with a more aggressive course
Gastric carcinoid	• Occurs almost exclusively in patients with MEN1 with a gastrinoma and associated Zollinger-Ellison syndrome • Multicentric, frequently metastasizing to local nodes and the liver • On fluoroscopy or cross-sectional imaging, it commonly presents as multiple masses with diffuse gastric wall thickening

Data from Scarsbrook AF, Thakker RV, Wass JA, et al. Multiple endocrine neoplasia: spectrum of radiologic appearances and discussion of a multitechnique imaging approach. Radiographics 2006;26(2):433–51.

Table 6
Features of MEN2 syndrome

	MEN2A	MEN2B	FMTC
Hereditary medullary thyroid cancer	Accounts for 80% of cases	Accounts for 5% of cases (but may be more aggressive)	Characterized by adult FMTC alone
Adrenal pheochromocytomas	Develop in 50% of patients	Develop in 40% of patients	Rare
Primary hyperparathyroidism	Occurs in 25% of patients (often mild, asymptomatic from hyperplasia)	Parathyroid hyperplasia is absent	Rare
Phenotype	Cutaneous lichen amyloidosis develops in 10% of patients	Hypertrophied lips, marfanoid habitus, ocular and musculoskeletal abnormalities, mucosal neuromas	Rare
Gastrointestinal manifestation	Hirschsprung disease may occur	Intestinal ganglioneuromas may occur	Rare

Data from Ganeshan D, Paulson E, Duran C, et al. Current update on medullary thyroid carcinoma. AJR Am J Roentgenol 2013;201(6):W867–76.

Pheochromocytomas also demonstrate avid enhancement on dynamic contrast-enhanced MR imaging, which is the modality of choice because of its lack of ionizing radiation and the additional information it provides, particularly T2 signal characteristics. Pheochromocytomas classically demonstrate "light bulb bright" T2 signal hyperintensity, although this is variable because of the degree of heterogeneity that is seen related to hemorrhage and/or necrosis (**Fig. 12**). Whole-body functional imaging with ^{123}I MIBG is useful for detecting a pheochromocytoma in the contralateral adrenal gland and identifying metastases[5] (**Tables 8** and **9**).

Table 7
Imaging features of medullary thyroid carcinoma

Size	• Tends to be larger than papillary thyroid cancer • Primary tumor size is useful for predicting nodal metastasis (20%–30% incidence of nodal metastasis in medullary thyroid carcinomas <1 cm in diameter but up to 90% in tumors measuring more than 4 cm)[17]
Echogenicity	• Hypoechoic • More often cystic than papillary thyroid cancer • Tends to have more homogeneous hypoechoic echotexture within solid components compared with papillary thyroid cancer
Suspicious features	Hypervascularity, spiculated margins, calcifications (microcalcifications and macrocalcifications), "taller than wide" orientation
Features of nodal metastases	Irregular margins or bulging contours, heterogeneous echotexture, calcifications (microcalcifications or macrocalcifications), cystic degeneration, hypervascularity
Distant metastases	• Liver: Metastases tend to be hyperechoic (but can be hypoechoic or mixed); dynamic contrast-enhanced liver MR imaging is the modality of choice for evaluation of liver metastases • Lung and bone metastases: CT or PET/CT is preferred for characterizing potential lung metastases, whereas MR imaging or bone scintigraphy is preferred for bony metastases

From Ganeshan D, Paulson E, Duran C, et al. Current update on medullary thyroid carcinoma. AJR Am J Roentgenol 2013;201(6):W867–76; with permission.

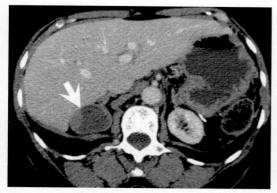

Fig. 11. Axial contrast-enhanced CT image showing an enhancing right adrenal mass with a large area of central necrosis (*arrow*). Pheochromocytomas demonstrate a wide array of appearances, including prominent necrosis as seen in this case.

Parathyroid tumors

Some patients with MEN2A develop primary hyperparathyroidism, most commonly in the setting of concomitant MTC. Hypercalcemia in these cases is usually mild and asymptomatic.[1]

MEN4 SYNDROME

MEN4 is a recently described form of MEN in patients with parathyroid and anterior pituitary tumors. Patients with MEN4 syndrome may also

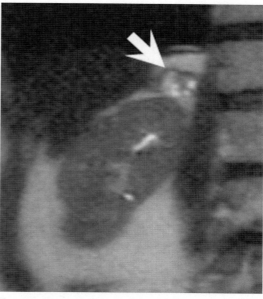

Fig. 12. Coronal T2-weighted MR image demonstrating a right adrenal mass with high T2 signal intensity, the so-called "light bulb bright" appearance that is seen with some pheochromocytomas.

Table 8	
Imaging findings of pheochromocytoma on CT and MR imaging	
Attenuation on CT	• May be homogeneous or heterogeneous (smaller tumors tend to be more homogeneous) • Solid or complex cystic • May have calcifications • Most have density values exceeding 10 HU, but some may be <10 HU because of the presence of intracellular fat (which can lead to a false diagnosis of an adrenal adenoma) • Macroscopic fat is rare but possible • Hemorrhage can also occur, leading to high unenhanced attenuation
Signal characteristics on MR imaging	• Typically hypointense on T1 weighted (presence of macroscopic fat or hemorrhage can produce T1 hyperintensity) • Typically hyperintense on T2 weighted • Signal voids on T1 and T2 weighted are seen because of the presence of tumor vessels, creating the "salt and pepper" appearance • Can show signal drop-out on opposed-phase T1 imaging in rare cases of pheochromocytomas containing intracellular fat
Enhancement	• Typically enhance avidly (density exceeding 100–120 HU) • Can enhance heterogeneously because of areas of cystic degeneration
Washout	• Typically show a relative washout rate of <40% and an absolute washout rate of <60%, thus distinguishing pheochromocytomas from adenomas • However, can show varying degrees of enhancement and washout, thus mimicking adenomas or metastases

Data from Blake MA, Kalra MK, Maher MM, et al. Pheochromocytoma: an imaging chameleon. Radiographics 2004;24 Suppl 1:S87–99.

Table 9
Imaging findings of pheochromocytoma on radionuclide imaging

[123]I MIBG	Near 100% specificity but limited sensitivity for localization of pheochromocytomas[18]
Octreotide	Pheochromocytoma localization is seen in <30% of cases[19]
[18]FDG PET	Pheochromocytomas demonstrate increased FDG uptake but findings overlap with uptake seen in adrenal metastases

Data from Blake MA, Kalra MK, Maher MM, et al. Pheochromocytoma: an imaging chameleon. Radiographics 2004;24 Suppl 1:S87–99.

develop bronchial and gastric carcinoids or gastrinomas leading to Zollinger-Ellison syndrome.[20–23]

MEN4 Tumors

Parathyroid tumors
A small sample size of patients with known MEN4 syndrome has demonstrated that benign parathyroid adenomas occur, resulting in primary hyperparathyroidism.[20–23]

Pituitary tumors
In the same small group of patients with MEN4, anterior pituitary tumors occurred in about half of the population. As with MEN1, these tumors include prolactinomas, somatotrophinomas, and adrenocorticotrophinomas.[20–23]

SUMMARY

MEN syndromes present as a group of genetically inherited disorders that manifest as tumors occurring in multiple endocrine organs. MEN1 and MEN2 occur most commonly, involving tumors of the parathyroid glands, pancreas, pituitary gland, thyroid gland, adrenal glands, and parathyroid glands, respectively. An understanding of the imaging features of these tumors is important for early detection of disease and accurate staging.

REFERENCES

1. Walls GV. Multiple endocrine neoplasia (MEN) syndromes. Semin Pediatr Surg 2014;23(2):96–101.
2. Farrell WE, Azevedo MF, Batista DL, et al. Unique gene expression profile associated with an early-onset multiple endocrine neoplasia (MEN1)-associated pituitary adenoma. J Clin Endocrinol Metab 2011;96(11):E1905–14.
3. Newey PJ, Jeyabalan J, Walls GV, et al. Asymptomatic children with multiple endocrine neoplasia type 1 mutations may harbor nonfunctioning pancreatic neuroendocrine tumors. J Clin Endocrinol Metab 2009;94(10):3640–6.
4. Trump D, Farren B, Wooding C, et al. Clinical studies of multiple endocrine neoplasia type 1 (MEN1). QJM 1996;89(9):653–69.
5. Scarsbrook AF, Thakker RV, Wass JA, et al. Multiple endocrine neoplasia: spectrum of radiologic appearances and discussion of a multitechnique imaging approach. Radiographics 2006;26(2):433–51.
6. Kalra MK, Maher MM, Mueller PR, et al. State-of-the-art imaging of pancreatic neoplasms. Br J Radiol 2003;76(912):857–65.
7. Thoeni RF, Mueller-Lisse UG, Chan R, et al. Detection of small, functional islet cell tumors in the pancreas: selection of MR imaging sequences for optimal sensitivity. Radiology 2000;214(2):483–90.
8. Angeli E, Vanzulli A, Castrucci M, et al. Value of abdominal sonography and MR imaging at 0.5 T in preoperative detection of pancreatic insulinoma: a comparison with dynamic CT and angiography. Abdom Imaging 1997;22(3):295–303.
9. Semelka RC, Custodio CM, Cem Balci N, et al. Neuroendocrine tumors of the pancreas: spectrum of appearances on MRI. J Magn Reson Imaging 2000;11(2):141–8.
10. d'Assignies G, Fina P, Bruno O, et al. High sensitivity of diffusion-weighted MR imaging for the detection of liver metastases from neuroendocrine tumors: comparison with T2-weighted and dynamic gadolinium-enhanced MR imaging. Radiology 2013;268(2):390–9.
11. Goudet P, Bonithon-Kopp C, Murat A, et al. Gender-related differences in MEN1 lesion occurrence and diagnosis: a cohort study of 734 cases from the Groupe d'etude des Tumeurs Endocrines. Eur J Endocrinol 2011;165(1):97–105.
12. Gatta-Cherifi B, Chabre O, Murat A, et al. Adrenal involvement in MEN1. Analysis of 715 cases from the Groupe d'etude des Tumeurs Endocrines database. Eur J Endocrinol 2012;166(2):269–79.
13. Waldmann J, Bartsch DK, Kann PH, et al. Adrenal involvement in multiple endocrine neoplasia type 1: results of 7 years prospective screening. Langenbecks Arch Surg 2007;392(4):437–43.
14. Becker-Weidman D, Kalb B, Mittal PK, et al. Differentiation of lipid-poor adrenal adenomas from non-adenomas with magnetic resonance imaging: utility of dynamic, contrast enhancement and single-shot T2-weighted sequences. Eur J Radiol 2015;84(11):2045–51.
15. Frank-Raue K, Rondot S, Raue F. Molecular genetics and phenomics of RET mutations: impact on prognosis of MTC. Mol Cell Endocrinol 2010;322(1–2):2–7.
16. American Thyroid Association Guidelines Task Force, Kloos RT, Eng C, et al. Medullary thyroid

cancer: management guidelines of the American thyroid association. Thyroid 2009;19(6):565–612.

17. Kim MJ, Kim EK, Park SI, et al. US-guided fine-needle aspiration of thyroid nodules: indications, techniques, results. Radiographics 2008;28(7):1869–86 [discussion: 1887].

18. Tenenbaum F, Lumbroso J, Schlumberger M, et al. Comparison of radiolabeled octreotide and meta-iodobenzylguanidine (MIBG) scintigraphy in malignant pheochromocytoma. J Nucl Med 1995;36(1):1–6.

19. van der Harst E, de Herder WW, Bruining HA, et al. [(123)I]metaiodobenzylguanidine and [(111)In]octreotide uptake in begnign and malignant pheochromocytomas. J Clin Endocrinol Metab 2001;86(2): 685–93.

20. Lee M, Pellegata NS. Multiple endocrine neoplasia syndromes associated with mutation of p27. J Endocrinol Invest 2013;36(9):781–7.

21. Lee M, Pellegata NS. Multiple endocrine neoplasia type 4. Front Horm Res 2013;41:63–78.

22. Marinoni I, Pellegata NS. p27kip1: a new multiple endocrine neoplasia gene? Neuroendocrinology 2011;93(1):19–28.

23. Pellegata NS, Quintanilla-Martinez L, Siggelkow H, et al. Germ-line mutations in p27Kip1 cause a multiple endocrine neoplasia syndrome in rats and humans. Proc Natl Acad Sci U S A 2006;103(42): 15558–63.

Imaging Manifestations of Thoracic Tuberculosis

Carlos Santiago Restrepo, MD*, Rashmi Katre, MD, Amy Mumbower, MD

KEYWORDS

- Tuberculosis • Pulmonary tuberculosis • Primary tuberculosis • Postprimary tuberculosis
- Miliary tuberculosis • Mycetoma

KEY POINTS

- Tuberculosis is one of the most prevalent infectious diseases in the world, with the second highest death rate among communicable diseases worldwide.
- Even though traditionally primary and postprimary tuberculosis are considered 2 different forms of the disease based on the time of exposure, this has been recently challenged based on molecular and DNA analysis, although this terminology is still useful to describe the morphologic and imaging manifestations of the disease.
- Imaging plays a very important role in the diagnosis and follow-up of primary and postprimary tuberculosis for both pulmonary and extrapulmonary forms of the disease.

INTRODUCTION

Tuberculosis (TB) is a disease likely as old as humanity itself.[1] Aristotle is credited as being the first to recognize the contagious nature of the disease, but discovery of the specific infectious agent, the tubercle bacillus (Mycobacterium tuberculosis), did not occur for several more centuries until it was isolated by Robert Koch in 1882.[2] Distinct differences in the epidemiology of TB are observed between developing and industrialized nations. In countries where the standard of living is low and health resources are sparse, the risk of infection is highest with 80% of cases involving persons in their productive years (15–59 years of age).[3] Among communicable diseases, TB is the second leading cause of death worldwide after human immunodeficiency virus (HIV)/AIDS, killing nearly 2 million people each year; approximately 13% of TB patients have coexistent HIV infection.[4] In the United States, the most important risk factors for development of disease are host immunodeficiency, immigration from or travel to an endemic area, close contact with a TB patient, exposure to untreated cases in crowded living facilities such as prisons or nursing homes, advanced age, residing in an inner city, or homelessness.[5]

Global emergence of multidrug-resistant (MDR) strains of M tuberculosis in recent years has greatly complicated the management and control of transmission of active cases.[3,4] MDR TB is no more infective than nonresistant TB; however, it is a more serious infection, which requires prolonged administration of more toxic medications associated with higher morbidity and mortality. In addition, these patients remain infectious for a longer period once treatment has been initiated.[6] MDR TB most commonly develops during the course of TB treatment, most frequently as a result of inappropriate treatment, patients missing doses, or patients failing to complete their treatment.[7,8]

In 2013, an estimated 9.0 million people developed TB and 1.5 million died of the disease, 360,000 of whom were HIV-positive. TB is slowly declining each year, and it is estimated that 37 million lives were saved between 2000 and 2013

Department of Radiology, The University of Texas Health Science Center at San Antonio, 7703 Floyd Curl Drive, Mail Code 7800, San Antonio, TX 78229-3900, USA
* Corresponding author.
E-mail address: restrepoc@uthscsa.edu

Radiol Clin N Am 54 (2016) 453–473
http://dx.doi.org/10.1016/j.rcl.2015.12.007

radiologic.theclinics.com

through effective diagnosis and treatment. However, given that most deaths from TB are preventable, the death toll from the disease remains unacceptably high, and efforts to combat the disease should continue to accelerate. Although most TB cases and deaths occur among men, the burden of disease among women remains high with an estimated 3.3 million cases and 510,000 TB deaths among women and an estimated 550,000 cases and 80,000 deaths among children reported in 2013.[9]

PATHOPHYSIOLOGY

M tuberculosis is a slightly curved bacillus that is an aerobic, nonmotile, non-spore-forming rod-shaped bacterium. The organism has a cell wall that has an unusually high lipid content that resists staining by the usual Gram method but accepts basic fuchsin dyes and is not easily discolorized, even with alcohol. This resistance to decolorization by acid-alcohol is termed acid-fast, a property shared only by members of the mycobacterial family and a few other organisms (*Nocardia*, *Rhodococcus*, and *Corynebacterium* species). These properties form the basis for the simple, rapid, and relatively specific traditional technique of identification by means of an acid-fast smear. In addition, of note, they are primarily intracellular pathogens with slow growth rates.[3]

Transmission of disease occurs as a result of contact to a source case in more than 80%, typically the result of exposure to sputum smear-positive cases, although smear-negative culture-positive cases have been responsible for up to 17% of new cases.[4] The presence of acid-fast bacilli in the sputum smear is the main indicator of potential for transmission. Additional source patient characteristics to consider, which increase the probability of transmission, include positive sputum culture, lung parenchymal cavitation on imaging, TB laryngitis, as well as high-volume and/or watery respiratory secretions.[3,10]

M tuberculosis is transmitted via airborne droplet nuclei produced when persons with pulmonary or laryngeal TB cough, sneeze, or speak. In a person with active pulmonary TB, a single cough can generate 3000 infective droplets, with as few as 10 bacilli needed to initiate infection. The droplets, which measure 1 to 5 μm in size and may contain up to 400 bacilli, can be kept airborne by normal air currents for prolonged periods of time, resulting in dispersion throughout a room or building. Infection occurs when a susceptible person inhales droplet nuclei that contain tubercle bacilli.[3,6] The distribution of inhaled droplet nuclei is determined by the ventilatory pattern and volumes of the various lobes of the lungs with the site of implantation preferentially in the middle and lower lung zones, although any lobe may be affected. Once lodged in the alveolus, *M tuberculosis* is ingested by alveolar macrophages. If the alveolar macrophage cannot destroy or inhibit *M tuberculosis*, the bacilli multiply within its intracellular environment, causing the host macrophage or its progeny to burst. The cycle continues as released bacilli are ingested by other alveolar macrophages and monocytes are recruited from the blood. During this period of rapid growth, tubercle bacilli are spread through lymphatic channels to regional hilar and mediastinal lymph nodes and through the bloodstream to more distant sites in the body.[3,11]

In most patients, the logarithmic phase of bacillary growth is arrested with the development of cell-mediated immunity and delayed-type hypersensitivity at 2 to 10 weeks after the initial infection.[3,12,13] Granuloma formation with a subsequent decrease in the number of bacilli is typically seen, and some of these bacilli remain viable but dormant for many years. This stage is called latent TB infection, which is generally an asymptomatic, radiologically undetected process in humans.[1,3] Sometimes, a primary complex (Ghon complex) can be seen radiographically and comprises the primary lesion and hilar adenopathy. Later, the primary lesion tends to become calcified and can be identified on chest radiographs for decades.[1,3,14] In approximately 5% of infected individuals, immunity is inadequate, and clinically active disease develops within 1 year of infection. HIV coinfection is the greatest risk factor for progression to active disease in adults, and the relation between HIV and TB has augmented the deadly potential of each disease. Other risk factors for progression to active disease include diabetes mellitus, renal failure, coexistent malignancies, malnutrition, silicosis, immunosuppressive therapies (including steroids and anti-tumor necrosis factor [TNF] drugs), and TNF receptor defects. In another 5% of the infected population, endogenous reactivation of latent infection occurs remote from time of initial infection, referred to as postprimary TB.[3,11,14]

TRADITIONAL VERSUS NEW CONCEPT OF ETIOPATHOGENESIS AND IMAGING MANIFESTATIONS OF TUBERCULOSIS

Traditionally, TB findings have been described as primary infection that occurs in patients who develop disease after the initial exposure to TB bacilli, whereas patients who develop disease as a result of reactivation of a previous focus of TB are considered to have reactivation or postprimary TB. Primary TB and secondary TB are thought to be 2 distinct entities on the basis of clinical, pathologic, and imaging findings. However, recently this concept has been challenged by the DNA fingerprinting and genotyping of *M tuberculosis* isolates.[15] A multicentric molecular study using restriction fragment length polymorphism analysis (DNA fingerprinting of *M tuberculosis* with IS6110 insertion sequence) by Geng and colleagues[15] concluded that the host immune mechanism is the most important and dependent factor to determine the imaging findings of TB. Patients with recently acquired infection characterized by identical DNA strains of *M tuberculosis* referred to as cluster cases distinguished from remotely acquired TB show similar radiographic features. Therefore, time from acquisition of infection to the development of clinical disease does not reliably predict the radiographic appearance of TB. However, because most of the current literature still uses the traditional TB lexicon as "primary" and "postprimary/reactivation" TB, they are discussed under these headings in this article.

TB may masquerade as any disease; therefore, tissue and microbiological as well as imaging assessment is very important in establishing the diagnosis. In daily practice, the radiologist should be familiar with the imaging features of pulmonary and extrapulmonary TB as well as manifestations of TB in immunocompromised patients. Chest radiographs remain the basic imaging modality for pulmonary TB, although computed tomography (CT), MR imaging, and nuclear medicine techniques, including PET/CT, may be helpful in the assessment of both pulmonary and extrapulmonary TB. It can sometimes be difficult to differentiate primary and postprimary TB both clinically and radiologically because their features can overlap. However, confirming the diagnosis is more important than identifying the subtype because it allows initiation of appropriate clinical management.[3,6]

PRIMARY TUBERCULOSIS

As the name indicates, primary TB is seen in patients not previously exposed to *M tuberculosis*. It is most common in infants and children and has the highest prevalence in children less than 5 years of age.[3,16,17] Of note, the prevalence of primary TB in adults is increasing, now accounting for 23% to 34% of all adult cases of TB. Chest radiography remains the mainstay of diagnosis; however, normal radiographic findings may be seen in up to 15% of patients with proven TB.[5,18]

At imaging, primary TB manifests as 4 main entities: lymphadenopathy, parenchymal disease, miliary disease, and pleural effusion.[6] Radiographic evidence of lymphadenopathy is seen in up to 96% of children and 43% of adults. Lymphadenopathy is typically unilateral and right-sided, involving the hilum and right paratracheal region, although it is bilateral in about one-third of cases. CT is better at detecting nodal disease, and oftentimes, nodes greater than 2 cm in diameter may display a low-attenuation center secondary to necrosis, sometimes with a peripheral rim of enhancement due to a rim of granulomatous inflammatory tissue (**Fig. 1**). These findings are highly suggestive of active disease.[6,11,19] Although lymphadenopathy is usually associated with other manifestations of TB, it may be the sole radiographic feature, a finding that is more common in infants and decreases in frequency with age.[6]

Typically, parenchymal disease manifests as dense, homogeneous consolidation in any lobe; however, predominance in the lower and middle lobes (areas of greatest ventilation) is suggestive of the disease, especially in adults. Patchy, linear, nodular, and masslike parenchymal opacities may also be encountered on both radiographs and CT scans.[3,5,11,16–18] Tuberculous consolidation is often indistinguishable from that of bacterial pneumonia; however, it can be differentiated from bacterial pneumonia on the basis of radiographic evidence of lymphadenopathy and the lack of response to conventional antibiotics (**Figs. 2–4**).[6]

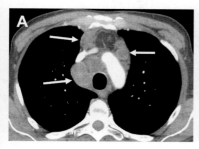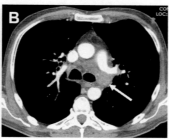

Fig. 1. TB lymphadenopathy in a 48-year-old man. Contrast-enhanced CT axial images at the level of the aortic arch (*A*) and carina (*B*) demonstrate enhancing lymph nodes in multiple mediastinal compartments (*arrows*).

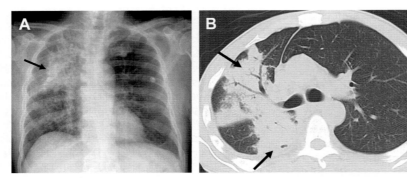

Fig. 2. Acute TB pneumonia in a 46-year-old man. (*A*) Multifocal opacities with denser airspace consolidation in the right upper lobe are noted in the chest radiograph (*arrow*). (*B*) Noncontrast CT shows air bronchogram in the right upper lobe and right lower lobe (*arrows*).

In children less than 2 years of age, lobar or segmental atelectasis is often seen, typically involving the anterior segment of an upper lobe or the medial segment of the middle lobe, usually a result of adjacent lymphadenopathy and compressive effects (**Fig. 5**).[3,16] In approximately two-thirds of cases, the parenchymal focus resolves without imaging sequelae, although this resolution can take up to 2 years.[6] In the remaining cases, a radiologic scar persists that can calcify in up to 15% of cases, an entity that is known as a Ghon focus (**Fig. 6**). In addition, masslike opacities called tuberculomas may be seen in approximately 9% of cases, which may cavitate and undergo calcification.[6,17–19] The combination of calcified hilar nodes and a Ghon focus is called a Ranke complex and is suggestive of previous TB, although it can also result from histoplasmosis (**Fig. 7**). With treatment, there is usually slower resolution of the lymphadenopathy than of the parenchymal disease, and nodal calcification may

develop. However, this calcification usually occurs 6 months or more after the initial infection. Miliary and pleural disease may also be encountered and are discussed later in this document.

REACTIVATION (POSTPRIMARY) TUBERCULOSIS: IMAGING FEATURES IN IMMUNOCOMPETENT HOSTS

Postprimary TB (PTB) is one of the many terms (including reactivation, secondary, or adulthood) applied to the form of TB that develops and progresses under the influence of acquired immunity.[20] The most commonly involved parts of the lung in postprimary TB are the apical and posterior segments of the upper lobe and superior segments of the lower lobes.[21] Parenchymal consolidations in these areas of the lungs are often associated with cavitation and are the characteristic radiographic manifestations (**Fig. 8**).[3,22] Parenchymal involvement occurs in more than

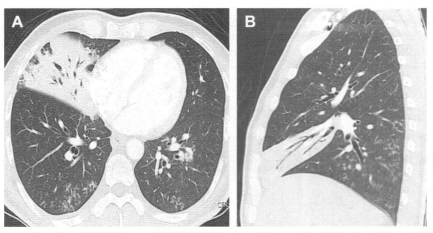

Fig. 3. Pulmonary TB with middle lobe syndrome in a 41-year-old man. CT of the chest (*A*) axial image and (*B*) sagittal reconstruction demonstrate the characteristic triangular opacity in the right middle lobe from atelectasis and consolidation as well as tree-in-bud nodular opacities in the bilateral lower lobes.

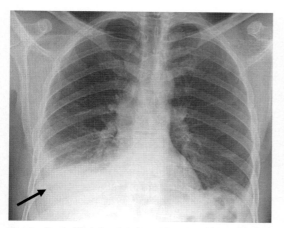

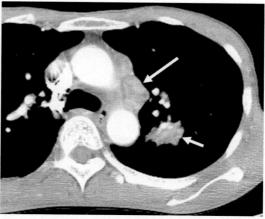

Fig. 4. Acute TB infection in a 30-year-old man. Chest radiograph shows an ill-defined right lower lobe opacity with an ipsilateral pleural effusion blunting the lateral costophrenic angle (*arrow*). Sputum analysis confirmed *M tuberculosis*.

Fig. 6. Ghon focus in a 33-year-old woman with *M tuberculosis* in sputum. Chest CT axial image at the level of the aortopulmonary window shows the left-side focal parenchymal opacity (*short arrow*) with ipsilateral lymphadenopathy (*long arrow*).

one segment in most cases.[3] Commonly, in addition to the aforementioned typical locations, consolidation and fibronodular opacities may occur in other lobes and segments of the lungs. Twenty percent to 45% of patients demonstrate cavitation, which is the hallmark of postprimary TB.[22] Walls of cavities may range from thin and smooth to thick and nodular.[22,23] Air-fluid levels have been reported to occur in 9% to 21% of tuberculous cavities.[22,23] After antituberculous chemotherapy, the tuberculous cavity may disappear; occasionally, the wall becomes paper thin and an air-filled cystic space remains (**Fig. 9**).[24] Serial imaging helps determine the stability or activity of pulmonary disease.

Tuberculoma may be a manifestation of either primary or postprimary TB. In postprimary TB, a tuberculoma is the salient or the only abnormality seen on chest radiographs in approximately 5% of patients.[22] Histologically, it consists of a central core of caseating necrosis with a surrounding wall

of a granulomatous reaction containing Langerhans giant cells, epithelioid histiocytes, and lymphocytes. Tuberculomas can be solitary or multiple and range in diameter from 0.5 to 4.0 cm or greater. Satellite nodules around the tuberculoma may be present in as many as 80% of cases. Typically, they have smooth or sharply defined margins. Twenty percent to 30% of tuberculomas may eventually calcify (**Fig. 10**).[19] When solitary, they may be mistaken for malignancy because active tuberculomas have fludeoxyglucose F18 (F18-FDG) PET uptake.[25] Kim and colleagues[26] evaluated the potential role of dual time point imaging with 18F-FDG PET in the differentiation of active pulmonary tuberculomas using maximum standardized uptake value (SUVmax) early and delayed imaging. The specificity and sensitivity were both 100% in detecting active granulomas when they used a cutoff of 1.05 SUV. The potential role of contrast-enhanced dynamic CT in diagnosing active tuberculomas has

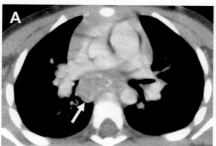

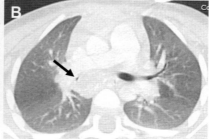

Fig. 5. Primary TB infection in a 3-year-old boy. Contrast-enhanced CT axial images with mediastinal window (*A*) and lung window (*B*). Large subcarinal and posterior mediastinal lymphadenopathy are seen (*white arrow*), with extrinsic compression of right lower lobe bronchus (*black arrow*).

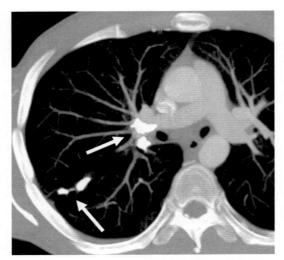

Fig. 7. Ranke complex. Maximum intensity projection axial image. Densely calcified granulomas are seen in the right lower lobe and right hilum (*arrows*).

been recently studied by Tateishi and colleagues[27] by using peak height and relative flow values.

Endobronchial spread of the disease occurs when an area of caseous necrosis or a caseous lymph node liquefies and communicates with the bronchial tree. Radiographically, bronchogenic spread manifests as multiple, ill-defined, 5- to 10-mm nodules distributed in a segmental or lobar distribution, distant from the site of cavity formation, typically involving the lower (dependent) lung zone.[28] High-resolution thin-section CT is the method of choice for revealing early endobronchial spread of disease, characterized by 2- to 4-mm centrilobular nodules and sharply marginated linear branching opacities described as "tree-in-bud pattern," which mimics the branching pattern of a budding tree.[28] These centrilobular small

nodules and Y-, V-shaped branching opacities represent caseous necrosis and granulomatous inflammatory products filling terminal and respiratory bronchioles as well as alveolar ducts and when identified is a good indicator of active disease (**Fig. 11**).[21]

Hilar and mediastinal lymphadenopathy are uncommon manifestations of postprimary TB seen in approximately 5% of cases.[22] Lymphadenopathy involving the right paratracheal region is most commonly seen on radiographs, although any node in the mediastinum can be affected. Usually, a node greater than 2 cm in diameter having a low-attenuation center secondary to necrosis at CT is highly suggestive of active disease.[18,29] Although lymphadenopathy is usually associated with extensive parenchymal consolidation, it can be the sole radiographic feature, especially common in infants, and decreases in frequency with age. As with the primary form of disease, CT is more sensitive than chest radiography for assessing lymphadenopathy. Similar to a parenchymal tuberculoma, lymph nodes calcify subsequently. Radiographic evidence of the original primary infection in the form of calcified lymph nodes and nodules and/or upper lobe fibrotic changes is found in approximately 20% to 40% of individuals with active, postprimary disease.[22,30]

Tuberculous pleural effusion (TPE) can be a manifestation of primary or postprimary TB. It may be associated with parenchymal abnormalities or can be the sole imaging finding (**Fig. 12**) and is thought to occur secondary to increased permeability of the pleural capillaries due to a compartmentalized inflammatory process.[31] In a few patients, a remote tuberculous pleurisy may cause a fibrous peel over the visceral pleura that prevents lung expansion ("trapped lung"), thereby creating a high negative pleural space pressure

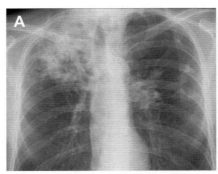
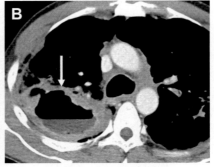

Fig. 8. Upper lobe cavitary lesion. (*A*) Chest radiograph shows an area of cavitation within an extensive opacity in the right upper lobe in a patient who also presents left-side nodular opacities and left hilar lymphadenopathy. (*B*) Contrast-enhanced CT axial image shows the irregular cavity with an air-fluid level in the posterior right upper lobe (*arrow*).

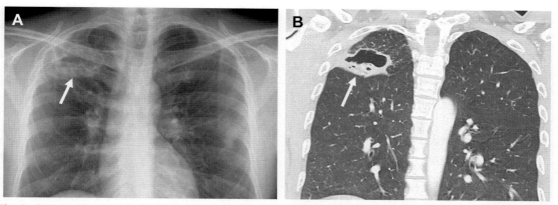

Fig. 9. Cavitary TB. Chest radiograph (*A*) and chest CT coronal reconstruction (*B*) in a young adult patient being treated for active TB with a residual cavity with slightly irregular wall is still present in the posterior right upper lobe (*arrows*).

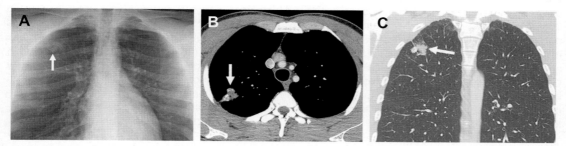

Fig. 10. Tuberculoma. Posterior left upper lobe tuberculoma in a 36-year-old man. (*A*) Chest radiograph, apical lordotic view, (*B*) contrast-enhanced CT with mediastinal window, and (*C*) lung window coronal reconstruction. There is lobulated and spiculated partially calcified nodule in the right upper lobe (*arrows*), which was proven to be TB infection.

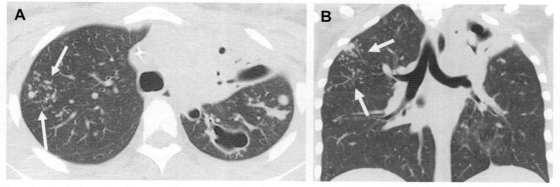

Fig. 11. Tree-in-bud in a 20-year-old woman with pulmonary TB. Chest CT axial (*A*) and coronal (*B*) images. There are cavitary lesions in the left lung with bronchogenic spread of the disease, which manifest as tree-in-bud nodular opacities in the right upper lobe (*arrows*).

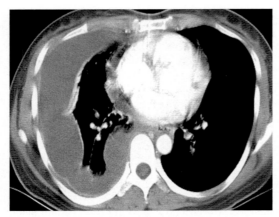

Fig. 12. Subacute TPE. Contrast-enhanced CT image shows a moderate size loculated right-side pleural effusion with mild pleural thickening in a young adult woman with pulmonary TB.

that fosters the development of chronic pleural effusion (**Fig. 13**). The fluid is invariably an exudate, with lymphocytic predominance in about 90% of cases.[32] The definitive diagnosis of TPE depends on the demonstration of *M tuberculosis* in the sputum, pleural fluid, or pleural biopsy specimens.[33] In the appropriate clinical setting, the diagnosis can also be established with reasonable certainty by demonstrating granuloma in the parietal pleura or an elevated adenosine deaminase level in pleural fluid.

TUBERCULOSIS WITH HUMAN IMMUNODEFICIENCY VIRUS COINFECTION

The diagnosis of TB in HIV-infected patients can be challenging. Up to 50% of AIDS patients with culture-proven TB have false-negative sputum

and bronchoalveolar lavage for *M tuberculosis* bacilli.[34] The clinical and imaging features depend on the level of immunosuppression and CD4 counts. Up to 10% patients with advanced AIDS and TB can have normal chest radiographs.[35] CT evaluation for pulmonary TB in HIV-seropositive persons with normal radiographs usually demonstrates subtle abnormalities.[36] Leung and colleagues[36] identified 3 patterns of disease on CT scans in patients with a normal chest radiograph. The dominant patterns (in the order of decreasing frequency) consisted of multiple nodules, tuberculoma, and lymphadenopathy (right paratracheal, hilar, and subcarinal stations). Persons with relatively intact cellular immune function demonstrate radiographic findings similar to those of non-HIV-infected individuals. On CT, HIV-seropositive patients with a CD4 T-lymphocyte count less than $200/mm^3$ characteristically demonstrate an atypical radiographic pattern, for example, middle and lower lung involvement, absence of cavity formation, presence of lymphadenopathy and pleural effusions, or a miliary pattern.[37,38] A study performed to determine the CT spectrum of PTB in HIV patients showed nodular opacities (in 78.5% of cases), consolidation (46.4%), lymphadenopathy (35.7%), pleural effusion (35.7%), ground glass opacity (21.4%), and cavitation (21.4%).[37,38] Patients with severe immunosuppression have an increased incidence of miliary pulmonary disease, with diffuse, randomly distributed nodules on CT (**Fig. 14**).

HIGHLY ACTIVE ANTIRETROVIRAL THERAPY AND IMMUNE RESTORATION SYNDROME

With the introduction of highly active antiretroviral therapy, a new clinical and radiographic entity has emerged in patients coinfected with HIV and

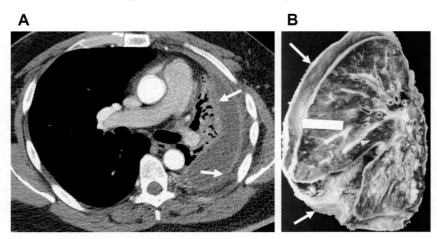

Fig. 13. Chronic tuberculous pleural infection. (*A*) Contrast CT axial image shows very thick visceral and parietal pleura (*arrows*) with extensive collapse of the left lung. (*B*) Autopsy specimen from a different patient with chronic TB demonstrates extensive pulmonary disease with severe pleural thickening (*arrows*).

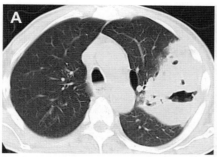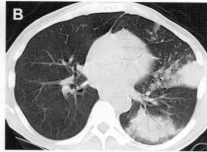

Fig. 14. Multilobar TB in a 29-year old man with AIDS. CT of the chest, axial images in the upper (*A*) and lower (*B*) lung zones demonstrates posterior left upper lobe consolidation and necrosis with airspace consolidation in the lingula and posterior left lower lobe.

TB characterized by paradoxic worsening of the patient's clinical status related to an increase in the CD4 counts and a decrease in the viral loads.[39] The patient's cellular inflammatory response to mycobacteria is restored. Typical imaging findings include intrathoracic or cervical lymphadenopathy in approximately 70% of patients, new or increasing areas of parenchymal consolidation, and pleural effusions in a febrile patient. Intraabdominal manifestations develop in approximately 40% of cases. Tuberculous meningitis and other central nervous system involvement may also complicate immune restoration syndrome, which in itself has a high morbidity and mortality.[40] Severely symptomatic patients may benefit from steroid administration.

MILIARY TUBERCULOSIS

Miliary TB refers to widespread dissemination of TB by lymphohematogenous spread from a pulmonary or extrapulmonary focus and embolization to various distant organs. Organs with high blood flow, for instance, liver, lungs, spleen, bone marrow, adrenals, and kidneys, are frequently affected.[41] The term "miliary" was coined by John Magnet in 1700 to describe the resemblance of gross pathologic findings of lungs to millet seeds in size and appearance.[41] The tuberculous granuloma is the histopathological hallmark of the disease. Up to 8% patients affected with all forms of TB show miliary pattern of disease.[24,41] It is usually seen in the elderly, infants, and immunocompromised persons.[6] Some of the important predisposing factors to the development of miliary disease are childhood infections, malnutrition, HIV/AIDS, alcoholism, diabetes mellitus, and immunosuppressive drugs.[41]

Initially, chest radiographs may be normal in 25% to 40% of cases.[11] The typical changes evolve over the course of the disease; hence, serial radiographs should be obtained when there is a high clinical suspicion. High-resolution CT is the modality of choice because it has high sensitivity for diagnosing miliary disease before it becomes radiographically apparent.[42] The characteristic CT findings consist of innumerable 1- to 3-mm-diameter nodules, randomly distributed throughout both lungs, often associated with intralobular and interlobular septal thickening.[3,43] However, in up to 10% of patients, the nodules may be greater than 3 mm in diameter.[41] These nodules may coalesce to form focal or diffuse consolidation (**Fig. 15**). The nodules usually resolve within 2 to 6 months with treatment, without scarring or calcification. Studies have shown that patients may have additional radiographic abnormalities in up to 69% of cases.[43,44] These radiographic abnormalities include consolidation (predominantly upper lobes), cavitation, pleural fluid, and necrotic lymphadenopathy (**Fig. 16**). Patients with superimposed ground glass opacities may represent impending adult respiratory distress syndrome.[45] Lymphadenopathy is seen more often in HIV-positive patients than HIV-negative patients.[43] Patchy areas of air trapping are also seen in some patients likely because of concomitant tuberculous bronchiolitis. Some of the dreaded clinical complications of miliary TB are acute respiratory distress syndrome, renal failure, myocarditis, infective endocarditis, mycotic aneurysms, meningitis, and hepatitis, which need prompt recognition and treatment.

MULTIDRUG-RESISTANT TUBERCULOSIS AND EXTENSIVELY DRUG-RESISTANT TUBERCULOSIS

MDR TB is defined as a strain of *M tuberculosis* resistant to at least isoniazid and rifampin.[46] Extensively drug-resistant (XDR) TB is a dreaded infection caused by a strain of *M tuberculosis*

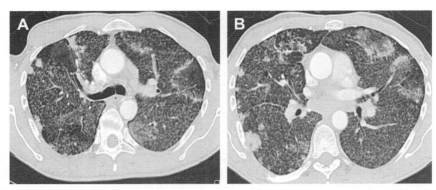

Fig. 15. Miliary TB in a 54-year-old man. Contrast-enhanced CT. Axial images at the carina (*A*) and lower lobes (*B*) reveal innumerable small pulmonary nodules scattered throughout the bilateral lungs, with areas of larger coalescent nodular opacities in the periphery.

that is resistant to any type of fluoroquinolone and at least 1 of the 3 following injectable drugs: amikacin, capreomycin, or kanamycin in addition to isoniazid and rifampin.[46] Up to 10% of MDR TB isolates are in fact found to be XDR strains.[47] Soman and colleagues[48] have coined the terms MDR+ and pe-XDR TB for patients who have intermediate spectrum of drug-resistance between MDR and XDR TB. Successful treatment of fully susceptible TB depends on the combination of drugs and duration of therapy, cost, and drug's side effects. Conversion of culture-positive to culture-negative sputum within 2 months and subsequent clearing of infiltrates on chest radiograph are positive signs, whereas positive sputum cultures after 4 months of multidrug therapy indicate treatment failure.[4,48] Incomplete and inappropriate therapy results in acquired resistance. Primary resistance occurs when the resulting *M tuberculosis* strain is transmitted to a new host, as it causes TB that is already resistant to the indicated

drug(s). The major concerns of drug resistance are fear regarding the spread of drug-resistant organisms and the ineffectiveness of chemotherapy in patients infected with them. In addition, MDR TB is a fatal disease because of the high mortality, depending on the underlying diseases, particularly in HIV-infected patients (40%–80% mortality).[49–51]

Prior studies have shown that the imaging findings of MDR TB are similar to those of drug-sensitive TB.[52–54] In patients with MDR TB, the most common radiographic and CT finding is multiple cavities. Fishman and colleagues,[54] in their study of HIV-TB coinfected patients, reported that most patients with primary drug resistance showed a primary pattern, such as noncavitary consolidation, pleural effusion, and lymphadenopathy, whereas cavitary disease was common in patients who acquired MDR TB secondary to noncompliance with therapy. However, Yeom and colleagues,[52] in their study of MDR TB in non-HIV-infected patients, observed that cavities

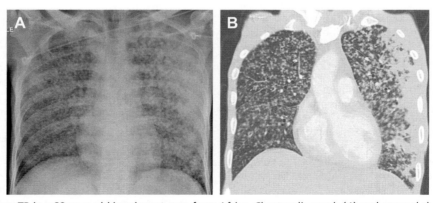

Fig. 16. Miliary TB in a 33-year-old immigrant man from Africa. Chest radiograph (*A*) and coronal chest CT image (*B*) demonstrate very extensive micronodular disease in the bilateral lung with more confluent disease and consolidation in the periphery of the left lung.

were more frequently seen in patients with primary MDR TB, and the mean number of cavities in patients with primary MDR TB was larger than that in patients with drug-susceptible TB. As stated earlier, findings in the Fishman study again could be related to integrity of the host immune response. Patients with severe immunocompromised status show a tendency to have the primary form of TB, whereas immunocompetent patients have the reactivation form of the disease.[15] Other imaging features that can be seen in patients with MDR TB are emphysema, bronchiectasis, bronchovascular distortion, and calcified granulomas.[53] Lee and colleagues[47] compared imaging features of XDR TB and non-XDR MDR TB patients. They found that in XDR-TB patients, CT features of micronodules, tree-in-bud pattern, consolidation, cavity, and bronchiectasis were larger and involved significantly more extensive lobes than MDR TB. Furthermore, a larger percentage of XDR-TB patients have pulmonary cavities than those with MDR TB and involve more pulmonary lobes (**Fig. 17**).[47]

COMPLICATIONS AND SPECIAL FORMS
Tracheobronchial Tuberculosis

Even though the incidence of tracheobronchial TB has declined compared with the preantibiotic era, this complication still affects patients with advanced disease, particularly in endemic areas. The most significant complication resulting from bronchial TB is bronchial stenosis with a prevalence ranging between 10% and 40%.[55] Mycobacterial implantation to the tracheobronchial wall in patients with TB may originate from infected sputum, extension from adjacent parenchymal infection, regional lymph nodes, or hematogenous spread. In the pathophysiology of central airway TB infection, peribronchial lymphatic spread seems to be more common than endobronchial spread from infected sputum.[56] The infectious process produces granulation tissue, fibrosis,

and airway wall destruction that may end with tracheobronchial stenosis. Isolated tracheal disease is rare with most patients presenting tracheobronchial disease that more often involves the distal trachea as well as the proximal right or left main stem bronchi. In patients with tracheal involvement, the carina is almost invariably affected.[57] CT is the best imaging modality for the evaluation of the trachea and airways and can readily demonstrate these abnormalities. Characteristic findings of tracheobronchial TB include irregular circumferential wall thickening with luminal narrowing, in some cases associated with increased mediastinal density consistent with active inflammation and enlarged mediastinal lymph nodes.[58,59] The coexistence of tracheobronchial disease and lymphadenopathy is particularly high in patients with active pulmonary TB.[57] The abnormal tissue producing bronchial wall thickening may present significant enhancement after iodine contrast administration in a substantial number of cases.[57,60] In patients with bronchial stenosis, postobstructive opacity with atelectasis and bronchial dilation with retained secretions may also be present (**Fig. 18**).[61]

Bronchopleural Fistula

Bronchopleural fistula, which consists of an abnormal communication between the pleural space and the bronchial tree, most often results as a postoperative complication after pulmonary surgery and resection, but may also result from a necrotizing lung infection such as TB. This relatively rare complication carries a high morbidity and mortality and has a variable clinical and imaging manifestation depending on whether it is an acute, subacute, or chronic form as well as the underlying condition. Imaging manifestations include tension pneumothorax, hydropneumothorax, lung abscess or cavitary lung lesion, peripheral bronchiectasis, and subcutaneous emphysema. The abnormal communication between the pleural

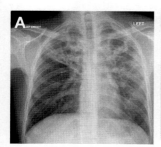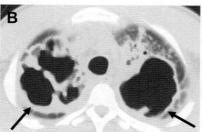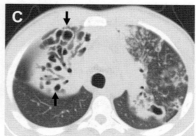

Fig. 17. MDR TB in a 28-year-old man. (*A*) Chest radiograph and chest CT axial images at 2 different levels (*B, C*) show extensive bilateral upper lobe disease with large irregular thick wall cavitary lesions (*long arrows*), bronchiectasis (*short arrows*), nodular opacities, and patchy consolidation.

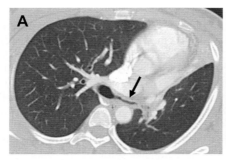
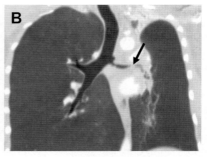

Fig. 18. Tracheobronchail TB in a 22-year-old woman. Contrast-enhanced chest CT axial image (*A*) and coronal minimum intensity projection at the level of the carina (*B*) show severe left-side bronchial wall thickening with long segment stenosis (*arrows*). Transbronchial biopsy confirmed necrotizing granulomas consistent with TB in the affected left main bronchus.

space and airways increases the risk for aspiration pneumonia and adult respiratory distress syndrome, which are common causes of death in affected patients. Multidetector CT with multiplanar reconstruction is the imaging modality of choice to demonstrate the location, number, and size of the abnormal communication between the bronchial tree and the pleural space (**Fig. 19**).[62,63]

Rasmussen Aneurysm

Rasmussen aneurysm is the name given to pulmonary artery pseudoaneurysm associated with pulmonary TB, caused by erosion into the artery by the adjacent tuberculous cavity. Fritz Valdemar Rasmussen, a Danish physician, was the first to describe the intimate relation between a pulmonary artery and the wall of a pulmonary cavity in patients with TB and hemoptysis.[64] In a subsequent large autopsy series published in 1939, the prevalence of Rasmussen aneurysm in chronic pulmonary TB was 4% and was associated with

significant mortality from massive bleeding.[64] Pulmonary TB remains the most important cause of hemoptysis in many developing countries and still remains a significant cause of hemoptysis (25%) in industrialized countries.[65] A common misconception is to consider hemoptysis in pulmonary TB as commonly associated with Rasmussen aneurysm. Pulmonary artery Rasmussen aneurysms are rare, and the most common source of hemoptysis in TB patients is from hypertrophic high-pressure systemic bronchial circulation (90%) and not from the low-pressure pulmonary vasculature (5%–7%).[66,67] Rasmussen aneurysms can vary in size and number but, most commonly, present as small (<1 cm) single lesions surrounded by a parenchymal opacity, a consolidation, or in the wall of a lung cavity, typically in the upper lobes or superior segment of a lower lobe (**Fig. 20**).[68,69] Rarely, multiple aneurysms may be seen in the same patient and occasionally giant aneurysms (>3 cm) may occur.[70,71] Signs of pulmonary arterial origin of hemoptysis seen on multidetector CT

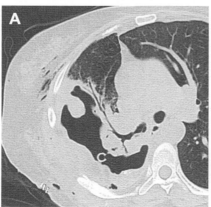
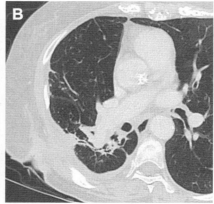

Fig. 19. Bronchopleural fistula. TB infection with right-side chronic bronchopleural fistula and chest wall infection in a 40 year-old woman. Chest CT axial image at the carina (*A*) and right infrahilar region (*B*). There is a right pneumothorax, severe pleural thickening, and extensive infection and inflammation in the right side chest wall.

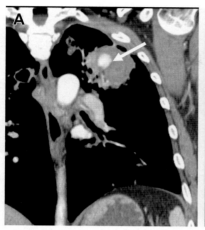
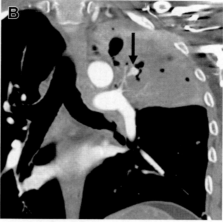

Fig. 20. Rasmussen aneurysm in 2 different patients. Coronal reconstruction after contrast-enhanced CT in 2 different patients with pulmonary TB and history of hemoptysis. (*A*) Saccular collection of contrast is seen in the left upper lobe round masslike opacity (*white arrow*). (*B*) An enhancing aneurysm is seen in the left upper lobe within an area of necrotizing consolidation (*black arrow*).

angiography include direct visualization of the focal contrast-enhancing dilation or outpouching arising from the pulmonary artery (75%), or the presence of a pulmonary artery in the inner wall of a pulmonary cavity (25%).[66] The potential causes of pulmonary artery pseudoaneurysms are numerous, and in addition to TB, include pyogenic pulmonary abscess, angioinvassive apergillosis, lung cancer, vasculitis (Behçet disease, Hughes-Stovin syndrome), penetrating and nonpenetrating trauma, Swan-Ganz catheter, and arteriovenous malformation.[64] Regardless, in patients with any infectious origin, the mechanism is the same, with erosion of the arterial wall and formation of the pseudoaneurysm.

Mycetoma

Pulmonary mycetomas develop from saprophytic infection of a pre-existing pulmonary cavity, cyst, or space, from previous pulmonary TB, sarcoidosis, bronchiectasis, or bullous emphysema, with the formation of an intracavitary fungus ball formed by a mass of tangled fungal hyphae, fibrin, epithelial cells, mucus, and cellular debris with blood cells.[72] In immunocompetent patients, TB is by far the most common cause of the pre-existing cavity (60%–80%), but in HIV-infected patients, pneumocystis pneumonia infection is a common predisposing condition (40%).[73–75] *Aspergillus fumigatus* is the most common fungal organism found in these cavitary lesions (70%), followed by *Aspergillus niger* (20%) and *Aspergillus flavus* (<10%).[76] Less common infecting organisms include *Mucor* species, *Nocardia*, and *Candida albicans*.[77,78] For this reason, these

mycetomas or fungus balls are also referred to as aspergillomas. Hemoptysis and productive cough are the 2 most common clinical manifestations in affected patients, who typically present in the fifth decade of life, with advanced underlying pulmonary disease, commonly with poor prognosis. Pseudostratified columnar or metaplastic squamous epithelium is the most common lining of these cavitary lesions, which in patients with TB may also have caseating granulomas with or without acid-fast organisms. The cavitary lesions tend to be complex (75%) with gross pulmonary disease in the surrounding parenchyma, more often than simple (25%), in which the lesion consists of an isolated thin-walled cyst. The upper lobe is the most common location (70%), with similar distribution between the right and left lung.[73] The classic radiographic appearance is a solid round, often mobile, irregular intracavitary mass located in the dependent portion of the cavity with a crescent of air between the fungus ball and the cavity wall, an imaging finding known as the "Monod or crescent sign" (**Fig. 21**).[79,80]

Empyema Necessitatis

A rare complication of pleural infection in which purulent fluid extends from the pleural space through the parietal pleura into the soft tissues of the chest wall resulting in abscess formation is known as empyema necessitatis or necessitans. Increased pressure within a loculated pleural collection facilitates chest wall extension with necrosis and migration of inflammatory exudates into the chest wall. This complication is more often seen as a result of inadequate treatment. The most

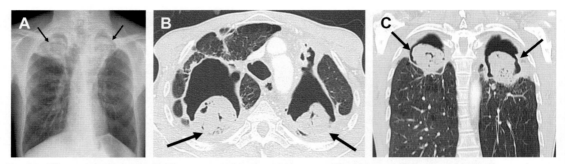

Fig. 21. Bilateral mycetomas. Sixty-two-year-old man with past medical history of TB presented with cough exacerbation and hemoptysis. (*A*) Chest radiograph, (*B*) chest CT axial image, (*C*) coronal reconstruction show biapical lung cavities with fungus balls that move freely with the patient's change in position (*arrows*).

common location is between the second and sixth intercostal spaces, but transdiaphragmatic extension to the abdomen or extension into the mediastinum may also occur. TB is still the most common cause, followed by actinomycosis, staphylococcus, streptococcus, and atypical mycobacteria.[81,82] The chest wall involvement may also affect the bones with rib, or sternal destruction associated with soft tissue mass and fluid. Imaging findings include chest wall fluid collection with peripheral enhancement, thick and occasionally calcified pleura as sequelae of chronic infection, and rib thickening from chronic periosteal reaction due to adjacent loculated pleural fluid collection (**Fig. 22**).[83,84]

Chest Wall Tuberculosis

TB of the chest wall is an uncommon manifestation of the disease, which constitutes less than 5% of all musculoskeletal TB, far less common than other skeletal sites more commonly affected, such as the spine, pelvis, hip, and knee joints. Excluding the spine, the most commonly affected

site is the ribs, but chest wall TB may affect the sternum, sternoclavicular joints, as well as soft tissue involvement including myositis, cellulitis, and breast infection. It is not clear whether chest wall infection occurs from reactivation of latent foci formed during hematogenous or lymphatic dissemination from the primary infection or from direct extension contiguous lung and pleura. Series with culture-proven chest wall infection in the absence of contiguous pleuro-pulmonary disease favor hematogenous/lymphatic route.[85] On the other hand, many cases of well-documented pleuropulmonary or mediastinal disease with adjacent chest wall infection favor a direct extension.[86] Most likely, both routes of chest wall infection exist. Concurrent lung infection is commonly seen in patients with chest wall infection (64%). Bone involvement more often manifests as bone erosion and destruction, with surrounding soft tissue mass and associated soft tissue abscess with peripheral enhancement (**Fig. 23**).[87] As in other bone infections, MR imaging is more sensitive for depicting bone marrow and soft tissue abnormalities, with involved structures appearing

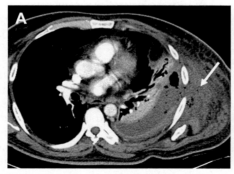
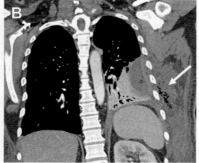

Fig. 22. Empyema necessitans. Adult woman with chronic TB empyema who presented with spontaneous drainage to the left-side chest wall. Contrast-enhanced CT of the chest axial image (*A*) and coronal reconstruction (*B*) show the left-side pleural thickening with fluid and gas extending through the intercostal space into the soft tissues of the chest wall (*arrows*).

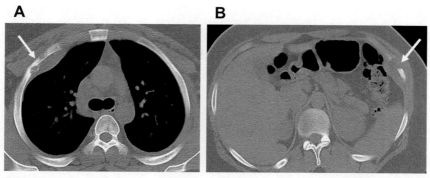

Fig. 23. Multifocal TB osteomyelitis in a 24-year-old man. Noncontrast chest CT axial image at the level of the carina (*A*) and lower chest wall (*B*) demonstrates right upper and left lower rib osteomyelitis with bone erosion and soft tissue mass (*arrows*).

hypointense on T1-weighted and hyperintense on T2-weighted sequences.[88]

Spinal Tuberculosis

Spinal TB (Pott spine or Pott disease) remains one of the most common forms of extrapulmonary TB and roughly accounts for 50% of all cases of skeletal TB infection. In 1779, Sir Percival Pott, a British physician, was the first to describe the destruction of disk space and adjacent vertebral bodies primarily in children who developed progressive kyphosis; hence, the condition subsequently became known as Pott disease. Spinal TB is uncommon in the western world, where *Staphylococcus* spp remains the most common cause of vertebral osteomyelitis, but still remains the most common cause in countries with high burden of pulmonary TB.[89] Spinal involvement typically results from hematogenous spread from a pulmonary, genitourinary, or gastrointestinal infection, via either arterial or venous route into the rich vasculature of the vertebral bodies. The destruction characteristically affects the intervertebral disc space and the adjacent vertebral bodies with usually slow and insidious collapse of the anterior elements, resulting in wedge deformity and gibbus formation. Neurologic manifestations are common and often signal the devastating complication of spinal cord involvement (pain, numbness, weakness, paraplegia, quadriplegia, weak, or absent reflexes). Kyphosis is the most common deformity resulting from vertebral body collapse, which can involve any spinal segment, but more commonly affects the lower thoracic spine or upper lumbar region.[90,91] Concomitant pulmonary TB is common (67%) in patients with spinal TB.[92] Imaging findings include bone destruction with osteolytic changes, occasionally in association with bone sclerosis, soft tissue involvement with paraspinal abscess that may present as a mediastinal mass. The presence of

calcification within a paraspinal abscess is fairly characteristic of TB infection (**Fig. 24**). Although contrast-enhanced CT is an excellent imaging modality for the evaluation of the bone and mediastinal disease, MR imaging is the imaging technology of choice for examination of the spine and spinal cord and should be always performed in patients with suspected neurologic involvement (**Fig. 25**).

Collapse Therapy

Before the advent of effective anti-TB antibiotics, different surgical procedures were developed as methods for inducing pulmonary cavity collapse and secondary sputum conversion, aiming to reduce the aerobic environment needed for the survival and growth of the bacteria. These surgical procedures included artificial pneumothorax, phrenic nerve crush, thoracoplasty, extrapleural plombage, and oleothorax. Because of the high complication rate, low efficacy, and development

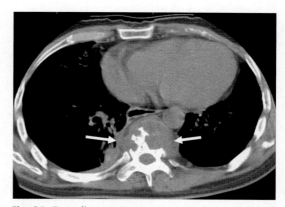

Fig. 24. Pott disease. Noncontrast CT shows vertebral body osteolytic lesions surrounded by a paraspinal abscess (*arrows*) and small right-side pleural effusion. Needle biopsy and aspiration confirmed *M tuberculosis* infection.

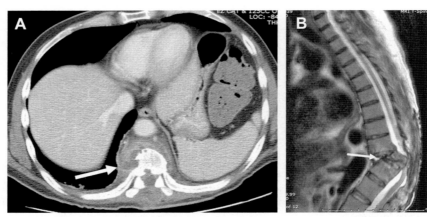

Fig. 25. Pott disease. Fifty-seven-year-old man with spinal TB who presented progressive back pain and neurologic symptoms from spinal cord compression that required wide laminectomy. Contrast-enhanced CT (*A*) shows vertebral body lytic lesions with paraspinal abscess (*arrow*). (*B*) Sagittal MR imaging better demonstrates the vertebral body collapse, kyphotic deformity, and spinal cord compression (*white arrow*).

of effective antituberclosis drugs, all these techniques were abandoned. Thoracoplasty consisted of surgical resection of multiple ribs, up to 8, depending on the degree of collapse required, and apposition of visceral and parietal pleura (**Fig. 26**). Plombage consisted of the insertion of an inert substance in the pleural, extrapleural, or extrafascial space to force lung collapse. Materials such as vegetable and mineral oil, fat (omentum), blood, bone, polythene bags, paraffin wax, silk, gelatin, gauze sponge, rubber balloons, and methyl methacrylate spheres (Lucite balls) were used (**Fig. 27**). Late complications included

pyogenic infection, superior vena cava obstruction, brachial plexus injury, bronchopleural fistula, foreign body migration, and malignancy (sarcoma).[93–96]

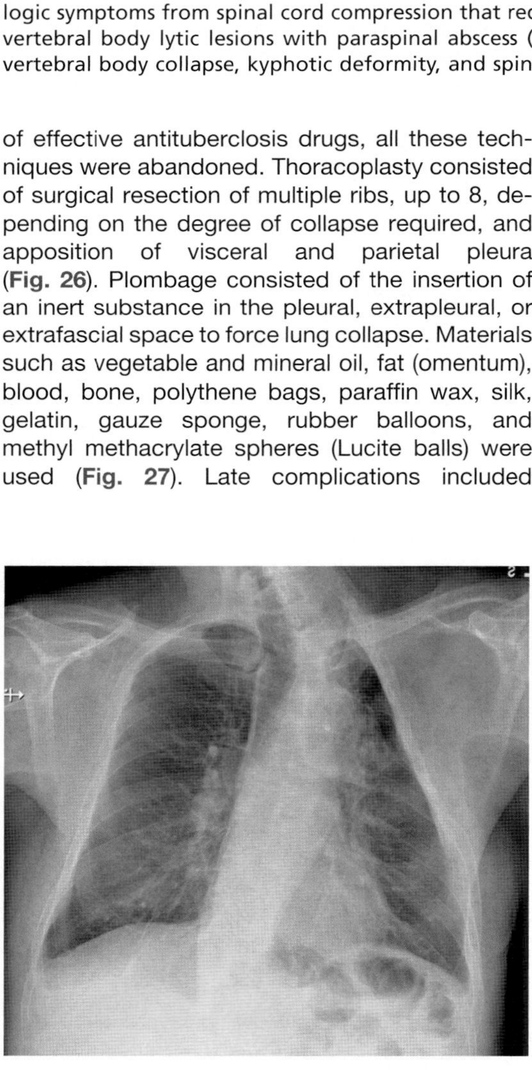

Cardiovascular Tuberculosis

Tuberculous pericarditis, the most common cardiovascular complication of TB, is found in 1% to 2% patients with pulmonary infection and remains the most common manifestation in countries with a high prevalence of TB.[97] Pericardial involvement may result from retrograde lymphatic spread from mediastinal lymph nodes or by hematogenous spread. Tuberculous pericarditis may present clinically as pericardial effusion, constrictive pericarditis, or as a combination, with effusive-constrictive pericarditis. In patients with acute or active disease, pericardial effusion should be suspected if chest radiograph reveals an enlarged cardiac silhouette. Tuberculous pericardial effusion, which is typically exudative with high protein content and increased leukocyte count, may manifest with cardiac tamponade (10%).[98] Fibrinous strands within a pericardial effusion on echocardiogram are very suggestive of TB infection.[99] Constrictive pericarditis is one of the most serious complications of tuberculous pericarditis, reported in as much as half of affected patients with TB pericardial infection.[100] Affected pericardium exhibits thickening (>3 mm) with fibrinous exudate (subacute variety), and occasionally in the chronic stage, focal or diffuse calcification is often seen at the atrioventricular groove (**Fig. 28**). The combination of pericardial inflammation, fibrosis, thickening, and calcification contributes to diastolic dysfunction with lower

Fig. 26. Elderly woman with remote history of TB treated with left-side thoracoplasty many years before. Chest radiograph demonstrates chest wall deformity from multiple left upper rib resection.

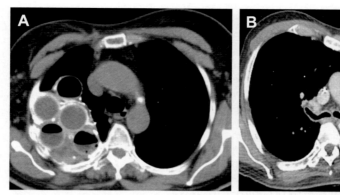

Fig. 27. Plombage for collapse therapy in 2 different patients. (*A*) Methyl methacrylate spheres (lucite balls) are seen in the upper right hemithorax. (*B*) Oval-shaped extrapleural calcified material, presumably polythene bag, is seen in the upper left hemithorax.

diastolic volume and stroke volume. In addition to the abnormal appearance of the pericardium, additional imaging findings include tubular configuration of the ventricles, sigmoid-shaped configuration of the interventricular septum, atrial enlargement and dilated inferior vena cava, superior vena cava, hepatic veins, and coronary sinus. In effusive-constrictive pericarditis, in addition to the constrictive changes, a variable amount of concomitant pericardial effusion coexists that may be associated with myocardial thinning.

Myocardial involvement by *M tuberculosis* is less common than pericardial disease, and before the cross-sectional imaging era, it was rarely diagnosed ante-mortem. It is usually due to tuberculomas that are commonly associated with miliary or extensive TB, which may present as a diffuse infiltrative process or as a nodular or mass-like lesion.[101] Myocardial involvement should be suspected in TB patients with arrhythmias, atrioventricular block, syncope, heart failure, or sudden cardiac death.[102] Another common presentation is as a superior vena cava syndrome, or as a right atrial mass or mass at the atrial-caval junction.[103] On contrast-enhanced cardiac MR imaging, cardiac tuberculomas are seen as low to isointense lesions on T1 and T2, with heterogeneous enhancement after contrast injection (see **Fig. 28**).[104,105]

Tuberculous aortitis is another rare complication of mycobacterial infection that invariably indicates disseminated disease. The affected aorta more often develops aneurysm or pseudoaneurysm, which may be associated with perforation and fistula formation to an adjacent organ. On CT, in addition to the abnormalities of the aorta, affected patients will also exhibit findings of tuberculous pulmonary or pericardial disease.[106] Aortic stenosis is a less common complication but may be an additional presentation of aortic wall tuberculous infection.[107]

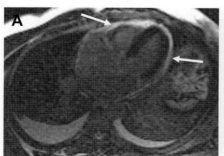
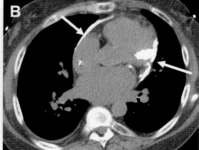

Fig. 28. (*A*) TB exudative pericarditis in a patient with fever, night sweats, and constrictive physiology. Cardiac MR delayed images after contrast injection demonstrates abnormal thickening and late gadolinium enhancement of the pericardium (*arrows*). (*B*) Chronic constrictive pericarditis in a patient with history of TB. Noncontrast CT shows abnormal thickening and calcification of the pericardium (*arrows*).

SUMMARY

Although clinical scenarios in which pulmonary TB can present are numerous, imaging examination is often performed both in the initial diagnosis and for follow-up. In addition, not infrequently it may be from the imaging studies that the possibility of TB is initially suspected. Although chest radiograph still has an essential role in the initial evaluation, advanced cross-sectional imaging, in particular MDCT, is critical for improved lesion detection, characterization, and disease extension assessment, both in limited and in advanced disease and also in detecting the presence of complications. The role of the radiologist is pivotal, and appropriate understanding of the pathophysiology with associated imaging manifestations allows the radiologist to narrow the differential diagnosis and, when appropriate, suggest management options, significantly impacting patient outcome.

REFERENCES

1. MacGregor RR. Tuberculosis: from history to current management. Semin Roentgenol 1993;28(2): 101–8.
2. Sepkowitz KA. Tuberculosis and the health care worker: a historical perspective. Ann Intern Med 1994;120(1):71–9.
3. Leung AN. Pulmonary tuberculosis: the essentials. Radiology 1999;210(2):307–22.
4. American Thoracic Society, Centers for Disease Control and Prevention, Infectious Diseases Society of America. American Thoracic Society/Centers for Disease Control and Prevention/Infectious Diseases Society of America: controlling tuberculosis in the United States. Am J Respir Crit Care Med 2005;172(9):1169–227.
5. Harisinghani MG, McLoud TC, Shepard JA, et al. Tuberculosis from head to toe. Radiographics 2000;20(2):449–70 [quiz: 528–9, 32].
6. Burrill J, Williams CJ, Bain G, et al. Tuberculosis: a radiologic review. Radiographics 2007;27(5): 1255–73.
7. Farmer P. The major infectious diseases in the world–to treat or not to treat? N Engl J Med 2001; 345(3):208–10.
8. Iseman MD. Treatment of multidrug-resistant tuberculosis. N Engl J Med 1993;329(11):784–91.
9. WHO. Global tuberculosis report; 2014. ISBN 978 92 4 156480 9.
10. Control of tuberculosis in the United States. American Thoracic Society. Am Rev Respir Dis 1992; 146(6):1623–33.
11. Jeong YJ, Lee KS. Pulmonary tuberculosis: up-to-date imaging and management. AJR Am J Roentgenol 2008;191(3):834–44.
12. Dannenberg AM Jr. Delayed-type hypersensitivity and cell-mediated immunity in the pathogenesis of tuberculosis. Immunol Today 1991;12(7):228–33.
13. Houben EN, Nguyen L, Pieters J. Interaction of pathogenic mycobacteria with the host immune system. Curr Opin Microbiol 2006;9(1):76–85.
14. American Thoracic Society. Diagnostic standards and classification of tuberculosis. Am Rev Respir Dis 1990;142(3):725–35.
15. Geng E, Kreiswirth B, Burzynski J, et al. Clinical and radiographic correlates of primary and reactivation tuberculosis: a molecular epidemiology study. JAMA 2005;293(22):2740–5.
16. Leung AN, Muller NL, Pineda PR, et al. Primary tuberculosis in childhood: radiographic manifestations. Radiology 1992;182(1):87–91.
17. Andreu J, Caceres J, Pallisa E, et al. Radiological manifestations of pulmonary tuberculosis. Eur J Radiol 2004;51(2):139–49.
18. Curvo-Semedo L, Teixeira L, Caseiro-Alves F. Tuberculosis of the chest. Eur J Radiol 2005; 55(2):158–72.
19. Kim HY, Song KS, Goo JM, et al. Thoracic sequelae and complications of tuberculosis. Radiographics 2001;21(4):839–58 [discussion: 59–60].
20. Van Dyck P, Vanhoenacker FM, Van den Brande P, et al. Imaging of pulmonary tuberculosis. Eur Radiol 2003;13(8):1771–85.
21. Lee KS, Im JG. CT in adults with tuberculosis of the chest: characteristic findings and role in management. AJR Am J Roentgenol 1995;164(6):1361–7.
22. Woodring JH, Vandiviere HM, Fried AM, et al. Update: the radiographic features of pulmonary tuberculosis. AJR Am J Roentgenol 1986;146(3): 497–506.
23. Miller WT, Miller WT Jr. Tuberculosis in the normal host: radiological findings. Semin Roentgenol 1993;28(2):109–18.
24. Winer-Muram HT, Rubin SA. Thoracic complications of tuberculosis. J Thorac Imaging 1990;5(2): 46–63.
25. Goo JM, Im JG, Do KH, et al. Pulmonary tuberculoma evaluated by means of FDG PET: findings in 10 cases. Radiology 2000;216(1):117–21.
26. Kim IJ, Lee JS, Kim SJ, et al. Double-phase 18F-FDG PET-CT for determination of pulmonary tuberculoma activity. Eur J Nucl Med Mol Imaging 2008;35(4):808–14.
27. Tateishi U, Kusumoto M, Akiyama Y, et al. Role of contrast-enhanced dynamic CT in the diagnosis of active tuberculoma. Chest 2002;122(4): 1280–4.
28. Hadlock FP, Park SK, Awe RJ, et al. Unusual radiographic findings in adult pulmonary tuberculosis. AJR Am J Roentgenol 1980;134(5):1015–8.
29. Im JG, Itoh H, Han MC. CT of pulmonary tuberculosis. Semin Ultrasound CT MR 1995;16(5):420–34.

30. Krysl J, Korzeniewska-Kosela M, Muller NL, et al. Radiologic features of pulmonary tuberculosis: an assessment of 188 cases. Can Assoc Radiol J 1994;45(2):101–7.

31. Porcel JM. Tuberculous pleural effusion. Lung 2009;187(5):263–70.

32. Lin MT, Wang JY, Yu CJ, et al. Mycobacterium tuberculosis and polymorphonuclear pleural effusion: incidence and clinical pointers. Respir Med 2009;103(6):820–6.

33. Gopi A, Madhavan SM, Sharma SK, et al. Diagnosis and treatment of tuberculous pleural effusion in 2006. Chest 2007;131(3):880–9.

34. Pepper T, Joseph P, Mwenya C, et al. Normal chest radiography in pulmonary tuberculosis: implications for obtaining respiratory specimen cultures. Int J Tuberc Lung Dis 2008;12(4):397–403.

35. Palmieri F, Girardi E, Pellicelli AM, et al. Pulmonary tuberculosis in HIV-infected patients presenting with normal chest radiograph and negative sputum smear. Infection 2002;30(2):68–74.

36. Leung AN, Brauner MW, Gamsu G, et al. Pulmonary tuberculosis: comparison of CT findings in HIV-seropositive and HIV-seronegative patients. Radiology 1996;198(3):687–91.

37. Atwal SS, Puranik S, Madhav RK, et al. High resolution computed tomography lung spectrum in symptomatic adult HIV-positive patients in South-East Asian Nation. J Clin Diagn Res 2014;8(6): RC12–6.

38. Feng F, Shi YX, Xia GL, et al. Computed tomography in predicting smear-negative pulmonary tuberculosis in AIDS patients. Chin Med J (Engl) 2013; 126(17):3228–33.

39. Fishman JE, Saraf-Lavi E, Narita M, et al. Pulmonary tuberculosis in AIDS patients: transient chest radiographic worsening after initiation of antiretroviral therapy. AJR Am J Roentgenol 2000;174(1): 43–9.

40. Shelburne SA 3rd, Hamill RJ, Rodriguez-Barradas MC, et al. Immune reconstitution inflammatory syndrome: emergence of a unique syndrome during highly active antiretroviral therapy. Medicine (Baltimore) 2002;81(3):213–27.

41. Sharma SK, Mohan A, Sharma A, et al. Miliary tuberculosis: new insights into an old disease. Lancet Infect Dis 2005;5(7):415–30.

42. Sharma SK, Mukhopadhyay S, Arora R, et al. Computed tomography in miliary tuberculosis: comparison with plain films, bronchoalveolar lavage, pulmonary functions and gas exchange. Australas Radiol 1996;40(2):113–8.

43. Kwong JS, Carignan S, Kang EY, et al. Miliary tuberculosis. Diagnostic accuracy of chest radiography. Chest 1996;110(2):339–42.

44. Proudfoot AT, Akhtar AJ, Douglas AC, et al. Miliary tuberculosis in adults. Br Med J 1969;2(5652):273–6.

45. Hong SH, Im JG, Lee JS, et al. High resolution CT findings of miliary tuberculosis. J Comput Assist Tomogr 1998;22(2):220–4.

46. Extensively drug-resistant tuberculosis (XDR-TB). recommendations for prevention and control. Wkly Epidemiol Rec 2006;81(45):430–2.

47. Lee ES, Park CM, Goo JM, et al. Computed tomography features of extensively drug-resistant pulmonary tuberculosis in non-HIV-infected patients. J Comput Assist Tomogr 2010;34(4):559–63.

48. Soman R, Pillai P, Madan S, et al. Successful management of highly drug resistant tuberculosis with individualised drug susceptibility testing. J Assoc Physicians India 2014;62(7):567–70.

49. Frieden TR, Sterling T, Pablos-Mendez A, et al. The emergence of drug-resistant tuberculosis in New York City. N Engl J Med 1993;328(8):521–6.

50. Goble M, Iseman MD, Madsen LA, et al. Treatment of 171 patients with pulmonary tuberculosis resistant to isoniazid and rifampin. N Engl J Med 1993;328(8):527–32.

51. Sacks LV, Pendle S, Orlovic D, et al. A comparison of outbreak- and nonoutbreak-related multidrug-resistant tuberculosis among human immunodeficiency virus-infected patients in a South African hospital. Clin Infect Dis 1999;29(1):96–101.

52. Yeom JA, Jeong YJ, Jeon D, et al. Imaging findings of primary multidrug-resistant tuberculosis: a comparison with findings of drug-sensitive tuberculosis. J Comput Assist Tomogr 2009; 33(6):956–60.

53. Kim HC, Goo JM, Lee HJ, et al. Multidrug-resistant tuberculosis versus drug-sensitive tuberculosis in human immunodeficiency virus-negative patients: computed tomography features. J Comput Assist Tomogr 2004;28(3):366–71.

54. Fishman JE, Sais GJ, Schwartz DS, et al. Radiographic findings and patterns in multidrug-resistant tuberculosis. J Thorac Imaging 1998; 13(1):65–71.

55. Jokinen K, Palva T, Nuutinen J. Bronchial findings in pulmonary tuberculosis. Clin Otolaryngol Allied Sci 1977;2(2):139–48.

56. Smith LS, Schillaci RF, Sarlin RF. Endobronchial tuberculosis. Serial fiberoptic bronchoscopy and natural history. Chest 1987;91(5):644–7.

57. Moon WK, Im JG, Yeon KM, et al. Tuberculosis of the central airways: CT findings of active and fibrotic disease. AJR Am J Roentgenol 1997; 169(3):649–53.

58. Kim Y, Lee KS, Yoon JH, et al. Tuberculosis of the trachea and main bronchi: CT findings in 17 patients. AJR Am J Roentgenol 1997;168(4): 1051–6.

59. Choe KO, Jeong HJ, Sohn HY. Tuberculous bronchial stenosis: CT findings in 28 cases. AJR Am J Roentgenol 1990;155(5):971–6.

60. Lee KS, Kim YH, Kim WS, et al. Endobronchial tuberculosis: CT features. J Comput Assist Tomogr 1991;15(3):424–8.

61. Cha JH, Han J, Park HJ, et al. Aneurysmal appearance of medium-sized bronchi: a peripheral manifestation of endobronchial tuberculosis. AJR Am J Roentgenol 2009;193(2):W95–9.

62. Lois M, Noppen M. Bronchopleural fistulas: an overview of the problem with special focus on endoscopic management. Chest 2005;128(6): 3955–65.

63. Seo H, Kim TJ, Jin KN, et al. Multi-detector row computed tomographic evaluation of bronchopleural fistula: correlation with clinical, bronchoscopic, and surgical findings. J Comput Assist Tomogr 2010;34(1):13–8.

64. Restrepo CS, Carswell AP. Aneurysms and pseudoaneurysms of the pulmonary vasculature. Semin Ultrasound CT MR 2012;33(6):552–66.

65. Khalil A, Fartoukh M, Parrot A, et al. Impact of MDCT angiography on the management of patients with hemoptysis. AJR Am J Roentgenol 2010; 195(3):772–8.

66. Khalil A, Parrot A, Nedelcu C, et al. Severe hemoptysis of pulmonary arterial origin: signs and role of multidetector row CT angiography. Chest 2008; 133(1):212–9.

67. Ramakantan R, Bandekar VG, Gandhi MS, et al. Massive hemoptysis due to pulmonary tuberculosis: control with bronchial artery embolization. Radiology 1996;200(3):691–4.

68. Picard C, Parrot A, Boussaud V, et al. Massive hemoptysis due to Rasmussen aneurysm: detection with helicoidal CT angiography and successful steel coil embolization. Intensive Care Med 2003; 29(10):1837–9.

69. Keeling AN, Costello R, Lee MJ. Rasmussen's aneurysm: a forgotten entity? Cardiovasc Intervent Radiol 2008;31(1):196–200.

70. Santelli ED, Katz DS, Goldschmidt AM, et al. Embolization of multiple Rasmussen aneurysms as a treatment of hemoptysis. Radiology 1994; 193(2):396–8.

71. Patankar T, Prasad S, Deshmukh H, et al. Fatal hemoptysis caused by ruptured giant Rasmussen's aneurysm. AJR Am J Roentgenol 2000;174(1): 262–3.

72. Daly P, Kavanagh K. Pulmonary aspergillosis: clinical presentation, diagnosis and therapy. Br J Biomed Sci 2001;58(3):197–205.

73. Lee JG, Lee CY, Park IK, et al. Pulmonary aspergilloma: analysis of prognosis in relation to symptoms and treatment. J Thorac Cardiovasc Surg 2009; 138(4):820–5.

74. Pratap H, Dewan RK, Singh L, et al. Surgical treatment of pulmonary aspergilloma: a series of 72 cases. Indian J Chest Dis Allied Sci 2007;49(1):23–7.

75. Greenberg AK, Knapp J, Rom WN, et al. Clinical presentation of pulmonary mycetoma in HIV-infected patients. Chest 2002;122(3):886–92.

76. Tomlinson JR, Sahn SA. Aspergilloma in sarcoid and tuberculosis. Chest 1987;92(3):505–8.

77. Butz RO, Zvetina JR, Leininger BJ. Ten-year experience with mycetomas in patients with pulmonary tuberculosis. Chest 1985;87(3):356–8.

78. Abel AT, Parwer S, Sanyal SC. Pulmonary mycetoma probably due to Candida albicans with complete resolution. Respir Med 1998;92(8):1079–80.

79. Lee SI, Shepard JA, Chew FS. Pulmonary fungus ball. AJR Am J Roentgenol 1998;170(2):318.

80. Nitschke A, Sachs P, Suby-Long T, et al. Monod sign. J Thorac Imaging 2013;28(6):W120.

81. Kono SA, Nauser TD. Contemporary empyema necessitatis. Am J Med 2007;120(4):303–5.

82. Ahmed SI, Gripaldo RE, Alao OA. Empyema necessitans in the setting of pneumonia and parapneumonic effusion. Am J Med Sci 2007;333(2):106–8.

83. Sahn SA, Iseman MD. Tuberculous empyema. Semin Respir Infect 1999;14(1):82–7.

84. Glicklich M, Mendelson DS, Gendal ES, et al. Tuberculous empyema necessitatis. Computed tomography findings. Clin Imaging 1990;14(1):23–5.

85. Grover SB, Jain M, Dumeer S, et al. Chest wall tuberculosis—a clinical and imaging experience. Indian J Radiol Imaging 2011;21(1):28–33.

86. Khalil A, Le Breton C, Tassart M, et al. Utility of CT scan for the diagnosis of chest wall tuberculosis. Eur Radiol 1999;9(8):1638–42.

87. Morris BS, Maheshwari M, Chalwa A. Chest wall tuberculosis: a review of CT appearances. Br J Radiol 2004;77(917):449–57.

88. Shah J, Patkar D, Parikh B, et al. Tuberculosis of the sternum and clavicle: imaging findings in 15 patients. Skeletal Radiol 2000;29(8):447–53.

89. Grammatico L, Baron S, Rusch E, et al. Epidemiology of vertebral osteomyelitis (VO) in France: analysis of hospital-discharge data 2002-2003. Epidemiol Infect 2008;136(5):653–60.

90. Garg RK, Somvanshi DS. Spinal tuberculosis: a review. J Spinal Cord Med 2011;34(5):440–54.

91. Ansari S, Amanullah MF, Ahmad K, et al. Pott's spine: diagnostic imaging modalities and technology advancements. N Am J Med Sci 2013;5(7): 404–11.

92. Schirmer P, Renault CA, Holodniy M. Is spinal tuberculosis contagious? Int J Infect Dis 2010; 14(8):e659–66.

93. Hicks A, Muthukumarasamy S, Maxwell D, et al. Chronic inactive pulmonary tuberculosis and treatment sequelae: chest radiographic features. Int J Tuberc Lung Dis 2014;18(2):128–33.

94. Deboisblanc BP, Burch WC Jr, Buechner HA, et al. Computed tomographic appearance of an oleothorax. Thorax 1988;43(7):572–3.

95. Weissberg D. Late complications of collapse therapy for pulmonary tuberculosis. Chest 2001; 120(3):847–51.

96. Moran A, Stableforth DE, Matthews HR. Treatment of late complications of plombage by simultaneous removal of plomb and decortication. Thorax 1989; 44(12):1051–2.

97. Fowler NO. Tuberculous pericarditis. JAMA 1991; 266(1):99–103.

98. Reuter H, Burgess LJ, Doubell AF. Role of chest radiography in diagnosing patients with tuberculous pericarditis. Cardiovasc J S Afr 2005;16(2): 108–11.

99. Liu PY, Li YH, Tsai WC, et al. Usefulness of echocardiographic intrapericardial abnormalities in the diagnosis of tuberculous pericardial effusion. Am J Cardiol 2001;87(9):1133–5. A10.

100. Sagrista-Sauleda J, Permanyer-Miralda G, Soler-Soler J. Tuberculous pericarditis: ten year experience with a prospective protocol for diagnosis and treatment. J Am Coll Cardiol 1988;11(4):724–8.

101. Jeilan M, Schmitt M, McCann G, et al. Images in cardiovascular medicine. Cardiac tuberculoma. Circulation 2008;117(7):984–6.

102. Liu A, Hu Y, Coates A. Sudden cardiac death and tuberculosis—how much do we know? Tuberculosis (Edinb) 2012;92(4):307–13.

103. Rao VR, Jagannath K, Sunil PK, et al. A rare disappearing right atrial mass. Interact Cardiovasc Thorac Surg 2012;15(2):290–1.

104. Dixit R, Chowdhury V, Singh S. Case report: myocardial tuberculosis—MRI. Indian J Radiol Imaging 2009;19(1):57–9.

105. Breton G, Leclerc S, Longuet P, et al. Myocardial localisation of tuberculosis: the diagnostic value of cardiac MRI. Presse Med 2005;34(4):293–6 [in French].

106. Choudhary SK, Bhan A, Talwar S, et al. Tubercular pseudoaneurysms of aorta. Ann Thorac Surg 2001; 72(4):1239–44.

107. Lin MM, Cheng HM. Images in cardiovascular medicine: tuberculous aortitis. Intern Med 2012; 51(15):1983–5.

Imaging Spectrum of Extrathoracic Tuberculosis

Abhijit A. Raut, MD[a],*, Prashant S. Naphade, MD, DNB[b],
Ravi Ramakantan, MD[a]

KEYWORDS

- Musculoskeletal TB • CNS TB • TB lymphadenitis • Abdominal TB • Genitourinary TB
- Peritoneal TB

KEY POINTS

- The incidence of extrathoracic tuberculosis (ETB) continues to increase slowly, especially in immunocompromised and multidrug-resistant tuberculosis (TB) patients.
- ETB has nonspecific clinical presentations, and being less frequent, is less familiar to most physicians.
- The most common sites of ETB include lymphadenopathy, peritoneum, ileocecal region, hepatosplenic, genitourinary, central nervous system (CNS), and musculoskeletal (MSK) regions; multisystem involvement is common.
- For early and correct diagnosis of ETB, imaging plays a vital role.
- Imaging modalities of choice are computed tomography (lymphadenopathy and abdominal TB) and MR imaging (CNS and MSK TB).

INTRODUCTION

Even today, tuberculosis (TB) remains a global health problem despite availability of effective antituberculous treatment. This global resurgence of TB is mainly owing to the AIDS epidemic, increasing migration from endemic areas to the developed world where TB is uncommon, and the increasing number of drug-resistant strains of *Mycobacterium tuberculosis*. Although pulmonary involvement is the most common form of TB, almost any organ can be involved by TB, particularly in immunocompromised patients.[1] The incidence of extrathoracic TB (ETB) continues to increase slowly, especially in immunocompromised and multidrug-resistant TB patients.[2,3] The most common sites of ETB include lymph nodes, ileocecal (IC) region, peritoneum, liver, spleen, genitourinary system, central nervous system (CNS), and musculoskeletal system.

The diagnosis of ETB may be missed or delayed owing to nonspecific patient symptoms as well as a lack of familiarity of protean manifestations to most physicians. ETB involves relatively inaccessible sites; thus, fewer bacilli can cause much greater damage. In addition, multisystem involvement is common with ETB. For early and correct diagnosis of ETB, imaging plays a vital role. In this article, we discuss the imaging features of ETB.

Funding Support: Nil.
The authors have nothing to disclose.
[a] Department of Radiology, Kokilaben Dhirubhai Ambani Hospital, Rao Saheb Achutrao Patwardhan Marg, Four Bunglows, Andheri West, Mumbai, Maharashtra 400053, India; [b] CT/MRI Department, ESIC Hospital, Central Road, Andheri East, Mumbai 400093, India
* Corresponding author.
E-mail address: abhijitaraut@gmail.com

Radiol Clin N Am 54 (2016) 475–501
http://dx.doi.org/10.1016/j.rcl.2015.12.013

CENTRAL NERVOUS SYSTEM TUBERCULOSIS

Tuberculous involvement of the CNS is a serious form of extrapulmonary disease accounting for 1% of all TB and 10% to 15% of extrapulmonary TB. CNS TB is a leading cause of morbidity and mortality in endemic regions, particularly in children.[4,5] Depending on the site of involvement and pathologic manifestations, varied forms of CNS TB have been described such as tuberculous meningitis (TBM) and its complications, focal cerebritis, tuberculoma, and tuberculous abscess (Table 1). Spinal infection is less common and causes either arachnoiditis and/or intramedullary tuberculomas. Imaging plays a vital role in diagnosis of CNS TB, in the detection of early complications and also in follow-up. Computed tomography (CT) and MR imaging are used in the diagnosis of CNS TB; however, MR has greater sensitivity and specificity than CT in detection of CNS TB.

Pathophysiology

TB bacilli reach the CNS by an hematogeneous route from distant active TB sites elsewhere in the body. During bacteremia, small Rich's focus develops in the meninges, in the subpial or subependymal surface of the brain or the spinal cord. It may remain dormant for a long period. Rupture of Rich's focus produces various types of CNS TB.[6] Infrequently, CNS TB can occur by direct spread from adjacent infected paranasal sinuses or mastoid air cells. Rupture of TB granuloma into the subarachnoid space and cerebrospinal fluid (CSF) results in leptomeningitis. Leptomeningitis can lead to obstructive hydrocephalus or vasculitis. Depending on the virulence of the

Table 1
Neurologic TB spectrum

Intracranial TB	Intraspinal TB
Meningeal TB	Intraspinal TBM
TBM	Tuberculous myelitis
Pachymeningitis	Intramedullary tuberculoma
Parenchymal TB	—
Tuberculoma	
Tuberculous abscess	
Tuberculous cerebritis	
Tuberculous encephalopathy	
Complications of TBM: vasculitis, hydrocephalus, cranial neuropathy	

Abbreviations: TB, tuberculosis; TBM, tuberculous meningitis.

organisms and host immunity, parenchymal cerebral tuberculous foci may develop into tuberculoma or tuberculous brain abscess.[7]

TUBERCULOUS MENINGITIS

In developing countries, TBM is the most common cause of chronic meningitis. The diagnosis of TBM is challenging and is based on a constellation of clinical features, imaging findings, and CSF abnormalities, which include detection of acid-fast bacilli by direct staining of CSF or positive CSF culture for bacilli and response (both clinical and CSF) to antituberculous medications.[8] However, the clinical features are often nonspecific and microbiological detection of the organisms is difficult owing to paucibacillary CSF. Imaging plays a crucial role in the diagnosis of TBM and early detection of its complications. Focal or diffuse cerebral atrophy, areas of gliosis secondary to infarcts, hydrocephalus, meningeal, or ependymal calcifications, and occasionally syringomyelia are the sequelae of TBM.

Imaging characteristics suggestive of TBM are basal meningeal enhancement, hydrocephalus, tuberculomas, and infarcts on CT and MR imaging (Figs. 1 and 2).[9,10] Basal exudates in TBM appear mildly hyperdense on plain scans and reveal intense homogenous postcontrast enhancement.[11] Basal exudates in TBM appear hyperintense on fluid-attenuated inversion recovery MR imaging and show intense enhancement on postcontrast T1-weighted images. Linear enhancement along the ventricular margins confirms ependymitis. MR imaging is superior to CT in diagnosing suspected meningitis and associated complications.[12] The magnetization transfer (MT) technique is reported to be superior in differentiating TBM from other nontuberculous causes of meningitis. Meninges appear hyperintense on precontrast T1-weighted MT images and enhance further on postcontrast T1-weighted MT images. MT ratio in TBM is significantly higher than in viral meningitis, and fungal and pyogenic meningitis show higher MT ratio compared with TBM.[13] Patients with acquired AIDS may show minimal or absent meningeal enhancement, likely owing to lack of immunologic response.[14]

TUBERCULOUS PACHYMENINGITIS

Chronic TBM can infrequently lead to localized or diffuse dura matter involvement and may present as tuberculous pachymeningitis. There may be pial or parenchymal extension. The cavernous sinuses, floor of middle cranial fossa, and tentorium are frequently involved. Tuberculous pachymeningitis

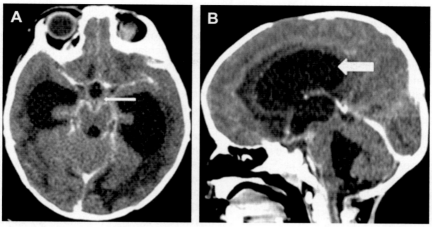

Fig. 1. Postcontrast axial (*A*) and sagittal (*B*) computed tomography images show enhancing basal exudates (*thin arrow*) and communicating hydrocephalus (*thick arrow*) in a proven case of tubercular meningitis.

appears hyperdense on plain CT scan and isointense to brain on T1-weighted imaging and isointense to hypointense on T2-weighted imaging. Postcontrast scan shows homogeneous enhancement. En plaque meningioma, dural carcinomatosis, neurosarcoidosis, lymphoma, and idiopathic progressive leptomeningeal fibrosis may show similar imaging features.[15] Tuberculous pachymeningitis responds well to antituberculous treatment.

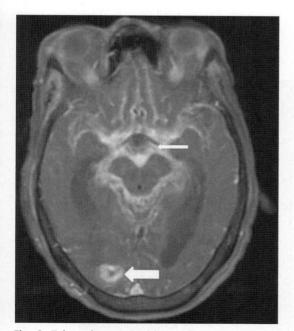

Fig. 2. Tubercular meningitis. Postcontrast axial T1-weighted MR image demonstrates extensive basal leptomeningeal enhancement (*thin arrow*) with dilated temporal horns. Ring enhancing tuberculoma (*thick arrow*) is seen in the right occipital lobe.

COMPLICATIONS OF TUBERCULOUS MENINGITIS
Hydrocephalus

Hydrocephalus is a frequent complication of TBM, especially in children, and carries a poor prognosis. It can be communicating, noncommunicating, or complex. Communicating hydrocephalus caused by obstruction to CSF flow in the basal cisterns by inflammatory exudates (see **Fig. 1**). It is the most common variety of hydrocephalus in TBM and accounts for 80% of the cases.[16] Obstruction at the fourth ventricular outlet foramina by basal exudates or tuberculoma or abscess or entrapment of ventricles by ependymitis results in noncommunicating hydrocephalus. Noncommunicating (obstructive) and communicating (defective absorption) hydrocephalus together are termed as complex hydrocephalus. A high incidence of complex hydrocephalus has been reported by Yadav and colleagues[17] and is a frequent cause of failure of endoscopic third ventriculostomy. By providing dynamic information, MR imaging CSF flowmetry is superior to CT in detecting this type of obstruction. Qualitative and quantitative analysis of CSF flow and dynamics is possible on MR imaging.

Vasculitis

Exudates along the basal cisterns cause an inflammatory response along the traversing blood vessels. To begin with, the inflammatory response occurs in the adventitial layer of the vessel; subsequently, the intima is affected and finally completely occludes the vessel. Contrast-enhanced CT and MR imaging angiography reveals small or long segment uniform narrowing and irregular beading or occlusion of affected arteries. Contrast-enhanced MR imaging is more sensitive for detection of small vessel involvement.[18] Multiple, bilateral infarcts located in the 'tuberculous zone' that is, caudate nucleus, anterior thalamus, anterior limb, and genu of the internal capsule, are seen in TB vasculitis (**Fig. 3**).[19] Diffusion-weighted MR imaging has an edge over conventional MR imaging and CT detecting early infraction in TB vasculitis. The medial striate, thalamotuberal, and thalamostriate arteries are often affected by TB exudates. Often these vessels are stretched by coexistent hydrocephalus.[19] Cortical stroke may also occur involving larger vascular territory supplied by middle, anterior, and posterior cerebral arteries.

Cranial Nerve Involvement

Cranial nerve involvement is seen in 17% to 40% of patients with TBM. It is owing to vascular compromise associated with TBM or entrapment of the nerves by the exudates.[20] Mass effect of the tuberculoma along the subarachnoid course of the nerve or direct involvement of the nerve nuclei owing to parenchymal TB are other less common causes. Fibrotic changes in the late stages can lead to permanent palsy. On imaging, the affected nerve is thickened and shows abnormal postcontrast enhancement. The proximal portion of the nerve near its root entry is most commonly affected.[21]

TUBERCULOMA

Tuberculoma occurs secondary to hematogeneous spread of infection and is the most common form of parenchymal TB. It comprises 15% to 50% of space-occupying lesions in endemic regions and can occur at any age. Infratentorial tuberculomas are more frequent in children, whereas in adults the supratentorial compartment is more commonly affected.[22] They can be solitary or multiple and can occur anywhere in the brain parenchyma. They are usually located in the corticomedullary junction corresponding to areas of narrowing of the arterioles at the gray/white matter junction.[23] Occasionally, intraventricular or meningeal tuberculomas may be seen. Extraaxial tuberculomas are rare and associated with widening of the basal foramen or adjacent bone destruction.[24] Hypophyseal tuberculoma is uncommon and shows thickening of the pituitary stalk.[25]

Imaging findings depend on the stage of tuberculoma—whether it is noncaseating or caseating and whether it has solid or liquid center. On MR imaging, noncaseating tuberculomas are hypointense on T1-weighted and hyperintense on T2-weighted images with homogeneous postcontrast enhancement. Caseating granulomas are isointense to hypointense on both T1-weighted and T2-weighted images with peripheral postcontrast enhancement (**Fig. 4**). Caseating granuloma may show central T2 hyperintensity owing to liquefaction. Associated TBM may be seen. In miliary TB, tiny 2- to 5-mm T2 hyperintense disc enhancing tuberculomas are seen with TBM. They are better visualized on MT spin echo T1-weighted images.[26] Healing stages of neurocysticercosis, fungal granulomas, pyogenic brain abscesses, lymphoma, metastases, and rarely glioma may resemble tuberculoma on

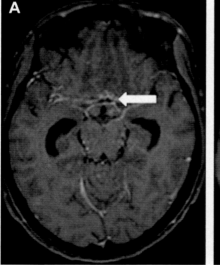
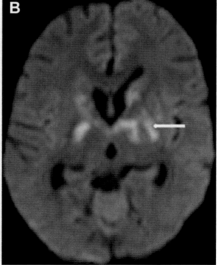

Fig. 3. Tubercular vasculitis. Axial postcontrast T1-weighted (*A*) and diffusion-weighted (*B*) MR images reveal enhancing basal exudates (*thick arrow*) with multiple, acute infarcts in bilateral gangliocapsular regions (*thin arrow*).

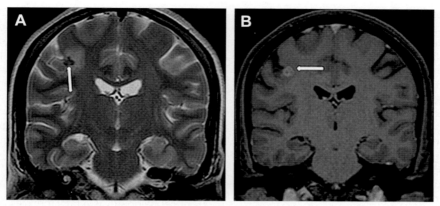

Fig. 4. Tuberculoma. Coronal T2-weighted (*A*) and postcontrast T1-weighted (*B*) MR images demonstrate small, confluent, T2-hypointense, ring enhancing lesions (*arrows*) in the right parietal lobe with mild perilesional edema.

imaging. Diffusion imaging, MR spectroscopy, and perfusion and MT imaging may differentiate these conditions from tuberculoma.

MT imaging improves the detectability of tuberculomas on precontrast T1-weighted MT spin echo images, compared with routine spin echo sequences. On noncontrast MT T1 images, the capsule of tuberculoma appears hyperintense and the solid caseation remains hypointense.[26] The core shows lower MT ratio than similar-resembling neurocysticerci lesions. MR spectroscopy is promising in the specific diagnosis of tuberculomas. Large lipid lactate peak at 1.3 ppm is characteristic, with associated reduced N-acetyl aspartate and/or slightly increased choline levels.

Postcontrast dynamic perfusion imaging allows differentiation of tuberculomas from other space occupying lesions with relative cerebral blood volume being the marker for perfusion. Tuberculomas usually appear hypoperfused (relative cerebral blood volume) compared with normal reference white matter with mildly increased relative cerebral blood volume along the peripheral wall (**Fig. 5**).[27]

TUBERCULOUS BRAIN ABSCESS

Tuberculous brain abscess is a relatively rare form of CNS TB accounting for 4% to 7% of cases in developing countries. A solitary, fairly large lesion with perilesional edema and mass effect is the

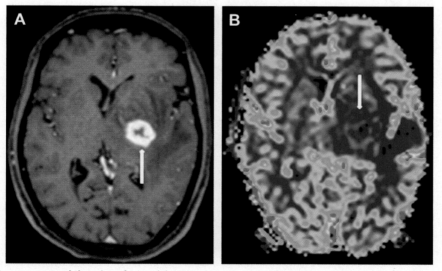

Fig. 5. Axial postcontrast (*A*) and perfusion (*B*) MR images show a left putaminal tuberculoma with a thick rind of enhancement. There is reduced relative cerebral blood volume (rCBV) of core with a thin peripheral rim of increased rCBV (*thin arrows*) as compared with normal reference white matter. Perilesional edema also shows reduced rCBV.

usual presentation. TB abscess is usually solitary and progresses rapidly compared with caseating tuberculoma. On imaging, it appears as a larger (typically >3 cm), multiloculated lesion with thin smooth enhancing walls, peripheral edema, and mass effect. Diffusion-weighted imaging in tuberculous abscesses show restricted diffusion with low apparent diffusion coefficient values (**Fig. 6**). On imaging, pyogenic and fungal abscesses may mimic tuberculous abscess. Tuberculous abscess shows large lipid lactate peak at 1.3 ppm on MR spectroscopy owing to presence of mycolic acid within mycobacterial walls (**Fig. 7**). Pyogenic brain abscesses reveal amino acid peak at 0.9 ppm, acetate peak at 1.9 ppm, and succinate peak at 2.4 ppm. Fungal abscesses may show amino acid and lipid lactate peaks, but a trehalose peak at 3.6 to 3.8 ppm is characteristic.[28]

TUBERCULOUS CEREBRITIS

Tuberculous cerebritis is a distinct form of CNS TB described by Jinkins, with specific clinical,

radiological, and histopathologic manifestations.[29] It is considered a precursor of tuberculoma formation and shows complete response if treated early. It shows typical cortical gyriform enhancement and angiographic blush on conventional angiography. CT shows intense focal postcontrast gyral enhancement and perilesional edema. On MR imaging, it appears hypointense on T1-weighted images and hyperintense on T2-weighted images with patchy postcontrast enhancement.

TUBERCULOUS ENCEPHALOPATHY

TB encephalopathy is a fatal form of CNS TB typically seen in infants and young children with pulmonary TB. A complex immunologic mechanism with delayed type IV hypersensitivity reaction by tuberculous protein is postulated for extensive damage of white matter with infrequent perivascular demyelination. Death usually occurs within 1 to 2 months of onset of illness despite antituberculous medication. Imaging shows extensive unilateral or bilateral brain edema.[21] No focal mass or

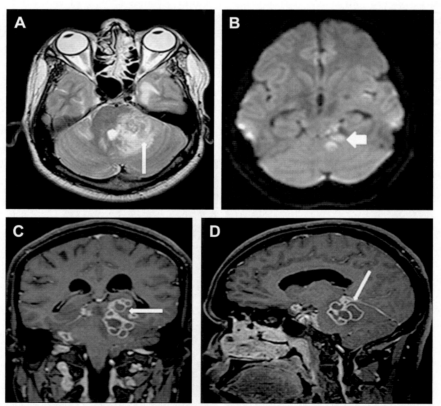

Fig. 6. Tubercular abscess. Axial T2-weighted image (*A*) reveals ill-defined, isointense to hypointense lesions (*thin arrow*) in the left cerebellar hemisphere and middle cerebellar peduncle with perilesional edema and mild mass effect on the fourth ventricle. Associated restricted diffusion (*thick arrow*) seen on diffusion-weighted image (*B*). The tubercular abscesses appear as confluent, multiloculated lesions with peripheral rim enhancement (*thin arrows, C* and *D*).

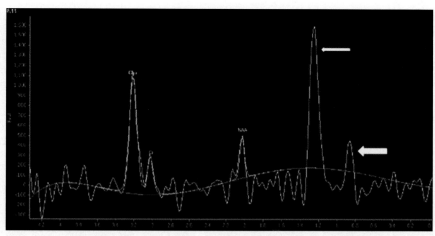

Fig. 7. Hydrogen 1 MR spectroscopy in a tubercular abscess reveals a large lipid lactate peak at 1.3 ppm (*thin arrow*) with markedly reduced *N*-acetyl aspartate (NAA). Additional lipid peak is seen at 0.9 ppm (*thick arrow*).

meningeal involvement is seen. Occasionally, perivascular demyelination or hemorrhagic leukoencephalopathy may be seen.

SPINAL CORD AND MENINGEAL INVOLVEMENT

Spinal TB commonly manifests as TBM and rarely intramedullary tuberculoma. MR imaging is the modality of choice for assessing spinal TB. Spinal TBM manifests as linear enhancing exudates along the spinal cord in the subarachnoid spaces and clumping of cauda equina nerve roots (**Fig. 8**). Intramedullary TB can present as myelitis without obvious focal granuloma or it can present as a T2 hypointense, ring-enhancing granuloma with perilesional edema similar to brain tuberculoma.

TUBERCULOUS LYMPHADENITIS

Tuberculous lymphadenitis (TBL) is a local manifestation of the systemic disease.[30] Lymphadenitis is the most common clinical presentation of extrapulmonary TB. TBL is seen in nearly 35% of extrapulmonary TB. TBL may occur during primary tuberculous infection or as a result of reactivation of dormant foci or direct extension from a contiguous focus. Cervical lymph nodes are the most common site of involvement and reported in 60% to 90% patients with or without involvement of other lymphoid tissue.[31] Mediastinal and axillary lymph node involvement is also common. An increased frequency of extrapulmonary TB, particularly lymphadenitis, is associated with human immunodeficiency virus infection.[32]

Superficial lymph node involvement is followed by progressive multiplication of *Mycobacterium tuberculosis*. Delayed hypersensitivity is accompanied by marked hyperemia, swelling, necrosis, and caseation of the center of the nodes followed by inflammation and matting with other nodes. Adhesion to the adjacent skin may result in induration and finally soft and caseous material may rupture into surrounding tissue through sinus tract formation. The clinical presentation of TBL is varied and may mimic neoplasm or sarcoidosis. Early diagnosis promotes effective treatment.

On ultrasonography of the neck, multiple hypoechoic and multiloculated conglomerate of cystic lymph nodes are seen with thick capsule and adjacent fat stranding. Ultrasonography is also useful in guided aspiration for cytology and biopsy. CT scan demonstrates conglomerate lymph nodes showing central lucency and a thick irregular rim of contrast enhancement (**Fig. 9**). Varying degrees of homogeneous enhancement can be seen in smaller lymph nodes. Overlying subcutaneous thickening with fat stranding can be seen. Lymphoma and metastatic lymphadenopathy may have similar imaging features. Histopathologic examination and culture are diagnostic of TBL.

ABDOMINAL TUBERCULOSIS

Abdominal TB is a common form of ETB with abdominal lymphadenopathy and peritoneal TB being the most common manifestations of abdominal TB. Brief imaging features of ileocecal, hepatosplenic, genitourinary, and adrenal TB are discussed below.

Abdominal Lymphadenopathy

TBL typically manifests as confluent, hypodense, centrally necrotic, peripherally enhancing abdominal lymph node masses with adjacent fat

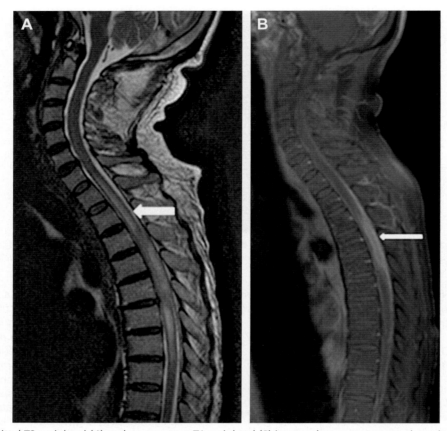

Fig. 8. Sagittal T2-weighted (*A*) and postcontrast T1-weighted (*B*) images demonstrate extensive spinal leptomeningeal enhancement in the cervicodorsal region with a peripherally enhancing, posterior subdural empyema (*thin arrow*) that indents the cord. Note the resultant abnormal T2 hyperintense signal of the cord signifying edema (*thick arrow*).

stranding. Although multiple, peripherally enhancing lymph nodes are a hallmark of TBL, nodal metastasis from testicular tumors, Whipple's disease, and rarely treated lymphoma may show similar pattern. Peripheral rim enhancement, nonhomogenous enhancement, homogenous enhancement, and homogenous nonenhancement are various CT patterns of TBL in order of decreasing frequency.[33] Calcification within the lymph nodes in the absence of malignancy is highly suggestive of TB. Mesenteric, periportal, omental, and upper paraaortic lymphadenopathy is seen commonly in abdominal TB (**Fig. 10**). Lower paraaortic lymph nodes are more frequent in lymphoma with typical homogenous postcontrast enhancement and encasement of blood vessels.

Peritoneal Tuberculosis

Peritonitis is the most common clinical manifestation of abdominal TB.[34] Infection of the peritoneum is usually secondary to hematogeneous spread from a pulmonary focus, from adjacent organs such as the intestine or the fallopian tube or ruptured necrotic lymph node. Liver cirrhosis, human immunodeficiency virus–positive, and chronic renal failure patients on continuous ambulatory peritoneal dialysis are at an increased risk for peritoneal TB.[35] Based on the pattern of ascites, omental and peritoneal tubercles, and associated inflammatory and fibrotic response, TB peritonitis has been traditionally classified into 3 categories (**Fig. 11**).[36]

Wet ascitic type

This is the most common variety of peritoneal TB seen among 90% of the cases with significant free or loculated high-density ascitic fluid on CT scan.

Fibrotic fixed type

This relatively less frequent variety of peritoneal TB is characterized by mesenteric and omental

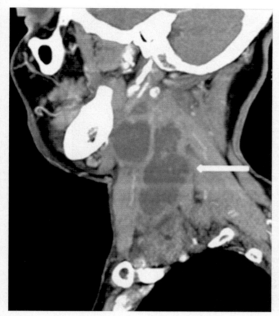

Fig. 9. Tubercular cervical lymphadenitis. Left parasagittal computed tomography image reveals a large conglomerate of necrotic jugular lymphadenopathy with peripheral rim enhancement (*white arrow*).

thickening, tuberculous deposits, and matted bowel loops.

Dry or 'plastic' type
This is a rare variety showing peritoneal nodules, fibrous peritoneal reaction, and dense adhesions. Ultrasonography can accurately demonstrate

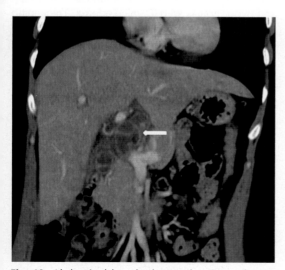

Fig. 10. Abdominal lymphadenopathy. Coronal postcontrast computed tomography image shows multiple, peripherally enhancing, centrally necrotic, confluent periportal lymph nodes (*white arrow*).

small quantities of loculated or free ascitic fluid. Multiple thin, complete or incomplete septae can be seen with echogenic debris being frequent in the loculated ascites. However, these features are can also be seen in malignancy, chronic infective peritonitis, and hemoperitoneum. CT scan shows loculated or free, high attenuation ascitic fluid (20–45 Hounsfield unites [HU]), omental thickening/nodularity, and thickened inflamed mesentery associated with mesenteric adenopathy. Diffuse smooth or nodular peritoneal thickening, adhesions, and bowel wall thickening/clumping are excellently demonstrated on CT scan.

Gastrointestinal Tract Tuberculosis

The common routes of spread of tubercle bacilli to the gastrointestinal tract (GIT) include hematogeneous spread from the primary lung lesion, ingestion of infected sputum from active pulmonary focus, direct spread from adjacent organs, or through lymphatic spread from infected lymph nodes. Although TB can involve any part of the GIT, the most common target site of involvement is the IC region. This is likely owing to several factors, including relative stasis, abundant lymphoid tissue, and closer contact of the bacilli with the mucosa in this region.[36] Variable sized confluent TB granulomas are seen in the mucosa or the Peyer's patches beneath the ulcer bed. TB ulcers are longitudinal in ileum and transverse in colon. Cicatricial healing of these circumferential ulcer leads to stricture formation. Tandon and Prakash[37] classified GIT TB as ulcerative and ulcerohypertrophic types. The ulcerative form is seen often among malnourished individuals and frequently leads to multiple strictures in the small intestine. The hypertrophic form is less common and usually seen in the IC region. This pattern is likely to be primary tuberculous infection.[38]

Esophageal tuberculosis
ETB constitutes 0.2% of cases of ETB.[39] Secondary involvement from the adjacent mediastinal adenopathy or pulmonary focus is commonly associated with ETB and frequently involves the middle one-third of the esophagus at the level of carina.[40]

Gastroduodenal tuberculosis
Gastroduodenal tuberculosis accounts for approximately 1% of cases of abdominal TB and may mimic peptic ulcer disease or cancer. Most patients present with duodenal obstruction owing to extrinsic compression of lymph nodes, rather than intrinsic duodenal lesion.

Ileocecal tuberculosis
The IC region is the most frequent site for bowel TB. The frequency of bowel involvement decreases

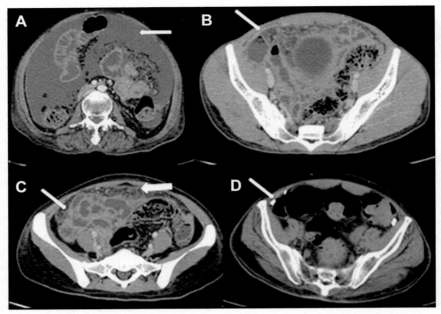

Fig. 11. Spectrum of peritoneal tuberculosis. Contrast-enhanced axial computed tomography images demonstrate ascites (*A*, wet peritoneal tuberculosis; *thin arrow*), peritoneal and bowel wall thickening (*B*, dry peritoneal tuberculosis; *thin arrow*), clumping of bowel loops (*thin arrow*) with omental and peritoneal thickening (*thick arrow*; *C*, fixed fibrotic peritoneal tuberculosis), and peritoneal calcifications (*D*, sequelae of peritoneal tuberculosis, *thin arrow*).

both proximally and distally from the IC region. Multiple strictures, adhesions, and bowel obstruction are the most the most common complications. Perforation followed by fistulae formation and intestinal bleeding may be seen but are uncommon.[39]

Colonic tuberculosis

The incidence of isolated colonic TB is around 9.2% of all the cases of abdominal TB and commonly involves the sigmoid, ascending, and transverse colon without IC TB. Multifocal colonic TB involvement is seen in one-third of cases. Minor or massive GIT bleeding is the most common complication of colonic TB.[39]

Plain radiography

Plain radiography of the abdomen is not specific and performed during acute exacerbation of the disease. Dilated bowel loops with multiple air–fluid levels suggest intestinal obstruction. Pneumoperitoneum may be seen in bowel perforation. A generalized increased density of abdomen and centrally placed gas-filled bowel loops is seen in ascites. Associated calcified mesenteric lymph nodes and hepatosplenomegaly may be seen.

Barium studies

Up until the recent past, barium contrast studies had been the mainstay for the diagnosis of intestinal TB. It has been documented that barium

studies are useful in 75% patients with suspected intestinal TB.[41] A barium esophagram delineates mucosal irregularity, ulceration, traction diverticulae, and stricture formation. Sinus tracts and fistulous communication with the mediastinum or tracheobronchial system may be demonstrated.[40]

Early manifestation of IC TB manifests as spasm and hypermotility with IC valve edema. Thickening of the IC valve may be associated with narrowing of the terminal ileum. The terminal ileal mucosa is thickened and appears nodular. As the disease progresses, the distal ileum becomes thick, rigid, and straight. Often, complete obliteration of the mucosal pattern is seen. The ileocecal valve becomes thickened and may project as a mass in the caecum. Owing to fixity of the bowel loops, there is loss of normal ileocecal angle. The IC valve becomes incompetent and widely opened. Associated granulation and ulceration distorts the valve. The edematous gaping ileocecal valve and developing stricture in the terminal ileum resembles inverted umbrella on barium examination, which is known as the Fleischner sign. The cecum becomes scarred, contracted, and conical. Direct passage of barium from affected ileum into ascending colon through widely opened IC valve is known as Stierlin sign (**Fig. 12**). The hypertrophic lesions on barium study resemble hourglass appearance with dilatation of proximal and distal normal bowel.

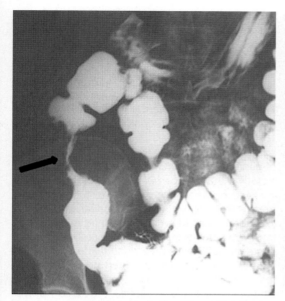

Fig. 12. Ileocecal tuberculosis. Small bowel barium examination image depicts cecal scarring/contraction and terminal ileal stricture (*black arrow*) with associated proximal ileal dilatation. (*Courtesy of* Department of Radiology, KEM Hospital, Mumbai, with permission.)

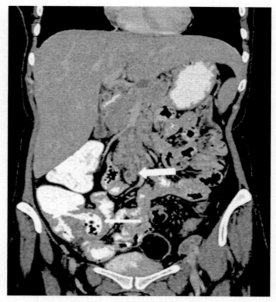

Fig. 13. Classic ileocecal tuberculosis. Coronal abdominal computed tomography image with oral and intravenous contrast shows circumferential wall thickening of the terminal ileum as well as a contracted cecum (*thin arrow*). Small, centrally necrotic, periportal and mesenteric lymph nodes are also seen (*thick arrow*).

Fluoroscopy and double contrast barium studies are more useful for assessing mucosal detail and visualization of ulceration in the early stages of the disease. On palpation during fluoroscopy, the bowel loops are fixed in position and remain unchanged in position during supine, prone, and standing examination. Fixed, dilated bowel loops show slow propagation of barium. Small bowel enteroclysis allows optimal distention of the small bowel lumen and delineation of mucosal detail is possible. Its advantage is detection and characterization of low-grade strictures.

Computed tomography scan

CT scan is the modality of choice for the evaluation of abdominal TB. Mural thickening of the IC region is frequent in GIT TB. It may be limited to the terminal ileum or caecum, or it may involve both (**Fig. 13**). The thickening may be symmetric or asymmetric. Asymmetric thickening of the IC valve and medial wall of the caecum may have an exophytic extension and this may engulf the terminal ileum. Fat stranding and inflammation is seen in the pericecal region and adjacent mesentery. There may be associated bowel obstruction and/or perforation. CT enteroclysis can excellently detect short segment strictures with concentric mural thickening with homogeneous mural enhancement (**Fig. 14**).[42] Abdominal CT findings supporting the diagnosis of TB include

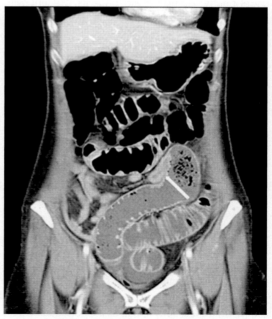

Fig. 14. Tubercular stricture. Coronal computed tomography postcontrast abdomen image demonstrates a short segment, high-grade small bowel stricture (*thin arrow*) causing small bowel obstruction.

high-density ascites, confluent necrotic abdominal lymphadenopathy, omental thickening/fat stranding, and hepatosplenic granulomas.

Hepatosplenic Tuberculosis

Hepatosplenic TB occurs secondary to hematogeneous spread of disease from active tuberculous focus elsewhere in the body. Commonly, it presents as miliary form in association with miliary pulmonary TB. Miliary TB manifests as hepatomegaly with multiple tiny low-attenuation foci without significant postcontrast enhancement on CT scan. The macronodular form of hepatosplenic TB is uncommon and manifests as a few hypodense lesions with ill-defined margins. These lesions may reveal minimal internal enhancement. Usually a thin peripheral postcontrast enhancement is seen (**Fig. 15**). Calcification of hepatosplenic granulomas can provide a clue to the diagnosis. On MR imaging, macronodular lesions appear T1 hypointense and T2 hypointense to hyperintense with thin peripheral and/or internal septal enhancement. Macronodular lesions can undergo liquefaction with formation of tuberculous abscess.

Adrenal Tuberculosis

Adrenal gland is the most common endocrine site involved by TB.[43] Hematogeneous dissemination of tubercle bacilli from primary active focus is the usual cause. Symptomatic patients present with adrenal insufficiency many years after initial infection. Early stage adrenal TB presents with bilateral asymmetric or unilateral adrenal enlargement with variable postcontrast enhancement (**Fig. 16**). Central necrotic areas may be seen. In advanced stages, atrophy and calcification are the usual imaging manifestations.[44]

Genitourinary Tuberculosis

The genitourinary system is one of the most common locations of ETB, contributing approximately 15% to 20% of cases.[45] The kidneys, prostate, and seminal vesicles are often the primary sites of genitourinary TB (GUTB). Other genital organs, including the epididymis and urinary bladder, are involved by ascent or descent of tubercle bacilli from elsewhere in the genitourinary tract.[46] It is infrequent in children and common in second to fourth decades of life.[47] Approximately 25% of patients of GUTB have prior documented pulmonary TB.[48] The symptoms are often nonspecific with resultant delayed diagnosis.[49] Patients may present with difficulty in voiding, dysuria, pyuria, microscopic or macroscopic hematuria, and back, flank, or abdominal pain apart from systemic symptoms. Demonstration of *M tuberculosis* in the urine by microbiological, cytopathologic, or histopathologic methods confirms the diagnosis of GUTB. Sterile pyuria is the classic finding.[50] The urine smear and culture often fail to demonstrate mycobacteria, most probably owing to the intermittent shedding of the bacilli in the urine and observer-dependent readings. Direct smears are positive only in 30% of patients and urine cultures require 6 to 8 weeks in special culture media.[51] Thus, in patients with suspected GUTB, imaging plays a major role in diagnosis.

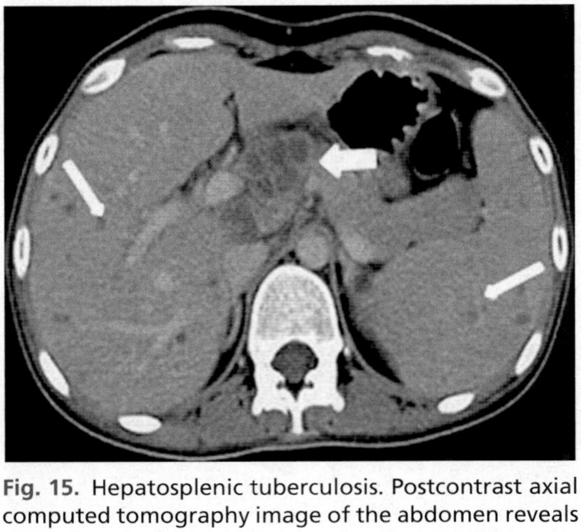

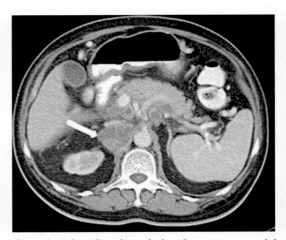

Fig. 15. Hepatosplenic tuberculosis. Postcontrast axial computed tomography image of the abdomen reveals multiple, hypodense, focal granulomas within the liver and spleen (*thin arrows*). Multiple conglomerate necrotic lymph nodes (*thick arrow*) are seen in the porta hepatis that indent the pancreas.

Fig. 16. Adrenal tuberculosis. Postcontrast axial computed tomography image of the abdomen shows a hypodense right adrenal lesion (*thin arrow*) and necrotic peripancreatic lymph nodes in a young patient with human immunodeficiency virus and tuberculous infection.

Pathophysiology

Hematogeneous dissemination of TB from a primary focus can involve the kidneys. Inflammatory response results in granuloma formation in the renal cortex. These granulomas may heal and form scars or may remain dormant for many years (5–40 years).[36] Depending on the virulence of the organism and host immune response, reactivation of these granulomas may occur and may subsequently enlarge and coalesce. Rupture of the granulomas into the proximal tubule and loop of Henle of nephron occurs. The organisms in the nephron are trapped at the loop of Henle where they grow and proliferate. Relatively poor blood flow, hypertonicity, and high ammonia concentration in the renal medulla/papilla help the organisms to grow and form medullary granulomas.[48] Subsequently, the granulomas rupture into the calyceal system with caseous necrosis, cavitation, and ulceration.

Extensive papillary necrosis may develop with frank cavities and destruction of the adjacent renal parenchyma. Healing in the kidneys results in fibrosis, calcium deposition, and stricture formation and subsequently leads to obstruction leading to renal dysfunction. Dystrophic calcification is the hallmark of the end-stage nonfunctional diseased kidney also called as putty or cement kidney. Dystrophic calcification is uncommon in early stage of the disease. Such lesions can harbor TB bacilli. Although granulomas develop in both the kidneys owing to hematogeneous spread, clinically significant disease is usually limited to 1 kidney.[52]

The organisms may be excreted in the urine and may affect the urothelial lining of the renal pelvis, ureter, urinary bladder, and urethra. Inflammatory response may lead to urothelial thickening. In advanced cases, ureteric stricture may be formed, which leads to obstructive uropathy. Ureteric strictures are common in the areas of physiologic narrowing of the ureter—the pelviureteric junction and the ureterovesical junction. Renal functional loss owing to ureteric stricture is more than parenchymal TB.[53] In the urinary bladder, the ureteral orifices are the most common sites of TB. The infection eventually may spread throughout the bladder with superficial ulceration and granuloma formation in all the layers. Healing by extensive fibrosis of the bladder wall results in small capacity bladder known as thimble bladder. Genital TB is common among men with TB of urinary tract. Epididymitis, prostatitis, and seminal vesicle and testicular involvement by TB is seen in approximately 70% to 80% of the men with urinary tract TB. In women, GUTB presents as salpingitis, complex tuboovarian masses, and endometritis and adhesions.

Plain radiography

Radiographic identification of calcification associated with renal TB is becoming less common.[53] On plain radiography, amorphous, granular or curvilinear, renal calcification can be seen in 24% to 44% of patients.[54] A granulomatous mass involving an entire renal lobe may appear as focal globular calcification.[54] Triangular ringlike calcification within the collecting system suggests papillary necrosis.[55] Calcified caseous tissue of homogeneous ground glass density is often referred to as putty kidney (**Fig. 17**).[56] The calcification may also be seen in the ureter. Upper ureteral calcification with other renal calcification strongly suggests GUTB.[53] Additional mesenteric lymph node calcification or spine TB on plain radiography may support to the diagnosis of GUTB. Renal calcification carries unfavorable prognosis and, if untreated, would lead to increasing calcification and deterioration of renal function.[57]

Intravenous urography

Depending on the severity of involvement of the kidneys, intravenous urography features can show a broad range of findings.[58] Up to 10% to 15% of active renal TB have normal intravenous urography findings. Minimal calyceal dilatation or mild loss of calyceal sharpness owing to mucosal edema may be seen in the initial stage on intravenous urography.[53] As the disease progresses, the calyceal outline becomes more irregular, fuzzy or ragged, and leads to a feathery and moth-eaten appearance owing to necrotizing papillitis.[54] Direct tissue destruction along with ischemia leads to papillary necrosis in GUTB. Small cavities in the

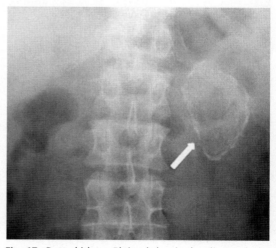

Fig. 17. Putty kidney. Plain abdominal radiograph depicts a calcified, atrophic left kidney owing to tuberculosis (*thin arrow*). (*Courtesy of* Department of Radiology, KEM Hospital, Mumbai, with permission.)

papillae progresses to medullary cavities that communicate with the adjacent collecting system, resulting in an irregular cavity filled with contrast (**Fig. 18**).[59] With papillary cavitation, the infection spreads to the urothelium and submucosa of the draining calix, which leads to calyceal infundibular stenosis.[48] Infundibular stenosis leads to localized calyectasis or incomplete opacification of the calyx and in advanced cases may lead to hydronephrosis. Sharp angulation of the renal pelvis develops owing to scarring of ureter.[36] Dilatation and mucosal irregularity (saw-tooth ureter) is seen in the initial stages, which may progress to strictures and ureteral shortening (pipe-stem ureter).[46] Multiple ureteric strictures resemble "beaded" or "corkscrew" ureter.[36]

Computed tomography

Cross-sectional imaging with CT is helpful in the evaluation of nonfunctional kidney, in the determination of the exact extent of the disease and perinephric spread. With multidetector CT scanners, multiphasic postcontrast imaging is possible with multiplanar reconstruction. CT urography gives better delineation of pathologic anatomy of the entire urinary tract. CT is also useful in detecting complications and other abdominal organ involvement. Fine calcifications that are unidentifiable on plain radiographs are much better seen with CT.[60]

Careful scrutiny of postcontrast corticomedullary and nephrographic phase images should be done for renal parenchymal and collecting system involvement in GUTB. TB granulomas are of variable size and appear as solid hypodense lesions with little or minimal peripheral enhancement on contrast scans. Associated changes in the collecting system may also be present (**Fig. 19**).[61] Sometimes on CT scan, larger nodules show mixed density and resemble renal neoplasms.[61] Rarely, renal TB resembles well-circumscribed cystic mass with enhancing septations.[62] Localized hypoperfusion owing to tissue edema and vasoconstriction similar to that in acute pyelonephritis may be seen in renal TB.[61]

Dilated calices filled with fluid, debris, or caseation (0 and 30 HU) may be seen on CT scan. One or more cavities adjacent to a calyx and thinning of the adjacent cortex were frequent findings (68%) in a series of 50 patients with GUTB.[63] TB renal abscesses appear hypodense (10–40 HU) and may show mild peripheral enhancement. The renal abscesses may rupture into the perinephric space or the calyceal system. Irregular parenchymal contrast filled cavities can be seen on excretory phase imaging.[61] Uneven calyectasis, if accompanied by uroepithelial thickening in the absence of other obstructing cause, should raise suspicion of GUTB (**Fig. 20**).[61] Focal or generalized cortical scarring and radiologically nonfunctioning kidney may be seen in advanced disease.[64] Pelviinfundibular strictures, papillary necrosis, cortical low-attenuating masses, scarring, and calcification are seen in various renal pathologies. However, the combination of 3 or more of these findings is highly suggestive of TB, even in the absence of documented pulmonary disease.[58] Merchant and colleagues[61] suggested that urothelial thickening should be added to this list. Chronic pyelonephritis, papillary necrosis, medullary

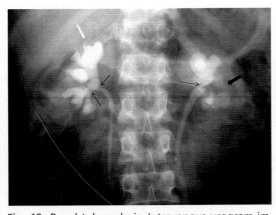

Fig. 18. Renal tuberculosis. Intravenous urogram image reveals uneven caliectasis in both kidneys with 'ballooning' of upper pole calyces and nonvisualization of interpolar calyces on the left side (*thick black arrow*). Bilateral infundibular and right pelvic strictures are seen (*thin black arrows*). Moth eaten appearance of the right upper pole calyx suggests papillitis and necrosis (*white arrow*). (*Courtesy of* Department of Radiology, KEM Hospital, Mumbai, with permission.)

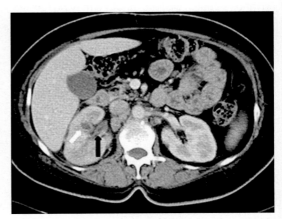

Fig. 19. Renal tuberculosis. Axial postcontrast computed tomography image of the abdomen demonstrates an oval hypodense medullary granuloma in the right kidney (*white arrow*) with urothelial thickening of the right renal pelvis (*black arrow*).

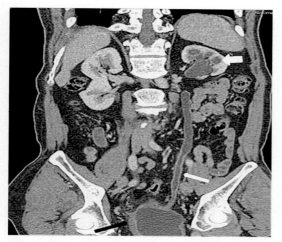

Fig. 20. Urinary tract tuberculosis. Coronal, postcontrast, abdominal computed tomography image shows left hydronephrosis (*thick white arrow*) and diffuse wall thickening of the left ureter (*thin white arrow*). Asymmetric, wall thickening of a reduced-capacity urinary bladder is also seen (*black arrow*).

sponge kidney, calyceal diverticulum, renal cell carcinoma, transitional cell carcinoma, and xanthogranulomatous pyelonephritis may resemble renal TB on imaging.[65]

Urinary bladder involvement is secondary to descending spread of infection along the urinary tract. The tuberculous bladder becomes distorted, ragged and shrunken. CT or MR imaging shows wall thickening and shrinkage.[66] In advanced cases owing to fibrosis at the ureteric orifice, vesicoureteric reflux develops with variable grades of hydroureteronephrosis.[67]

MR imaging
MR imaging may be used for characterizing the lesion in pediatric or pregnant patients or when ionizing radiation and iodinated contrast are contraindicated. MR imaging can provide morphologic details of the kidneys, delineation of pelvicalyceal system/ureter, bladder, and genital organs. Noncontrast MR urography is helpful in evaluating abnormalities of pelvicalyceal system and ureters in patients with renal failure.[50]

Genital Tuberculosis

Male genital TB results from hematogeneous spread or direct extension from urinary TB. It can manifest as epididymoorchitis with infection beginning in the tail of epididymis, seminal vesicle/vas deferens involvement, and prostatic abscess formation. Epididymoorchitis manifests as heterogeneous echogenicity of enlarged epididymis and testis.[68] On MR imaging, involved

structures reveal T2 intermediate to hypointensity. Prostatic abscess appears as a hypoattenuating, peripherally enhancing fluid collection on postcontrast CT scan (**Fig. 21**). Calcifications may be seen.

Female genital TB is usually secondary to hematogeneous spread to bilateral Fallopian tubes from an active primary focus or secondary to spread from adjacent organs. Infertility is a common clinical presentation. Lesions may present as tuboovarian abscesses (**Fig. 22**) or bilateral salpingitis with beaded appearance on hysterosalpingogram. The latter is owing to multiple strictures and/or hydrosalpinx. Endometrial involvement is seen as deformed endometrial cavity with endometrial adhesions.[69]

MUSCULOSKELETAL TUBERCULOSIS

Musculoskeletal TB is an uncommon form of extrapulmonary TB, constituting 1% to 3% of tuberculous infections.[70,71] Tuberculous spondylitis is the most common form of musculoskeletal TB constituting approximately 50% of patients. Extraspinal forms of musculoskeletal TB include peripheral tuberculous arthritis (60%), osteomyelitis (38%), and soft tissue TB including tenosynovitis and bursitis.[72–76]

Pathogenesis

Musculoskeletal TB is most commonly caused by *M tuberculosis*. Rarely, *M bovis* and atypical mycobacteria are the causative agents. Musculoskeletal TB occurs secondary to hematogeneous or lymphatic spread of mycobacteria from primary or reactivated focus of infection. Other possible mechanisms include direct inoculation by infected

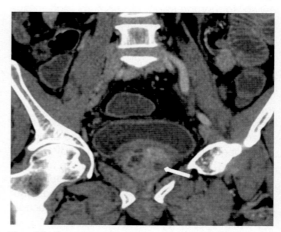

Fig. 21. Prostatic tubercular abscess. Postcontrast, coronal computed tomography image of the pelvic depicts prostatomegaly with multiple, small, low-density abscesses (*white arrow*).

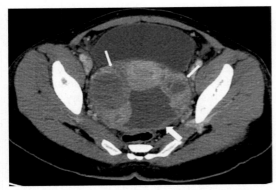

Fig. 22. Tuboovarian tubercular abscesses. Postcontrast axial computed tomography image of the pelvis reveals bilateral complex tuboovarian masses with thick peripheral enhancement (*thin arrows*) and an adjacent, thick-walled, loculated fluid collection (*thick arrow*).

syringes and reactivation of dormant infective foci by trauma.

Tuberculous Spondylitis

Tuberculous spondylitis is the most common form of musculoskeletal TB constituting 50% of cases.[45,46,71] It represents 1% of all tuberculous infections.[77] The thoracolumbar junction is the most common site of involvement, with L1 being the most commonly involved vertebra. Vertebral body involvement is more common than involvement of posterior elements with the anterior part of the vertebral body being most commonly involved.[66] Patients usually present with a long history of back pain, although an associated low-grade fever, weight loss, and neurologic deficit owing to compression by epidural soft tissue may be present. Posterior element TB can present with posterior paraspinal swelling owing to abscess formation.

Tuberculous spondylitis occurs secondary to hematogeneous dissemination of tubercle bacilli from primary focus through anterograde arterial route or retrograde spread via Batson's venous plexus. The most common site of infection is an anterior vertebral body adjacent to the endplate. Subsequently, the entire vertebral body can be involved. The infection spreads into the adjacent intervertebral disc via destruction of endplates or subligamentous spread of anterior or posterior longitudinal ligament. Extension commonly occurs to paraspinal and epidural soft tissues.

Plain radiographs
Plain radiographs are less sensitive for early detection of tuberculous spondylitis; at least 30% to 50% bone destruction is required before osteolytic changes are appreciated. Early changes include ill-defined appearance of endplates with loss of sclerotic margins and irregularity or erosions of endplates. Lytic lesion in the vertebral body typically lacks peripheral sclerosis.[45,66] Disc involvement is characterized by decreased disc space. Two adjacent vertebral bodies and intervening disc are commonly involved. As the disease progresses, anterior wedging and collapse of vertebral body occurs with resultant characteristic gibbus deformity. Subligamentous spread can cause scalloping of anterior margins of vertebral bodies. Paravertebral soft tissue is seen as displacement of paraspinal lines in thoracic region and outward convexity or ill-defined margins of psoas shadow. Calcification of paraspinal abscess, when seen, is pathognomic for tuberculous infection.[46]

Ultrasonography
Ultrasonography is useful in the diagnosis and percutaneous drainage of iliopsoas and paraspinal muscle abscesses.

Computed tomography scan
CT scan is useful for the evaluation of early bone destruction, pattern of destruction (fragmented bone destruction is more common), and calcification in associated hypodense paraspinal soft tissue (diagnostic of TB; **Figs. 23** and **24**).[78] CT is frequently used for guided transpedicular vertebral biopsy for histopathology and for culture/sensitivity evaluation. If multiple contiguous vertebral bodies are collapsed, CT is extremely useful for accurate demonstration of involved vertebral bodies by counting the posterior elements without corresponding vertebral bodies. CT is also useful in the evaluation of spinal deformities.

MR imaging
MR imaging is the modality of choice for evaluation of tuberculous spondylitis because it detects early marrow and paraspinal soft tissue changes with multiplanar capabilities and excellent soft tissue contrast resolution. Early changes include focal T2 hyperintense and T1 hypointense bone marrow edema in the anterior part of vertebral body adjacent to endplates with patchy postcontrast enhancement. Gradually, the destruction of the cortex and endplates occurs with resultant subligamentous spread, disc involvement, and contiguous vertebral body involvement. The involved disc space is reduced in height with abnormal T2 hyperintense signal (**Fig. 25**). Subligamentous spread may affect multiple contiguous vertebrae with preservation of intervening disc spaces. It is associated commonly with paravertebral and

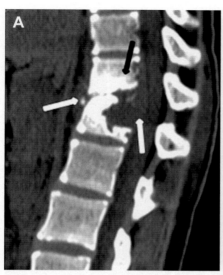
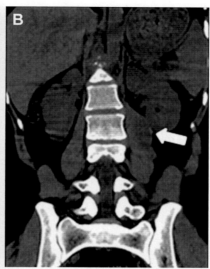

Fig. 23. Sagittal computed tomography (CT) image (*A*) shows irregular destruction of the adjoining endplates of T11 and T12 vertebral bodies with reduced height of T11 to T12 intervertebral disc and mild adjacent sclerosis (*black arrow*) in a young woman on treatment for tubercular spondylitis. Associated, abnormal, prevertebral and epidural soft tissue is seen (*thin white arrows*). Coronal CT image (*B*) shows a small, peripheral calcific focus in the left psoas abscess (*thick white arrow*), pathognomic of tubercular etiology.

epidural collections, which appear T2 hyperintense and T1 hypointense with thin smooth peripheral postcontrast enhancement (**Fig. 26**).[77,79] Multifocal TB, compression of the spinal cord, abnormal T2 hyperintense signal in the spinal cord, and neural foraminal and neural compromise secondary to epidural collections are excellently demonstrated on MR imaging (**Fig. 27**).[78] The complete extent of iliopsoas and paraspinal abscess can be demonstrated on MR imaging, which

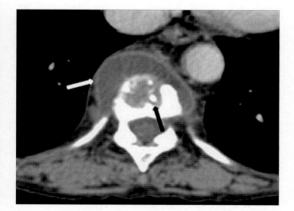

Fig. 24. Tubercular spondylitis with paravertebral abscess. Axial postcontrast computed tomography image demonstrates an ill-defined lytic lesion in the T8 vertebral body with destruction of the anterior cortex (*black arrow*). Prevertebral and bilateral paravertebral abscesses with thin smooth peripheral enhancement are seen (*white arrow*).

can reach up to the proximal thigh. Posterior element involvement is not uncommon. Cross-sectional imaging (CT and MR imaging) is extremely useful in detecting small foci of infection in posterior elements (**Fig. 28**).

Pyogenic spondylitis is the most important differential diagnosis. Features suggestive of tuberculous rather than pyogenic spondylitis include thin smooth peripheral enhancement of paraspinal collections, well-defined paraspinal soft tissue, subligamentous extension to 3 or more vertebral levels, involvement of multiple vertebrae, skip lesions, relative late disc destruction, absence of sclerosis, thoracic spine disease, and calcification in paraspinal abscess (pathognomic).[79] Other atypical infections, including brucellosis/fungal infections and sarcoidosis, may present with imaging findings similar to that of tuberculous spondylitis. When the infective process is limited to the vertebral body and paraspinal soft tissue, the differential diagnosis includes metastasis, myeloma, and lymphoma.

Tuberculous Arthritis

Tuberculous arthritis is the most common extraspinal form of musculoskeletal TB. Tuberculous arthritis is monoarticular in 90% cases, with the knee and hip joints being most commonly involved.[75,76] Other joints affected by tuberculous arthritis include the sacroiliac joint, shoulder, elbow, and ankle joints. TB arthritis usually present

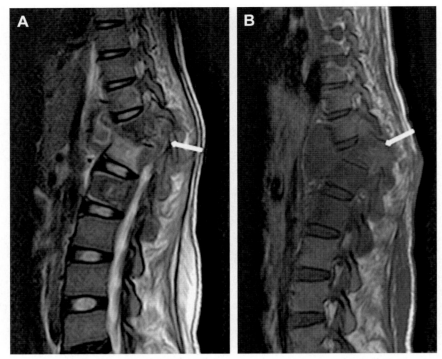

Fig. 25. Tubercular spondylodiscitis. Sagittal T2-weighted (*A*) and T1-weighted (*B*) images reveal irregular destruction with marked collapse of T10 and T11 vertebral bodies as well as abnormal T2-hyperintense and T1-hypointense signal (*thin arrows*). Resultant kyphotic deformity of the thoracic spine is seen. Abnormal T2 hyperintense signal is also seen in intervening T10 to T11 and T11 to T12 discs.

with nonspecific symptoms of chronic joint pain and swelling with resultant delay in diagnosis. TB arthritis may result from hematogeneous spread of tubercle bacilli through subsynovial vessels or secondary to tuberculous osteomyelitis foci in epimetaphysis eroding into the joint space. Secondary joint involvement is more common. Epiphyseal involvement is more common in adults and metaphyseal involvement is more common in children. Transphyseal spread of infection seen in TB is uncommon in pyogenic infections. Tuberculous arthritis starting as synovial infection causes synovial thickening with bone erosions at attachment sites. Articular cartilage destruction occurs late in the disease process with formation of rice bodies in the joint space. Tuberculous arthritis starting as epiphyseal/metaphyseal infection causes local hyperemia and focal bone destruction with or without periostitis. As the infection reaches the subchondral bone, articular cartilage undergoes necrosis owing to loss of nutrition. Ultimately, the infective focus ruptures into the joint space.

Plain radiographs and computed tomography scan

Classic plain radiographic findings of tuberculous arthritis are periarticular osteopenia, peripheral

bone erosions, and gradual loss of joint space (Phemister's triad; **Fig. 29**).[71] Phemister's triad is not pathognomonic for tuberculous arthritis and can be seen in rheumatoid arthritis and fungal diseases.[46] Peripheral osseous erosions are more common in weight-bearing joints such as the hip, knee, and ankle. Other common abnormalities include focal lytic lesions in epiphysis/metaphysis, periostitis (uncommon), periarticular soft tissue, and joint effusion. Periostitis, sequestration, and marginal sclerosis are usually not seen. However, these abnormalities are not diagnostic of tuberculous etiology and confirmation with biopsy and culture is usually required. The advanced stage of the disease reveals irregular bone destruction and sclerosis. Fibrous ankylosis is seen in end-stage tuberculous arthritis as compared with the bony ankylosis seen in pyogenic arthritis. CT scan excellently depicts bone destruction, bone erosions, status of subchondral bone, joint effusion, and periarticular collections.

Ultrasonography

Ultrasonography is useful in assessing joint effusion, synovial thickening, and periarticular soft tissue collections. Its main role, however, is in the guidance for synovial biopsy and percutaneous

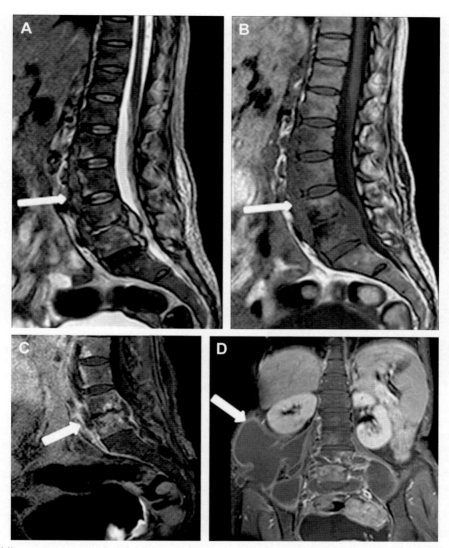

Fig. 26. Subligamentous spread and paraspinal abscess. Sagittal T2-weighted (*A*) and T1-weighted (*B*) images show tubercular spondylodiscitis at L4 to L5 level with T2-hyperintense and T1-isointense epidural soft tissue indenting the cauda equina. Contiguous L1, L2, and L3 vertebral bodies are involved secondary to subligamentous spread (*thin arrows*) with preserved intervening discs. Postcontrast T1-weighted sagittal (*C*) and coronal (*D*) images show thin smooth peripheral enhancement of prevertebral, epidural, and bilateral iliopsoas abscesses (*thick arrows*) characteristic of tuberculosis.

aspiration of effusion for histopathologic examination and culture and sensitivity testing.

MR imaging

MR imaging is the modality of choice for the evaluation of tuberculous arthritis with excellent demonstration of synovial and articular cartilage abnormalities. Synovial thickening in tuberculous arthritis is uniform, appearing intermediate to hypointense or hyperintense on T2-weighted images with intermediate signal on T1-weighted images.[71,75,76,80] It shows intense homogenous postcontrast enhancement. Hypointense T2 signal intensity of the synovium owing to caseation necrosis is characteristic of tuberculous arthritis and allows differentiation from other inflammatory synovial arthropathies. However, T2 hypointense synovial thickening can also be seen in pigmented villonodular synovitis and hemophilic arthropathy with blooming on gradient images owing to hemosiderin deposition.[71] Peripheral large bone erosions are seen with peripheral enhancement.[80] Joint effusion is common. Articular cartilage and subchondral bone erosions are seen. Periarticular

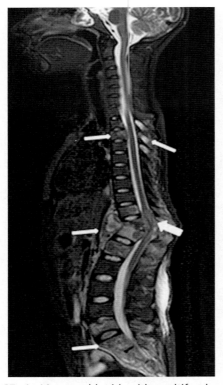

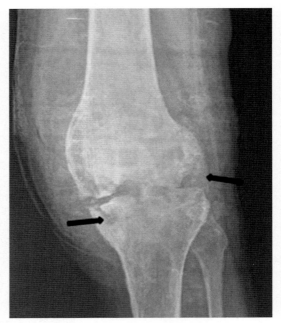

Fig. 29. Tubercular arthritis. Plain radiograph of the knee joint reveals periarticular osteopenia, large irregular peripheral erosions (*black arrows*), and relatively preserved joint space, constituting the classic Phemister's triad of tubercular arthritis.

Fig. 27. A 14-year old girl with multifocal spinal tuberculosis (TB). Sagittal short T1 inversion recovery image demonstrates multifocal spinal TB involving multiple dorsal, lumbar, and sacral vertebral bodies and posterior elements (*thin white arrows*) with lower thoracic cord compression and abnormal T2 signal in the cord (*thick white arrow*) owing to gibbus deformity and epidural soft tissue.

abscesses characteristically reveal minimal peripheral T1 hyperintense rim. Sinus tracts may extend from the collections up to the skin surface with peripheral postcontrast enhancement.

The differential diagnosis includes other infective arthritis (pyogenic or fungal), pauciarticular rheumatoid arthritis, and juvenile idiopathic arthritis. Synovial biopsy or joint fluid aspiration should be performed to confirm the diagnosis. Bone erosions are more common in tuberculous arthritis as compared with pyogenic arthritis. Extraarticular collections reveal thin smooth margins

bones reveal abnormal T2 hyperintense and T1 hypointense signal. Periarticular fluid collection or abscess can be seen with thin smooth peripheral enhancement (**Figs. 30** and **31**). Tuberculous

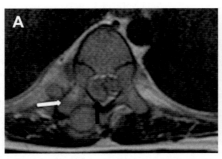

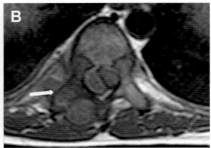

Fig. 28. Isolated posterior element tuberculosis in an 8-year-old boy who presented with lower dorsal posterior paraspinal swelling and back pain. Abnormal T2-weighted (*A*) and T1-weighted (*B*) intermediate signal intensity is seen in the right pedicle, transverse process and lamina of T8 vertebra on axial images (*white arrows*). The vertebral body is not involved. Abnormal right posterior paraspinal and epidural soft tissue is seen causing mild indentation on the thoracic cord (*black arrow*).

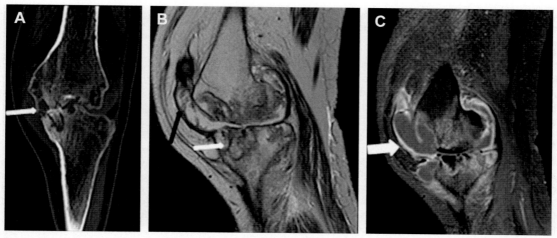

Fig. 30. Tubercular arthritis. A 37-year-old woman presented with long history of left knee pain. Coronal computed tomography (*A*), sagittal T2-weighted (*B*), and postcontrast T1-weighted (*C*) MR images show large subchondral peripherally enhancing erosions (*thin white arrows*), destruction of the cartilage, joint effusion and T2 intermediate synovial thickening (*black arrow*) with thin, smooth contrast enhancement (*thick white arrow*).

in tuberculous arthritis as compared with thick irregular margins in pyogenic arthritis.[80] MR imaging features, which are suggestive of tuberculous arthritis rather than pauciarticular rheumatoid arthritis, include large bone erosion with peripheral enhancement, uniform synovial thickening, and numerous extraarticular collections.[81]

Tuberculous Osteomyelitis

Tuberculous osteomyelitis is less common as compared with arthritis and represents less than 20% of musculoskeletal TB. Long bones are commonly involved with more common involvement of the femur and tibia.[46,71] Tuberculous osteomyelitis can also involve the small bones of the hands and feet, particularly in children. Calvarium and ribs can also be affected by tuberculous osteomyelitis. Solitary lesion is more common;

multifocal involvement is more common in immunocompromised patients and children.

Tuberculous osteomyelitis occurs from hematogeneous of spread of tubercle bacilli with resultant granuloma formation in the medullary cavity of metaphysis. Resultant focal osteopenia and bone destruction occurs. It commonly presents with history of chronic pain and swelling over a period of months as compared with acute pyogenic osteomyelitis, which presents within a few weeks.

Plain radiographs and computed tomography scan

Tuberculous osteomyelitis presents with a focal ill-defined lytic lesion in the metaphysis with or without cortical breakthrough. Associated periosseous soft tissue can be seen. Reactive sclerosis, sequestration and periostistis are

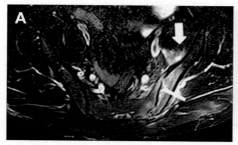
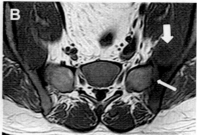

Fig. 31. Sacroiliac joint tubercular arthritis. Axial short T1 inversion recovery (*A*) and T1-weighted (*B*) MR images demonstrate subchondral erosions in the left sacroiliac joint with periarticular marrow edema (*thin arrows*). Edema is seen in adjacent soft tissues with a small collection in the left iliacus muscle (*thick arrows*) in a proven case of left sacroiliac joint tuberculosis.

uncommon.[45,75] CT scan is useful for early bone destruction and evaluation of calvarial TB.

Ultrasonography

Ultrasonography is useful for the evaluation of the soft issue component and abscess formation in addition to providing image guidance for aspiration and biopsy for histopathologic examination and culture/sensitivity.

MR imaging

MR imaging is the modality of choice for tuberculous osteomyelitis because it demonstrates early marrow involvement. Marrow changes appear hyperintense on T2-weighted images and hypointense on T1-weighted images with homogenous or heterogenous postcontrast enhancement. Bone necrosis appears as nonenhancing areas on postcontrast scan. Associated collections appear hyperintense on T2-weighted images and hypointense on T1-weighted images with minimal T1 hyperintense wall and thin peripheral postcontrast enhancement (**Figs. 32** and **33**). Associated sinus tract is excellently demonstrated on MR imaging.

Tuberculous Dactylitis

Tuberculous dactylitis occurs predominantly in children less than 6 years owing to the presence of hematopoietic marrow.[82,83] It usually presents with painless swelling over a period of months. Classical description of tuberculous dactylitis is spina ventosa (spina, *short bone* + ventosa, *inflated with air*).[84] Bones of the hand are more commonly affected than the feet, with the most common involvement of the proximal phalanx of

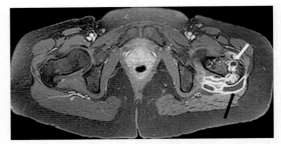

Fig. 33. Tubercular osteomyelitis with trochanteric bursitis. Postcontrast T1-weighted axial image shows a peripherally enhancing, centrally necrotic lesion in the left greater trochanter with cortical breach along the posteromedial aspect (*white arrow*). Associated trochanteric bursitis is also seen (*black arrow*).

the index and middle fingers. Diffuse osteopenia of involved phalanx/metacarpal is seen owing to medullary destruction by tuberculous granuloma with resorption of inner part cortex and expansion of bone. Cortical destruction may be seen with associated periosseous soft tissue component (**Fig. 34**). Periosteal reaction and sequestrum formation are classically absent. Sclerosis may be seen in long-standing disease and in the healing phase.[82,83,85] Bone density may return to normal on treatment with antituberculous therapy. Sequelae of tuberculous dactylitis include shortening of bone and deformity. In adults, tuberculous dactylitis usually affects flexor tendon sheaths with sparing of bone and joint.[85] The differential diagnosis includes pyogenic osteomyelitis (sequestrum common, painful swollen finger), syphilitic dactylitis (bilateral symmetric, periostistis,

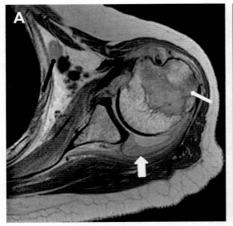
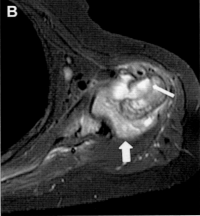

Fig. 32. Tubercular osteomyelitis with intraarticular extension. Axial T2-weighted (*A*) and short T1 inversion recovery (STIR) (*B*) MR images (STIR image at lower level) reveal abnormal T2 intermediate signal in the left humeral head, neck, and tuberosities with cortical breach along the anterior aspect (*thin white arrows*). Resultant glenohumeral arthritis is seen with abnormal synovial thickening and effusion (*thick white arrow*). Enlarged left axillary lymph node (*black arrow*) is also seen.

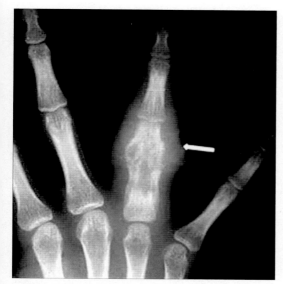

Fig. 34. Spina ventosa. Plain radiograph of the hand reveals a lytic expansile lesion in the proximal phalanx of the ring finger with associated soft tissue swelling (*arrow*). (*Courtesy of* Department of Radiology, KEM Hospital, Mumbai, with permission.)

absence of diffuse osteopenia and soft tissue swelling), enchondroma (punctate calcification), sarcoidosis (lytic lesions without bone expansion), leukemia, and hyperparathyroidism.[84,85] Associated present or past pulmonary TB may be seen. Confirmation usually requires biopsy with histopathologic demonstration of caseating granulomatous inflammation, polymerase chain reaction, and culture.

Calvarial Tuberculosis

Calvarial TB occurs secondary to hematogeneous spread of tuberculous bacilli in the diploic space. Destruction of both tables occurs, although outer table is affected first.[86] It occurs predominantly in young patients (<20 years) presenting with painless scalp swelling and/or discharging sinus. Neurologic deficit may be present in cases with significant epidural soft tissue and associated brain parenchymal TB. On plain radiographs and CT scan, it can present as a well-defined lytic lesion involving both inner and outer tables of skull with associated soft tissue swelling, diffuse lytic destruction of the inner table with epidural soft tissue, and a lytic lesion with peripheral sclerosis. Parietal and frontal bones are most commonly affected as expected, owing to the greater amount of cancellous bone.[86–89] CT scan and MR imaging permit excellent demonstration of the extent of bone destruction, subgaleal and epidural peripherally enhancing soft tissue, calcified foci in soft tissue, and associated brain parenchymal edema/tuberculoma and meningitis (**Fig. 35**). The destructive process is not limited by sutures.[86,88,90] The dura matter acts as a strong barrier for subdural and parenchyma extension of soft tissue. The soft tissue appears hypointense to intermediate intensity on T1-weighted imaging and intermediate to hyperintense on T2-weighted

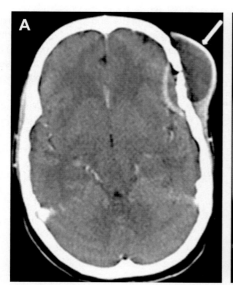
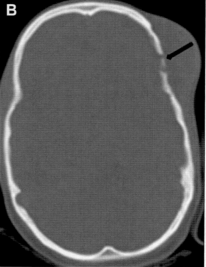

Fig. 35. Calvarial tuberculosis. Axial postcontrast soft tissue (*A*) and bone window (*B*) computed tomography images demonstrate bilobed, peripherally enhancing collection (*white arrow*) centered around ill-defined lytic destruction in the left frontal bone (*black arrow*). (*Courtesy of* Dr Darshana Sanghvi, Mumbai.)

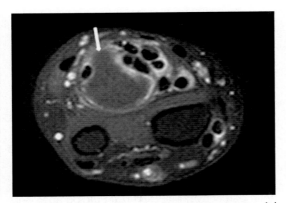

Fig. 36. Tubercular tenosynovitis. Postcontrast axial T1-weighted MR image depicts a thin, smooth, peripherally enhancing, large collection involving the flexor tendon sheath (*white arrow*).

images. An increased erythrocyte sedimentation rate and strongly positive Mantoux skin test are highly suggestive of calvarial TB.[88] Treatment consists of antituberculous therapy with surgical intervention only in cases of extensive bone destruction/sequestrum formation and associated large epidural soft tissues causing mass effect.

Soft Tissue Tuberculosis

Soft tissue TB is the least frequent form of musculoskeletal TB. It includes myositis with abscess formation, tenosynovitis, bursitis, and breast TB. Tuberculous myositis with abscess formation and bursal involvement is usually secondary to spread from adjacent osteomyelitis, arthritis and lymphadenopathy. The psoas muscle is commonly involved secondary to tuberculous spondylitis. The chest, abdominal wall, and extremity muscles may also be involved. Trochanteric, olecranon, prepatellar, and subacromial bursae are commonly involved.[71,76] These lesions reveal thin smooth peripheral enhancement (see **Fig. 33**). Tuberculous tenosynovitis most commonly involves flexor tendons of dominant hand with thickening of tendon/synovial sheath and minimal fluid collection.[91] T2 hypointense synovial thickening with thin homogenous contrast enhancement are characteristic of tuberculous etiology (**Fig. 36**).

SUMMARY

The incidence of ETB continues to increase slowly, especially in immunocompromised and multidrug-resistant TB patients. ETB manifests with nonspecific clinical symptoms, and being less frequent, is less familiar to most physicians. Imaging modalities of choice are CT (lymphadenopathy and abdominal TB) and MR imaging (CNS and

musculoskeletal system TB). ETB commonly involves multiple organ systems with characteristic imaging findings that permit accurate diagnosis and timely management.

ACKNOWLEDGMENTS

Authors thank Mr Sateesh K.D. for technical assistance in the preparation of the figures.

REFERENCES

1. Maclean KA, Becker AK, Chang SD, et al. Extrapulmonary tuberculosis: imaging features beyond the chest. Can Assoc Radiol J 2013;64(4):319–24.
2. Rafique A. The spectrum of tuberculosis presenting at a London district general hospital. West Lond Med J 2009;1(No 4):19–38.
3. Alrajhi AA, Al-Barrak AM. Extrapulmonary tuberculosis, epidemiology and patterns in Saudi Arabia. Saudi Med J 2002;23(5):503–8.
4. Garg RK. Classic diseases revisited: tuberculosis of the central nervous system. Postgrad Med J 1999; 75:133–40.
5. Thwaites GE, Tran TH. Tuberculous meningitis: many questions, too few answers. Lancet Neurol 2005;4: 160–70.
6. Rich AR, McCordock HA. Pathogenesis of tubercular meningitis. Bull Johns Hopkins Hosp 1933; 52:5–13.
7. Sheller JR, Des Prez RM. CNS tuberculosis. Neurol Clin 1986;4:143–58.
8. Galimi R. Extrapulmonary tuberculosis: tuberculous meningitis new developments. Eur Rev Med Pharmacol Sci 2011;15(No. 4):365–86.
9. Roos KL. Pearls and pitfalls in the diagnosis and management of central nervous system infectious diseases. Semin Neurol 1998;18(No. 2):185–96.
10. Kumar R, Kohli N, Thavnani H, et al. Value of CT scan in the diagnosis of meningitis. Indian Pediatr 1996; 33:465–8.
11. Przybojewski S, Andronikou S, Wilmshurst J. Objective CT criteria to determine the presence of abnormal basal enhancement in children with suspicious tuberculous meningitis. Pediatr Radiol 2006; 36:687–96.
12. Jinkins JR, Gupta R, Chang KH, et al. MR imaging of central nervous system tuberculosis. Radiol Clin North Am 1995;33:771–86.
13. Gupta RK, Kathuria MK, Pradhan S. Magnetization transfer MR imaging in CNS tuberculosis. AJNR Am J Neuroradiol 1999;20:867–75.
14. Villoria MF, de la Torre J, Fortea F, et al. Intracranial tuberculosis in AIDS: CT and MRI findings. Neuroradiology 1991;34:11–4.
15. Callebout J, Dormont D, Dubois B, et al. Contrast enhanced MR imaging of tuberculous pachymeningitis

cranialis hypertrophica: case report. AJNR Am J Neu-roradiol 1990;11:821–2.

16. Celso L, Domingues RC. Intracranial infections. In: Atlas SW, editor. Magnetic resonance imaging of the brain and spine. Philadelphia: Lippincott-Raven; 1996. p. 738–42.

17. Yadav YR, Mukerji G, Parihar V, et al. Complex hydrocephalus (combination of communicating and obstructive type): an important cause of failed endoscopic third ventriculostomy. BMC Res Notes 2009; 2:137.

18. Gupta R, Lufkin RB. MR imaging and spectroscopy of Central Nervous System Infections. New York: Kluwer Academic / Plenum publishers; 2001.

19. Misra UK, Kalita J, Maurya PK. Stroke in tuberculous meningitis. J Neurol Sci 2011;303(1–2):22–30.

20. Gupta RK. Tuberculosis and other non-tuberculous bacterial granulomatous infections. In: Gupta RK, Lufkin RB, editors. MR imaging and spectroscopy of central nervous system infection. New York: Kluwer Academic/Plenum Publishers; 2001. p. 95–145.

21. Patkar D, Narang J, Yanamandala R, et al. Central nervous system tuberculosis: pathophysiology and imaging findings. Neuroimaging Clin N Am 2012; 22(4):677–705.

22. Garcia-Monco JC. Central nervous system tuberculosis. Neurol Clin 1999;17:737–59.

23. Dastur DK, Manghani DK, Udani PM. Pathology and pathogenetic mechanisms in neurotuberculosis. Radiol Clin North Am 1995;33:733–52.

24. Kesavadas C, Somasundaram S, Rao RM, et al. Meckel's cave tuberculoma with unusual infratemporal extension. J Neuroimaging 2007;17:264–8.

25. Salem R, Khochtali I, Jellali MA, et al. Isolated hypophyseal tuberculoma: often mistaken. Neurochirurgie 2009;55:603–6.

26. Gupta RK, Kumar S. Central nervous system tuberculosis. Neuroimaging Clin N Am 2011; 21(4):795–814. vii-viii.

27. Naphade PS, Raut AA, Pai BU. Magnetic resonance perfusion and spectroscopy in a giant tuberculoma. Neurol India 2011;59(6):913–4.

28. Luthra G, Parihar A, Nath K, et al. Comparative evaluation of fungal, tubercular, and pyogenic brain abscesses with conventional and diffusion MR imaging and proton MR spectroscopy. AJNR Am J Neuroradiol 2007;28(7):1332–8.

29. Jinkins JR. Focal tuberculous cerebritis. AJNR Am J Neuroradiol 1988;9(1):121–4.

30. Kent DC. Tuberculous lymphadenitis: not a localized disease process. Am J Med Sci 1967;254:866–74.

31. Manolidis S, Frenkiel S, Yoskovitch A, et al. Mycobacterial infections of the head and neck. Otolaryngol Head Neck Surg 1993;109(3 Pt 1):427–33.

32. Finfer M, Perchick A, Burstein DE. Fine needle aspiration biopsy diagnosis of tuberculous lymphadenitis in patients with and without the acquired

immune deficiency syndrome. Acta Cytol 1991;35: 325–32.

33. Pombo F, Rodriguez E, Mato J, et al. Patterns of contrast enhancement of tuberculous lymph nodes demonstrated by computed tomography. Clin Radiol 1992;46:13–7.

34. Hanson RD, Hunter TB. Tuberculous peritonitis: CT appearance. Am J Roentgenol 1985;144:931–2.

35. Sanai FM, Bzeizi KI. Systematic review: tuberculous peritonitis–presenting features, diagnostic strategies and treatment. Aliment Pharmacol Ther 2005; 22(8):685–700.

36. Leder RA, Low VH. Tuberculosis of the abdomen. Radiol Clin North Am 1995;33(4):691–705.

37. Tandon HD, Prakash A. Pathology of intestinal tuberculosis and its distinction from Crohn's disease. Gut 1972s;13(4):260–9.

38. Carrera GF, Young S, Lewicki AM. Intestinal tuberculosis. Gastrointest Radiol 1976;1(2):147–55.

39. Sharma MP, Bhatia V. Abdominal tuberculosis. Indian J Med Res 2004;120(4):305–15.

40. Ramakantan R, Shah P. Tuberculous fistulas of the pharynx and esophagus. Gastrointest Radiol 1990; 15(2):145–7.

41. Bhargava DK, Shriniwas, Chopra P, et al. Peritoneal tuberculosis; laparoscopic pattern and its diagnostic accuracy. Am J Gastroenterol 1992;87: 109–12.

42. Kalra N, Agrawal P, Mittal V, et al. Spectrum of imaging findings on MDCT enterography in patients with small bowel tuberculosis. Clin Radiol 2014;69(3): 315–22.

43. Kelestimur F. The endocrinology of adrenal tuberculosis: the effects of tuberculosis on the hypothalamo-pituitary-adrenal axis and adrenocortical function. J Endocrinol Invest 2004;27(4):380–6.

44. Upadhyay J, Sudhindra P, Abraham G, et al. Tuberculosis of the adrenal gland: a case report and review of the literature of infections of the adrenal gland. Int J Endocrinol 2014;2014:876037.

45. Burrill J, Williams CJ, Bain G, et al. Tuberculosis: a radiologic review. Radiographics 2007;27(5): 1255–73.

46. Engin G, Acunas B, Acunas G, et al. Imaging of extrapulmonary tuberculosis. Radiographics 2000;20: 471–88.

47. Tonkin AK, Witten DM. Genitourinary tuberculosis. Semin Roentgenol 1979;14:305–18.

48. Pasternak MS, Rubin RH. Urinary tract tuberculosis. In: Schrier RW, editor. Diseases of the kidney and urinary tract. 7th edition. Philadelphia: Lippincott Williams & Wilkins; 2001. p. 1017–37.

49. Wang LJ, Wong YC, Chen CJ, et al. CT features of genitourinary tuberculosis. J Comput Assist Tomogr 1997;21:254–8.

50. Kapoor R, Ansari MS, Mandhani A, et al. Clinical presentation and diagnostic approach in cases of

genitourinary tuberculosis. Indian J Urol 2008;24(3): 401–5.

51. Negi SS, Khan SF, Gupta S, et al. Comparison of the conventional diagnostic modalities, bactec culture and polymerase chain reaction test for diagnosis of tuberculosis. Indian J Med Microbiol 2005;23:29–33.

52. Medlar EM. Cases of renal infection in pulmonary tuberculosis: evidence of healed tuberculosis lesions. Am J Pathol 1926;2:401–13.

53. Merchant S, Bharati A, Merchant N. Tuberculosis of the genitourinary system-urinary tract tuberculosis: renal tuberculosis—Part I. Indian J Radiol Imaging 2013;23(1):46–63.

54. Kollins SA, Hartman GW, Carr DT, et al. Roentgenographic findings in urinary tract tuberculosis: a 10 year review. Am J Roentgenol Radium Ther Nucl Med 1974;121:487–99.

55. Davidson AJ, Hartman DS, Choyke PL, et al. Parenchymal disease with normal size and contour. In: Davidson AJ, editor. Davidson's radiology of the kidney and genitourinary tract. 3rd edition. Philadelphia: Saunders; 1999. p. 327–58.

56. Premkumar A, Lattimer J, Newhouse JH. CT and sonography of advanced urinary tract tuberculosis. AJR Am J Roentgenol 1987;148:65–9.

57. Gow JG. Renal calcification in genito-urinary tuberculosis. Br J Surg 1965;52:283–8.

58. Kenney PJ. Imaging of chronic renal infections. AJR Am J Roentgenol 1990;155:485–94.

59. Elkin M. Urogenital tuberculosis. In: Pollack HM, editor. Clinical urography. Philadelphia: WB Saunders; 1990. p. 1020–52.

60. Becker JA. Renal tuberculosis. Urol Radiol 1988;10: 25–30.

61. Merchant S, Bharati A, Merchant N. Tuberculosis of the genitourinary system—urinary tract tuberculosis: renal tuberculosis-Part II. Indian J Radiol Imaging 2013;23(1):64–77.

62. Gurski J, Baker KC. An unusual presentation: renal tuberculosis. ScientificWorldJournal 2008;8:1254–5.

63. Lu P, Li C, Zhou X. Significance of the CT scan in renal tuberculosis. Zhonghua Jie He Hu Xi Za Zhi 2001;24:407–9.

64. Kawashima A, Sandler CM, Ernst RD, et al. Renal inflammatory disease: the current role of CT. Crit Rev Diagn Imaging 1997;38:369–415.

65. Narayana A. Overview of renal tuberculosis. Urology 1982;19:231–7.

66. Harisinghani MG, McLoud TC, Shepard JA, et al. Tuberculosis from head to toe. Radiographics 2000;20:449–70.

67. Kim SH. Genitourinary tuberculosis. In: Pollack HM, Dyer R, McClennan BL, editors. Clinical urography. 2nd edition. Philadelphia: Saunders; 2000. p. 1193–228.

68. Michaelides M, Sotiriadis C, Konstantinou D, et al. Tuberculous orchitis US and MRI findings. Correlation with histopathological findings. Hippokratia 2010;14(4):297–9.

69. YY1 Jung, Kim JK, Cho KS. Genitourinary tuberculosis: comprehensive cross-sectional imaging. AJR Am J Roentgenol 2005;184(1):143–50.

70. Abdelwahab IF, Bianchi S, Martinoli C, et al. Atypical extraspinal musculoskeletal tuberculosis in immunocompetent patients, a review. Part I: atypical osteoarticular tuberculosis and tuberculous osteomyelitis. Can Assoc Radiol J 2006;57(2):86–94.

71. Andronikou S, Bindapersad M, Govender N, et al. Musculoskeletal tuberculosis - imaging using low-end and advanced modalities for developing and developed countries. Acta Radiol 2011;52(4):430–41.

72. Suh JS, Lee JD, Cho JH, et al. MR imaging of tuberculous arthritis: clinical and experimental studies. J Magn Reson Imaging 1996;6:185–9.

73. Jaovisidha S, Chen C, Ryu KN, et al. Tuberculous tenosynovitis and bursitis: imaging findings in 21 cases. Radiology 1996;201:507–13.

74. Martini M, Adjrad A, Boudjemaa A. Tuberculous osteomyelitis: a review of 125 cases. Int Orthop 1986;10:201–7.

75. De Backer AI, Mortelé KJ, Vanhoenacker FM, et al. Imaging of extraspinal musculoskeletal tuberculosis. Eur J Radiol 2006;57(1):119–30.

76. De Backer AI, Vanhoenacker FM, Sanghvi DA. Imaging features of extraaxial musculoskeletal tuberculosis. Indian J Radiol Imaging 2009;19(3):176–86.

77. Lee KY. Comparison of pyogenic spondylitis and tuberculous spondylitis. Asian Spine J 2014;8(2):216–23.

78. Sinan T, Al-Khawari H, Ismail M, et al. Spinal tuberculosis: CT and MRI feature. Ann Saudi Med 2004; 24(6):437–41.

79. Jung NY, Jee WH, Ha KY, et al. Discrimination of tuberculous spondylitis from pyogenic spondylitis on MRI. AJR Am J Roentgenol 2004;182(6):1405–10.

80. Hong SH, Kim SM, Ahn JM, et al. Tuberculous versus pyogenic arthritis: MR imaging evaluation. Radiology 2001;218(3):848–53.

81. Choi JA, Koh SH, Hong SH, et al. Rheumatoid arthritis and tuberculous arthritis: differentiating MRI features. AJR Am J Roentgenol 2009;193(5):1347–53.

82. Andronikou S, Smith B. "Spina ventosa"–tuberculous dactylitis. Arch Dis Child 2002;86(3):206.

83. Bhaskar, Khonglah T, Bareh J. Tuberculous dactylitis (spina ventosa) with concomitant ipsilateral axillary scrofuloderma in an immunocompetent child: a rare presentation of skeletal tuberculosis. Adv Biomed Res 2013;2:29. eCollection 2013.

84. Singhal S, Arbart A, Lanjewar A, et al. Tuberculous dactylitis - a rare manifestation of adult skeletal tuberculosis. Indian J Tuberculosis 2005;52:218–9.

85. Hassan FO. Tuberculous dactylitis pseudotumor of an adult thumb: a case report. Strateg Trauma Limb Reconstr 2010;5(1):53–6.

86. Diyora B, Kumar R, Modgi R, et al. Calvarial tuberculosis: a report of eleven patients. Neurol India 2009; 57(5):607–12.

87. Singh Jain R, Prakash S, Mathur T, et al. Calvarial tuberculosis with intracranial tuberculomas: a rare association. J Neurol Res 2013;3(3–4):130–2.

88. Raut AA, Nagar AM, Muzumdar D, et al. Imaging features of calvarial tuberculosis: a study of 42 cases. AJNR Am J Neuroradiol 2004;25(3):409–14.

89. Safia R, Zeeba J, Sujata J. Calvarial tuberculosis: a rare localisation of a common disease. Ann Trop Med Publ Health 2013;6:309–11.

90. Rajmohan BP, Anto D, Alappat JP. Calvarial tuberculosis. Neurol India 2004;52(2):278–9.

91. Hoffman KL, Bergman AG, Hoffman DK, et al. Tuberculous tenosynovitis of the flexor tendons of the wrist: MR imaging with pathologic correlation. Skeletal Radiol 1996;25:186–8.

Multidetector Computed Tomography and MR Imaging Findings in Mycotic Infections

Niranjan Khandelwal, MD, Dip NBE, FICR, FAMS[a],*,
Kushaljit Singh Sodhi, MD, PhD, MAMS, FICR[a],
Anindita Sinha, MD[a], Jyothi G. Reddy, DNB[b],
Eshwar N. Chandra, MD, DNB, FRCR, FICR[b,1]

KEYWORDS

• CT • MR imaging • Fungal • Imaging • Opportunistic • Infections

KEY POINTS

- Human fungal infections vary from simple colonizations, as in an aspergilloma, to frank invasive infections.
- Imaging characteristics are variable and depend on the type of fungal infection as well as the host response.
- Common imaging features of fungal infection on multidetector computed tomography and MR imaging are highlighted in this article to familiarize readers with characteristic imaging features that facilitate early and accurate diagnosis.

INTRODUCTION

The global incidence of fungal infections continues to increase, particularly in patients with compromised immune function and chronic systemic disorders. Among the pathogenic fungi, there are 2 distinct groups:

1. Primary pathogens that most frequently infect healthy individuals. These include species like *Blastomyces*, *Coccidioides*, *Histoplasma*, and *Paracoccidioides*.
2. Opportunistic invaders. These fungi invade debilitated or immunocompromised individuals. Fungal infections in individuals with human immunodeficiency virus (HIV) infection and organ/stem cell transplant recipients

on immunosuppressive therapy are prototype examples. Prototype examples of opportunistic fungi include *Aspergillus*, *Candida*, and *Cryptococcus*.[1,2]

Knowledge of the spectrum of imaging findings that support the diagnosis helps in prompt treatment. This article therefore reviews predisposing factors, epidemiology, pathogenicity, clinical manifestations, and imaging morphology of different fungal infections.

CENTRAL NERVOUS SYSTEM INFECTION

Fungal infections of the central nervous system (CNS) are rare and occur mostly in immunocompromised patients, especially those with HIV

Disclosure Statement: The authors have nothing to disclose.
[a] Department of Radiodiagnosis, Post Graduate Institute of Medical Education & Research, Sector 12, Chandigarh 160012, India; [b] Department of Radiology, Kamineni Academy of Medical Sciences & Research Centre, LB Nagar, Hyderabad, Telangana 500068, India
[1] Present address: Plot No. 81, Road No. 6, Arunodayanagar, Nagole, Hyderabad, Telangana 500068, India.
* Corresponding author.
E-mail address: khandelwaln@hotmail.com

Radiol Clin N Am 54 (2016) 503–518
http://dx.doi.org/10.1016/j.rcl.2015.12.002
0033-8389/16/$ – see front matter © 2016 Elsevier Inc. All rights reserved.

infection and transplant recipients. Select CNS fungal infections such as mucormycosis are seen most frequently in patients with long-standing and uncontrolled diabetes mellitus (**Fig. 1**). In addition, some fungal infections are endemic to specific geographic areas: coccidioidomycosis, blastomycosis, and histoplasmosis are endemic in the southwest, Midwest, and the northeastern parts of the United States respectively.

On magnetic resonance (MR) imaging, fungal abscesses appear as solid or ring-enhancing lesions. On diffusion-weighted imaging (DWI), low apparent diffusion coefficient has been found in fungal abscesses.[3] The fungal abscesses typically show restricted diffusion caused by high viscosity and cellularity; the pattern of diffusion restriction may be heterogeneous or peripheral ringlike.[3] On MR spectroscopy, fungal lesions show increased levels of lipids, lactate, alanine, acetate, succinate, and choline. Unidentified multiple signals between 3.6 and 3.8 ppm are caused by the presence of trehalose sugar in the fungal wall.[4]

The common fungi to affect the brain include *Aspergillus*, *Mucor*, *Cryptococcus*, *Candida*, and *Blastomyces* species.

Aspergillosis

Invasive aspergillosis is seen in patients on chemotherapy and immunosuppressive therapy after solid organ or bone marrow transplant. Intracranial aspergillosis may occur from hematogenous spread, CSF seeding, or contiguous extension from adjacent tissues. The 2 main types of aspergillosis are rhinocerebral and cerebrovascular forms. Rhinocerebral aspergillosis results from contiguous spread of infection from the nasal cavity and paranasal sinuses to the brain. Hematogenous seeding leads to occlusion of large and medium-sized arteries by the hyphal forms.

Imaging patterns consist of infarcts, single or multiple ring-enhancing lesions caused by abscess formation, and dural or parenchymal infiltration caused by contiguous spread from paranasal sinuses or orbital infections. The *Aspergillus* species are angioinvasive; they produce elastase that digests the vessel wall, thereby causing microhemorrhage. Vessel wall weakening may lead to development of mycotic aneurysms.

Hematogenous Spread

Acute infarcts are an early manifestation, and are best detected by using DWI. Involvement of the basal ganglia is a characteristic finding. Cerebritis is usually located in the basal ganglia and deep white matter and does not show enhancement. An abscess most often results in the infarcted brain.

Fungal abscesses typically show an irregular outer margin of the wall and peripheral rim enhancement. A nonenhancing intracavitary projection caused by fungal elements containing paramagnetic substances is also typically seen. Restricted diffusion is common in the projections and the walls of the abscess. Fungal vasculitis may lead to mycotic aneurysm formation.[5,6]

Rhinocerebral Spread

Initial manifestation may show nonspecific mucosal thickening with enhancement of the sinuses on computed tomography (CT) or MR imaging. Infiltration and erosion of the bone with

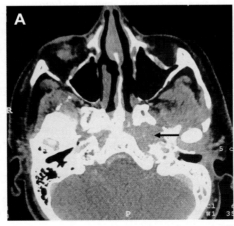
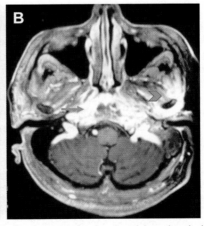

Fig. 1. A 52-year-old uncontrolled diabetic with *Aspergillus fumigatus* infection involving the skull base. Axial contrast-enhanced CT scan (*A*) shows infiltrative soft tissue (*arrow*) destroying the left petrous apex. Axial postcontrast T1 fat-suppressed magnetic resonance (MR) image (*B*) shows extensive infiltrative enhancing soft tissue in the skull base involving clivus (*arrow in B*) and bilateral petrous apex and extending into left masticator space and left temporomandibular joint (*arrowhead in B*).

localized meningitis and parenchymal involvement occurs late.

Parenchymal involvement is characterized by signal abnormality commonly in basifrontal or anterior temporal lobes that are contiguous with the adjacent rhinosinus disease.

On imaging, aspergillosis shows T1 hypointensity, T2-hyperintense center with hypointense wall, and mild to moderate ringlike contrast enhancement.

Cryptococcosis

Cryptococcosis is the most common opportunistic fungal infection of the CNS in patients with HIV. Infection usually starts as meningitis with a propensity to spread along the Virchow-Robin spaces. Parenchymal involvement present as cryptococcomas, dilated Virchow-Robin spaces, or enhancing cortical nodules that are most commonly distributed in the midbrain and the basal ganglia[7] (**Fig. 2**).

Cryptococcal lesions may have high or low attenuation on CT. MR imaging shows T1 and T2 prolongation, no diffusion restriction, and variable enhancement. Enhancement is more common in immunocompetent hosts, because of the presence of an effective inflammatory response. Meningoencephalitis manifests as T2 hyperintensity within the region of involvement; meningeal enhancement may be seen. MR spectroscopy shows marked increase in lactate level with decrease in N-acetyl aspartate, choline, and creatine levels.[8]

Mucormycosis

Mucormycosis is an acute and often lethal opportunistic infection, typically affecting immunocompromised patients or those with uncontrolled

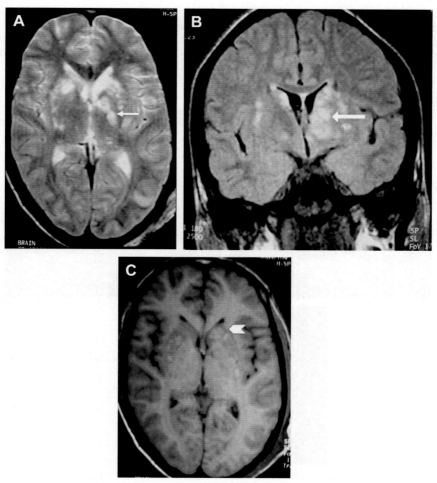

Fig. 2. Cryptococcomas. T2-weighted axial (*A*), fluid-attenuated inversion recovery (FLAIR) coronal (*B*) and T1 axial postcontrast images (*C*) in an immunocompromised patient. The lesions are hyperintense on T2 and FLAIR (*arrows in A and B*) with ring-enhancing/disc-enhancing lesions (*arrowhead in C*) in bilateral basal ganglia.

diabetes. The fungi cause a necrotizing vasculitis that extends rapidly into deep face, orbits, and brain through the skull base and neural foramina[9] (**Fig. 3**). Cerebral angioinvasion may lead to mycotic aneurysms, dissection, or thrombosis of the internal carotid artery with subsequent cerebral infarction.[9]

IMAGING

CT shows mucosal thickening, opacification of the affected paranasal sinuses, and periorbital tissue destruction. On MR imaging, sinus disease shows hypointensity on T1-weighted imaging (T1WI) and T2-weighted imaging (T2WI). Intracranial manifestations include high T2-weighted signal in the basal portions of the frontal and temporal lobes with mild mass effect that represents a combination of inflammation and infarction secondary to vascular invasion. Thrombosis of the cavernous portion of the internal carotid artery is well detected on MR angiography. A less common clinical manifestation includes hematogenous spread leading to central infarcts or granulomas.

Candidiasis

Candidiasis is caused by the pathogenic yeast, *Candida albicans*. The gastrointestinal tract is the site of entry for patients with diabetes mellitus and lymphoproliferative diseases. Intravenous drug abusers and patients in intensive care units may develop the disease after iatrogenic inoculation by way of indwelling catheters. Primary CNS candidiasis is rare, mostly secondary to hematogenous dissemination. Although neonates typically manifest acutely progressive meningitis, candidiasis in adults has a chronic course. Other patterns of CNS involvement include microabscesses and small hemorrhagic infarcts caused by arterial thrombosis.

CT shows hypodense foci that on contrast examination may show nodular or ring enhancement. MR imaging shows abnormal meningeal enhancement, which appears as thicker, lumpy, or nodular enhancement in the subarachnoid space. Microabscesses are seen as areas of hypointensity on T1-weighted images; lesions appear as nodular or ring-enhancing lesions. They are more common in the territory of the anterior or middle cerebral

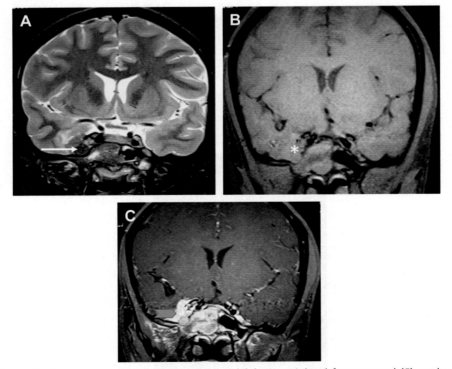

Fig. 3. Rhinocerebral mucormycosis. Coronal T2-weighted (*A*), T1-weighted fat-saturated (*B*), and postcontrast T1-weighted (*C*) images on a 3-T MR system of a 16-year-old shows a predominantly hypointense lesion on T2-weighted images (*arrow in A*) in the right cavernous sinus and Meckel cave. The lesion is isointense on T1-weighted images (*asterisk in B*) and shows heterogeneous contrast enhancement (*arrowhead in C*).

arteries and present at the junction of gray-white matter.[10]

Blastomycosis

Blastomycosis rarely affects the CNS. Most cases present as features of chronic meningitis.

Occasionally, extra-axial, plaquelike lesions that are hypointense on T1WI and T2WI are seen. These show significant contrast enhancement that mimic en plaque meningiomas on imaging.

HEAD AND NECK

Fungal involvement of the head and neck can manifest as ulceration of the mucosal surfaces, lymph-nodal enlargement, and most commonly as sinonasal disease.[11,12]

Fungal sinusitis can have variable imaging features depending on host immunity and the tissue response. Fungal sinusitis can be invasive or noninvasive. Invasive fungal sinusitis manifests as acute or chronic invasive disease or a chronic granulomatous disease. Noninvasive fungal sinusitis presents as an allergic sinusitis syndrome or with mycetoma formation. The most common species include *Aspergillus* and *Mucor*.

Acute Invasive Sinusitis

It is typically seen in immunosuppressed patients, often with hematological malignancies or uncontrolled diabetes mellitus. The hallmark of the disease is angioinvasion with extensive tissue destruction and a poor prognosis. *Aspergillus* and *Mucor* species are the most commonly implicated organisms. On CT, it appears as unilateral,

marked, soft tissue thickening of the nasal cavity (**Fig. 4**). Associated sinus mucosal thickening, soft tissue attenuation, as well as bone destruction with orbital or intracranial extension may be seen.

MR imaging is superior to CT in showing intraorbital and intracranial extension. Periantral fat obliteration should be diligently assessed for an early diagnosis.[13] In late stages, cerebritis, abscesses, granulomas, cavernous sinus thrombosis, and infarcts may be noted.

Chronic Invasive Sinusitis

Chronic invasive sinusitis is most often caused by *Aspergillus fumigatus* and typically occurs in immunocompetent individuals, although diabetic patients are more susceptible. Mucosal thickening is seen in the sinuses with lysis of the bony walls and extrasinus extension. Sclerosis of the bony walls may be present in some instances. In invasive disease, differentiation from malignancy may not be possible at imaging.[14]

Chronic Granulomatous Fungal Sinusitis

This condition is caused by *Aspergillus flavus* and is found in limited geographic locations, predominantly in Africa and Southeast Asia.[15] The disease usually manifests in immunocompetent individuals. The disease shows a slowly progressive course with invasion of the sinus walls, and intraorbital and intracranial extension.

Noninvasive Fungal Sinusitis

The most common pattern of fungal sinusitis is allergic fungal sinusitis, which develops in patients with asthma or atopy. On CT, there is involvement

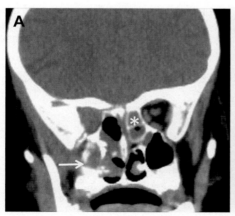
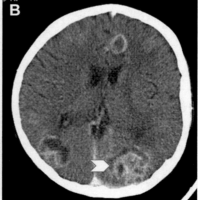

Fig. 4. Fungal sinusitis caused by mucormycosis in a 7-year-old with leukemia. (*A*) Noncontrast CT scan of the paranasal sinuses shows mucosal thickening of ethmoidal sinuses (*asterisk*) and right maxillary sinus (*arrow*) with sclerosis as well as areas of bone rarefaction and destruction. (*B*) Contrast-enhanced CT scan of fungal abscesses in a different neutropenic patient showing multiple ring-enhancing lesions with conglomerate lesions in left occipital lobe (*arrowhead*).

of multiple sinuses and nasal cavities with expansion and hyperattenuating soft tissue. MR imaging shows variable signal on T1WI and hypointensity on T2WI. Low T2 attenuation is attributed to the presence of high protein content, low water content, and the presence of various metals.[16]

Mycetoma is usually caused by *A flavus* or *A fumigatus* and consists of a fungal ball, most often in the maxillary sinus with little inflammatory reaction. The lesion appears hyperattenuating at CT because of the presence of hyphae.[17]

PULMONARY FUNGAL INFECTION

Knowledge of the background history of the patient is crucial in arriving at a possible causal diagnosis in pulmonary fungal infections. History of living in an endemic region or recent travel history to an endemic region may provide a clue to the diagnosis. Recent studies have highlighted the role of MR imaging, which has shown similar accuracy to high-resolution CT (HRCT) in detecting pulmonary infiltrates in neutropenic patients with leukemia.[18,19]

Opportunistic infections such as aspergillus, mucormycosis, and candida predominate in patients with neutropenia.[20,21] *Cryptococcus neoformans*, *Histoplasma capsulatum*, *Coccidioides immitis*, and *Blastomyces dermatitidis* are most common in patients with T-lymphocyte defects.[22] *Pneumocystis jiroveci* can occur in acquired immunodeficiency syndrome (AIDS), patients with cancer, organ transplant recipients, and in those on immunosuppressive therapy.[23,24]

Aspergillosis

The most important *Aspergillus* species from a human infectious disease point of view is *A fumigatus*. This article discusses 5 forms of pulmonary aspergillosis.[25]

Saprophytic aspergillosis (aspergilloma)

Although many patients are asymptomatic, the most common presentation of an aspergilloma is hemoptysis.[25] Aspergilloma usually appears as a soft tissue density mass within a cavity, creating the characteristic air-crescent sign, and often shows mobility with decubitus imaging[25] (**Fig. 5**).

Hypersensitivity reaction (allergic bronchopulmonary aspergillosis)

Allergic bronchopulmonary aspergillosis (ABPA) is a hypersensitivity reaction that is characterized by eosinophilia, asthma, central bronchiectasis, mucoid impaction, atelectasis, and consolidation.[25–27] Clinical features include wheezing, low-grade fever, cough, and productive sputum. Patients with chronic ABPA may also have a history of recurrent pneumonia. HRCT findings of ABPA include central bronchiectasis (usually varicose or cylindrical), bronchial occlusion caused by mucous plugging, and bronchial wall thickening. High attenuation of the impacted mucus or frank calcification is present in 30% patients[25] (**Fig. 6**). A tree-in-bud appearance and centrilobular nodules resulting from mucus filling the bronchioles may be seen, but in most patients with ABPA the peripheral airways appear normal. Parenchymal abnormalities, including consolidation, collapse, cavitation, and bullae, may be identified in as many as 40% of cases, particularly in the upper lobes. High-attenuation mucus and central bronchiectasis have been shown to be predictors of relapse as well as of immunologic severity.[26]

Semi-invasive (chronic necrotizing) aspergillosis

This form of aspergillosis is characterized by the presence of tissue necrosis and granulomatous inflammation simulating reactivated tuberculosis.[25] Predisposing factors include advanced age, chronic obstructive pulmonary disease, low-dose

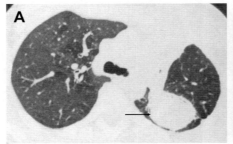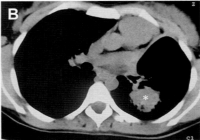

Fig. 5. Aspergilloma. Axial CT scan of the chest of an 18 year old female with past history of pulmonary tuberculosis and present complaints of hemoptysis and fever. A cavitary lesion is seen in the left upper lobe with an air crescent and intracavitary soft tissue (*arrow in A*). Hyperdense foci (*asterisk in B*) are seen within the soft tissue on Non Contrast CT, probably due to active haemorrhage. Total IgE (18061IU/mL) as well as *Aspergillus* specific IgE levels (31.6) were raised and *Aspergillus* skin test was positive.

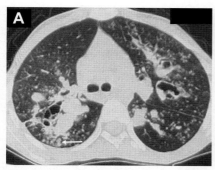
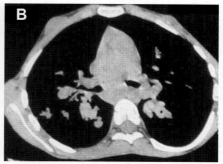

Fig. 6. Allergic bronchopulmonary aspergillosis. Axial HRCT chest lung (*A*) and mediastinal window (*B*) in a 12-year-old girl with increasing cough and breathlessness over the previous 2 years. Absolute eosinophil count was 330/μL and IgE levels were 25,000 IU/mL with increased *Aspergillus*-specific IgE level. Bilateral central bronchiectasis with bronchial plugging (*asterisk*) and hyperdense soft tissue are present. Centrilobular nodules and tree-in-bud opacities are also seen in bilateral lungs (*arrow*).

corticosteroid use, alcoholism, tuberculosis, diabetes mellitus, collagen-vascular diseases, and preexisting structural lung disease, such as pneumoconioses or prior radiation. Clinical presentation is nonspecific, consisting of low-grade fever with productive cough and occasionally hemoptysis. Imaging features of semi-invasive aspergillosis mimic active tuberculosis. Radiological features include multifocal segmental consolidation with or without cavitation and adjacent pleural thickening. Necrotizing aspergillus bronchitis may appear as an endobronchial mass with distal atelectasis or obstructive pneumonitis[25] (**Fig. 7**).

Airway-invasive aspergillosis
Aspergillus within airways may invade the airway wall and peribronchial or peribronchiolar lung, a condition known as airway-invasive aspergillosis or aspergillus bronchopneumonia.

This condition occurs most commonly in immunosuppressed patients and manifests as acute tracheobronchitis, bronchiolitis, and bronchopneumonia.[25] Patients with acute tracheobronchitis usually have normal radiological findings. Bronchiolitis presents on HRCT as patchy centrilobular nodules that in places may show tree-in-bud configuration. Bronchopneumonia usually presents with peribronchial consolidation. Radiologically, it cannot be differentiated from bronchopneumonia caused by other organisms. Obstructing bronchopulmonary aspergillosis is a noninvasive disease characterized by the presence of massive intraluminal overgrowth of *Aspergillus* species, usually in patients with AIDS.[25] Clinical presentation comprises cough with expectoration of fungal casts of bronchi, fever, new-onset asthma, and sometimes severe hypoxemia.[25] Imaging features mimic ABPA with bronchiectasis, bronchiolectasis, mucoid impaction, and lower lobe consolidation.

Angioinvasive aspergillosis
Aspergillus hyphae may invade the pulmonary vasculature, causing thrombosis, pulmonary hemorrhage, and infarction. This condition, known as angioinvasive aspergillosis, is almost exclusively seen in severely neutropenic patients. Characteristic CT findings include presence of the halo

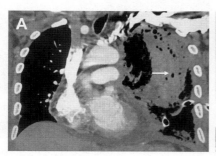
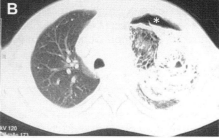

Fig. 7. Semi-invasive aspergillosis. Extensive necrotizing pneumonia on contrast-enhanced CT mediastinal (*A*) and lung window (*B*) with consolidation and multiple intraparenchymal mottled lucencies (*arrow*) replacing the left upper lobe in a 70-year-old man with a 3-month history of cough and occasional hemoptysis. The patient also had pericardial effusion and left-sided pneumothorax (*asterisk*).

sign, which signifies a nodule surrounded by a halo of ground-glass opacity caused by hemorrhage and peripheral wedge-shaped consolidation with or without areas of internal breakdown representative of pulmonary infarcts.[28]

Pneumocystis jiroveci (Pneumocystis carinii)

P jiroveci, previously known as *Pneumocystis carinii*, was initially classified as a protozoan but is now thought to be a fungus. It commonly occurs in HIV-positive patients with a CD4+ cell count less than 200 cells/mm^3.[29] It may also occur in other immunosuppressed patients, such as transplant recipients on immunosuppression or corticosteroid therapy. Infection in immunocompetent patients may also occur infrequently.

HRCT findings include extensive ground-glass opacities without pleural effusion. Crazy-paving pattern and consolidation develops later; the latter being more common in immunocompetent patients, reflecting damage caused by host immune response.[30] Some patients show the presence of lung cysts or pneumatoceles, which predisposes the patients to pneumothorax.

Zygomycosis

Zygomycosis encompasses the spectrum of fungal diseases caused by *Rhizopus*, *Rhizomucor*, and *Mucor*. Mucormycosis is the most important fungal disease. Predisposing factors include poorly controlled diabetes mellitus, especially in the setting of ketoacidosis, organ transplant, chronic renal failure, chemotherapy, corticosteroid therapy, AIDS, and hematologic malignancies.[31] Radiological findings are nonspecific and include multifocal airspace consolidations, single discrete nodules/masses or multiple, ill-defined nodules or masses (**Figs. 8** and **9**). Reverse halo sign and bird's nest sign have been described in mucormycosis; the former represents peripheral consolidation surrounding a central area of ground-glass opacity, and the latter represents associated irregular and intersecting areas of stranding or irregular lines within the area of ground-glass opacity.[32] These signs have also been described in aspergillosis. Pleural effusions and lymphadenopathy may also occur.

Cryptococcosis

C neoformans is found worldwide, especially in soil contaminated by bird excreta. Although the CNS is the most common affected organ system, pulmonary cryptococcal infections are also common. Typical patients have AIDS, with CD4 counts less than 100 cells/mm^3.[31] Immunocompetent patients with the disease are either asymptomatic or

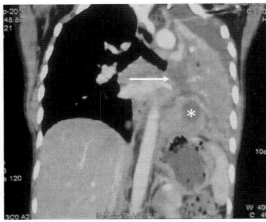

Fig. 8. Mucormycosis. Contrast-enhanced CT scan of the chest (coronal multiplanar reconstruction [MPR]) in an immunocompetent 25-year-old woman shows hypodense contents within left main bronchus (*arrow*) extending contiguously to the left upper and lower lobe bronchus. An abscess (*asterisk*) is seen in the lower lobe of the collapsed left lung. Bronchoscopic aspirate yielded mucormycosis. Patient also had occlusion of the left descending pulmonary artery (not shown).

present with mild flulike symptoms. Clinical features of cryptococcosis include fever, cough, dyspnea, sputum production, and pleuritic chest pain, which may be associated with symptoms caused by associated meningitis like headache and neck rigidity. Host factors determine imaging findings. Immunocompetent patients may manifest one or more lung nodules or airspace consolidation

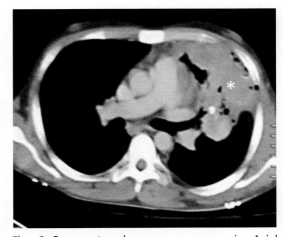

Fig. 9. Recurrent pulmonary mucormycosis. Axial contrast-enhanced CT of the chest of a 25-year-old renal transplant recipient presenting as a peripheral left lung mass (*asterisk*) because of mucormycosis after resection for the same disease 3 months ago.

usually without cavitation. In patients with AIDS, an interstitial pattern of disease characterized by reticular or reticulonodular pattern is the usual presentation. The latter pattern is often indistinguishable from *P jiroveci* pneumonia.[31] Lymphadenopathy and pleural effusion are infrequent (**Fig. 10**).

Histoplasmosis

H capsulatum is by far the most important *Histoplasma* species from a human disease perspective. Infection with *H capsulatum* is usually asymptomatic, but clinically overt infection may result from overwhelming inoculation or infection in immunocompromised patients.[33] Imaging features of histoplasmosis are nonspecific; multifocal consolidations may be found. Severe cases may simulate bacterial pneumonia. Mediastinal lymphadenopathy is common. Pleural effusion is rarely seen. If the exposure is large and/or the patient's immune status is poor, diffusely scattered nodules of varying sizes and miliary pattern are seen. Nodules eventually calcify with healing. Chronic pulmonary histoplasmosis may present as upper lobe fibrocavitary consolidation that is often indistinguishable from postprimary pulmonary tuberculosis. Acute disseminated histoplasmosis usually occurs in very young children or in severely immunocompromised individuals. The typical radiographic appearance is that of a miliary pattern of lung involvement with concomitant involvement of liver, spleen, lymph nodes, adrenal glands, and bone marrow, and often runs a fulminant course. The mediastinal lymph-nodal involvement by *H capsulatum* usually causes necrosis and

fibrosis of affected lymph nodes. Fibrosing mediastinitis may be a sequela of histoplasmosis that may lead to superior vena caval obstruction with extensive chest wall collateralization, pulmonary artery encasement, bronchial stenosis, and esophageal obstruction. Extensive lymph node calcification may be seen.[34]

Candidiasis

Among the *Candida* species capable of causing human disease, *C albicans* is the most common. *Candida* is a normal flora of gastrointestinal tract and skin; however, clinically overt pulmonary candidiasis commonly occurs in the setting of immunosuppression.[30] Associated multiple organ involvement is common. Imaging features include multiple nodules with ground-glass opacities and multifocal consolidation. Cavitation and lymphadenopathy are usually not seen.

Coccidioidomycosis

C immitis is endemic in the southwestern United States, northern Mexico, and areas of Central and South America. Depending on the clinicoradiological manifestation, pulmonary coccidioidomycosis is categorized into acute, disseminated, and chronic forms.[35] The clinical and radiological features are summarized in **Table 1**.

North American Blastomycosis

North American blastomycosis is caused by *Blastomyces dermatitidis* and is considered endemic to specific regions of North America. Clinical manifestations range from asymptomatic infection to a progressive fulminant course. Imaging features are also variable and can include airspace consolidation, focal masses, intermediate-sized nodules, interstitial disease, miliary disease, and cavitary lesions.[36]

South American Blastomycosis

South American blastomycosis is a similar infection caused by the fungus Paracoccidioides brasiliensis. It is considered to be an AIDS-defining illness.[36] Patients may be asymptomatic or present with a flulike illness. Disseminated disease occurs in immunocompromised patients. Imaging features include multifocal consolidation, one or more nodules that may cavitate, and associated lymphadenopathy.

INTRA-ABDOMINAL FUNGAL INFECTIONS

Virtually any abdominal organ or system can be involved by fungal infection.

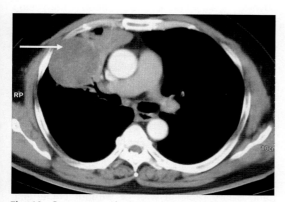

Fig. 10. Cryptococcosis. Parenchymal involvement in a 48-year-old smoker with cough, shortness of breath, and loss of weight over the previous 3 months. Axial contrast-enhanced CT scan of the chest shows a well-defined, hypodense, round, smoothly marginated mass in the right upper lobe (*arrow*) with collapse of adjacent anterior segment. Fine-needle aspiration from the mass revealed cryptococcosis.

Table 1
Clinical and imaging findings in the 3 forms of pulmonary coccidioidomycosis

Disease Form	Clinical Presentation	Imaging Findings
Acute/primary coccidioidomycosis	Mild flulike illness to acute pneumonia	• Parenchymal abnormalities: consolidation, nodules, cavities, and peribronchial thickening • Intrathoracic adenopathy • Pleural effusion
Disseminated coccidioidomycosis	Systemic features like fever, joint pain, and increased erythrocyte sedimentation rate predominate Acute respiratory distress syndrome can set in	• Parenchymal abnormalities: miliary nodules often progressing to confluent opacities • Hilar and mediastinal adenopathy
Chronic pulmonary coccidioidomycosis	Clinical symptoms or imaging abnormalities persist beyond 6 wk	• Parenchymal abnormalities: residual nodule, chronic cavity. grape-skin cavity refers to thin-walled cavity developing in a site of prior consolidation • Intrathoracic adenopathy • Pleural effusion

Adapted from Jude CM, Nayak NB, Patel MK, et al. Pulmonary coccidioidomycosis: pictorial review of chest radiographic and CT findings. Radiographics 2014;34:912–25.

Intra-abdominal fungal infection can arise in 2 settings:

1. Localized infections following surgery, trauma, or placement of foreign devices like peritoneal dialysis catheters
2. Disseminated infection in the background of immunocompromised state[37]

Liver and Spleen

Fungal infections of liver and spleen usually occur as a part of disseminated fungal disease in immunocompromised patients. The hepatosplenic involvement in fungal diseases is characterized by the presence of microabscesses, which are usually caused by *C albicans*.[38] Other fungus-related significant hepatosplenic diseases include cryptococcus infection, histoplasmosis, and mucormycosis.

Imaging features of all types of fungal disease are similar[38] (**Figs. 11** and **12**). Ultrasonography and CT are the routine imaging tools used for evaluation of hepatosplenic fungal infections. However, some investigators have suggested that MR imaging is superior to ultrasonography and CT for detection of fungal microabscesses.[39] Hepatosplenic candidiasis is characterized by formation of microabscesses, which on contrast-enhanced CT (CECT) appear as centrally enhancing, multiple, discrete hypoattenuating lesions of a size ranging from 2 mm to 20 mm.[39] Semelka and colleagues[40] described the features of different stages of

hepatic fungal microabscesses on contrast-enhanced MR imaging and these are summarized in **Table 2**.

Involvement of liver and spleen is common in disseminated histoplasmosis; associated primary pulmonary infection is usually seen. In the acute setting, imaging findings include hepatosplenomegaly with presence of ill-defined, diffusely scattered, parenchymal nodules that appear hypodense on CECT.[39] Locoregional necrotic lymphadenopathy may be found. In healed stages, small, punctate, diffusely scattered parenchymal calcifications are seen mimicking tuberculosis.

Biliary System

Fungal infection of the biliary system is also increasing, with *C albicans* being the most common fungus.[41] Clinical manifestations include the syndrome of ascending cholangitis and acute acalculous cholecystitis, which may progress to abscesses or gangrenous cholecystitis.[37,41] Microbiological analysis of bile aspirates remains the gold standard for establishing diagnosis. Ultrasonography and CECT may show dilated intrahepatic biliary radicles with or without cholangitic abscesses. MR cholangiopancreatography may be useful for the demonstration of ductal dilation and the level of obstruction. Endoscopic retrograde cholangiopancreatography is highly accurate for diagnosis of biliary mycosis and also provides the additional advantage of bile collection for establishing a definitive diagnosis.[41]

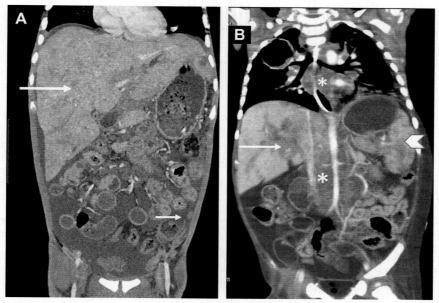

Fig. 11. Cryptococcosis. (*A*) A 25-year-old patient with HIV with infiltrative liver lesions (*long arrow in A*) with ascites and peritoneal nodules (*small arrow*) on coronal MPR CT scan. (*B*) A 2-year-old with disseminated cryptococcosis with peribiliary infiltration (*arrow*) and splenic lesions (*arrowhead*). Necrotic mediastinal and abdominal nodes (*asterisks*) are also seen on contrast-enhanced CT scan. A cavitary lesion is also present in right upper lobe.

Pancreas

The most common cause of pancreatic fungal infections is *Candida* species, most notably *C albicans*, followed by *Torulopsis* species belonging to the family Cryptococcaceae. The incidence of pancreatic infection after an episode of pancreatitis is usually between 6% and 10%.[42] The 3 common recognizable forms of pancreatitic fungal infections are pancreatic necrosis, infected pseudocyst, and pancreatic abscesses.[42] CECT helps in assessment of the extent of intrapancreatic and peripancreatic necrosis and fluid collections. In addition, CT-guided needle aspiration from the target areas aids in collecting samples for establishing microbiological diagnosis and for image-guided drainage.

Adrenal Glands

Pathogenic fungi are known to affect adrenal glands in both immunocompromised and immunocompetent individuals.[40] Adrenal involvement most frequently occurs in the setting of disseminated disease. Fungi commonly implicated include *H capsulatum* and *P jiroveci*.[43,44] In disseminated histoplasmosis, CT typically shows symmetric enlargement of bilateral adrenal glands with central hypoattenuation and peripheral areas of contrast enhancement. Depending on the stage of the disease, variable degrees of calcification may be seen (**Fig. 13**). Noncontrast CT may show punctate or coarse calcifications in adrenal glands in *P jiroveci* infection.

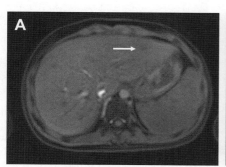

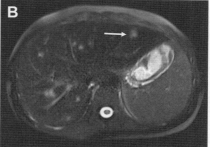

Fig. 12. An 18-year-old woman with leukemia and fungal liver lesions. T1-weighted MR axial image (*A*) shows hypointense lesions (*arrow*) that are bright on T2-weighted MR image (*arrow in B*) with a peripheral dark rim.

Table 2
Different stages and MR imaging characteristics of hepatic fungal microabscesses

Stage of Disease	T1	T2	Postgadolinium
Untreated nodules <1 mm in size	Minimally hypointense	Markedly hyperintense	Minimally hypointense with mild to moderate enhancement
Posttreatment subacute disease[a]	Mildly to moderately hyperintense	Mildly to moderately hyperintense	Significant enhancement
Completely treated lesions	Minimally hypointense	Isointense to mildly hyperintense	Moderately hypointense on early gadolinium-enhanced images, and minimally hypointense on delayed gadolinium-enhanced images

[a] A dark ring is usually seen around the lesions with all sequences in this stage as macrophages containing iron start appearing along the periphery of the lesions.

Adapted from Semelka RC, Kelekis NL, Sallah S, et al. Hepatosplenic fungal disease: diagnostic accuracy and spectrum of appearances on MR imaging. Am J Roentgenol 1997;169:1311–6.

Urogenital Tract

Upper urinary tract fungal infections are usually seen in patients with immunosuppression, diabetes mellitus, or urinary tract obstruction, and in those on prolonged antibiotic or steroid therapy.[45] The usual causative organism is *C albicans*. Infection may be acquired by hematogenous route or by an ascending urinary tract infection. Clinical features are similar to acute pyelonephritis with development of multiple renal abscesses if untreated.

CECT commonly shows striated nephrogram similar to acute bacterial pyelonephritis. Renal abscesses may be seen as multiple small, hypoattenuating cortical lesions. Fungal balls or mycetoma may be seen as irregularly marginated, soft tissue masses appearing as filling defects within the pelvicalyceal system on excretory phase CECT.[45]

Renal Aspergillosis

Renal aspergillosis is a rare entity occurring in immunosuppressed patients. On CECT, single or multiple complex cystic masses or abscesses may be seen with delayed enhancement of renal parenchyma and features of accompanying local pyelonephritis.[45] Diagnosis is made by urinalysis and aspiration of the lesion for microscopy and culture[45] (**Fig. 14**).

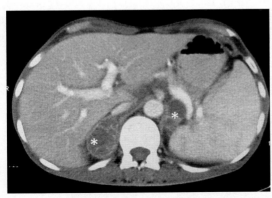

Fig. 13. Histoplasmosis. Axial CECT. A 35-year-old man with malaise and weight loss. Bilateral adrenal glands are enlarged, lobulated, and hypodense with thin septae (*asterisks*). Aspiration cytology yielded histoplasmosis.

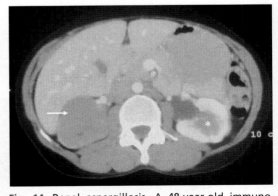

Fig. 14. Renal aspergillosis. A 48-year-old immunocompetent patient with right lumbar pain and a palpable mass. Axial CECT scan of the abdomen shows an infiltrative lesion replacing the right kidney (*arrow*). A smaller lesion is also seen in the left kidney (*asterisk*). Fine-needle aspiration yielded fungus and serology showed both *A fumigatus* and *A flavus*.

Renal Pneumocystis jiroveci Infection

Renal *P jiroveci* infection occurs secondary to hematogenous/lymphatic spread of pulmonary infection in patients with AIDS. On CT scan usually it presents as renal cortical calcification.[46]

Renal Mucormycosis

Renal mucormycosis is a rare condition and usually occurs as a part of disseminated disease. The fungal hyphae are known for involvement of blood vessels leading to hemorrhage, thrombosis, and ultimately infarction[47] (**Fig. 15**). Incidence among people infected with HIV is low, particularly if confined to kidneys; however, a higher incidence is seen among intravenous drug abusers and in patients with low CD4+ cell count.[47] Typically unilateral renal involvement is seen; however, bilateral involvement is associated with poor prognosis.[47] CT shows a large kidney with architectural distortion. Hypodense areas seen on CT are suggestive of infarcts or abscesses[47] (see **Fig. 15**). Vascular thrombus and perinephric fluid collections may also be seen. Although no calculi are seen, CT findings may mimic xanthogranulomatous pyelonephritis.[47]

Fungal Cystitis and Prostatitis

Fungal cystitis is a rare entity and is usually caused by *C albicans*. It can be diagnosed by demonstration of hyphae on urine microscopy or by urine culture sensitivity. Radiological features are nonspecific. Ultrasonography may show diffuse bladder wall thickening.

Mycotic granulomatous prostatitis may be associated with systemic mycoses such as coccidioidomycosis, cryptococcosis, histoplasmosis, paracoccidioidomycosis, blastomycosis, and candidiasis.[48] Imaging features are nonspecific.

Gastrointestinal Tract

Fungal infection of the gastrointestinal tract is uncommon. The most common fungus implicated is *C albicans*. Candida esophagitis is a well-known condition. Predisposing factors include diabetes mellitus, malignant neoplasms, administration of immunosuppressive agents, chemotherapy or radiation therapy, AIDS, scleroderma, strictures, achalasia, and previous fundoplication.[49] Barium studies show longitudinally oriented, plaquelike lesions within the upper esophagus and midesophagus.[50] Involvement of small and large bowel by *Candida*, *Aspergillus*, and other fungi have been described in literature and usually presents with features of typhlitis, colonic ulcers, and gastrointestinal bleeding.[37] Radiological features are nonspecific and may show dilated, edematous bowel loops with the presence of multifocal ulcerations.

Peritonitis

The most important cause of fungal peritonitis is *C albicans*. Risk factors include hollow viscus perforation, abdominal and thoracic surgery, surgical drains, intravenous and urinary catheters, peritoneal dialysis catheter, severe sepsis, and extensive *Candida* colonization.[37] Imaging features are nonspecific. CECT shows peritoneal fluid collections with patchy areas of enhancement. CT also helps in delineating the extent of localized collections for aspiration or catheter drainage.

MUSCULOSKELETAL

Musculoskeletal manifestation of fungal infection may occur as a part of disseminated disease or as a result of contiguous spread or inoculation. Common fungi are *Candida* and *Aspergillus*. Fungi such as *Coccidioides*, *Histoplasma*, *Blastomyces*,

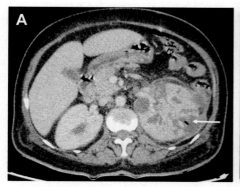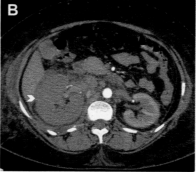

Fig. 15. Renal mucormycosis. Axial CECT in 2 different patients. The left kidney is enlarged with multiple abscesses (*A*) with small air foci (*arrow*). The entire right kidney is infarcted and nonenhancing (*arrowhead in B*). Doppler (not shown) showed thrombus in right renal vein.

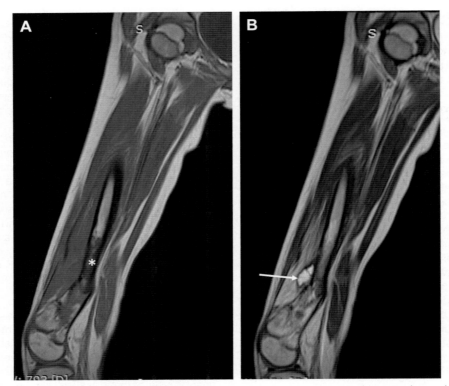

Fig. 16. Aspergillus osteomyelitis. T1-weighted (*A*) and T2-weighted (*B*) MR coronal images show a hypointense intramedullary diaphyseal lesion (*asterisk in A*) in the femur with hyperintense abscess anteriorly (*arrow in B*) with a pathologic fracture.

and *Sporothrix* may be causative organisms in endemic areas.[51] In the peripheral skeleton, imaging appearance often mimics chronic pyogenic osteomyelitis (**Fig. 16**). Spinal involvement is characterized by spondylodiscitis with large paravertebral fluid collections mimicking spinal tuberculosis. Intervertebral discs may be relatively spared. Hypointensity within the paravertebral collections on T2WI is common.[52] Involvement of the vertebral bodies may lead to vertebral compression fractures and gross deformity of the spine.[53] Multifocal infection is common in hematogenous dissemination. Neonates admitted to the intensive care unit are at risk of iatrogenic disseminated candidiasis, which might involve multiple joints and bones causing multifocal osteomyelitis.

SUMMARY

There is a wide spectrum of fungi that cause human infections involving multiple organ systems. Mycotic infections commonly occur in the background of compromised immune function. They present a diagnostic as well as therapeutic challenge to clinicians and radiologists. A high degree of clinical suspicion in the appropriate clinical setting and supportive imaging evidence may lead to early institution of therapy and reduce morbidity. CT and MR imaging are useful not only for early diagnosis and disease localization but also to evaluate response to therapy.

REFERENCES

1. Seaton A, Seaton O, Leitch AG. Actinomycotic and Fungal Diseases. In: Crofton and Douglas's respiratory diseases. 4th edition. Delhi (India): Oxford University Press; 1989. p. 448–75.
2. Fraser RS, Pare JAP, Eraser RG, et al. Infectious disease of the lung. In: Synopsis of diseases of the Chest. 2nd edition. Philadelphia: WB Saunders; 1994. p. 332–54.
3. Luthra G, Parihar A, Nath K, et al. Comparative evaluation of fungal, tubercular, and pyogenic brain abscesses with conventional and diffusion MR imaging and proton MR spectroscopy. AJNR Am J Neuroradiol 2007;28:1332–8.
4. Himmelreich U, Dzendrowoskyj TE, Allen C, et al. Cryptococcomas distinguished from gliomas with MR spectroscopy: an experimental rat and cell culture study. Radiology 2001;220:122–8.

5. Ho CL, Deruytter MJ. CNS aspergillosis with mycotic aneurysm, cerebral granuloma and infarction. Acta Neurochir (Wien) 2004;146:851–6.

6. Haris M, Gupta RK, Husain N, et al. Measurement of DTI metrics in hemorrhagic brain lesions: possible implication in MRI interpretation. J Magn Reson Imaging 2006;24:1259–68.

7. Takasu A, Taneda M, Otuki H, et al. Gd-DTPA-enhanced MR imaging of cryptococcal meningoencephalitis. Neuroradiology 1991;33:443–6.

8. Chang L, Miller BL, McBride D, et al. Brain lesions in patients with AIDS: H-1 MR spectroscopy. Radiology 1995;197:525–31.

9. McLean FM, Ginsberg LE, Stanton CA. Perineural spread of rhinocerebral mucormycosis. AJNR Am J Neuroradiol 1996;17:114–6.

10. Khandelwal N, Gupta V, Singh P. Central nervous system fungal infections in the tropics. Neuroimaging Clin N Am 2011;21:859–66.

11. Thrasher RD, Kingdom TT. Fungal infections of the head and neck: an update. Otolaryngol Clin North Am 2003;36:577–94.

12. Aribandi M, McCoy VT, Bazan C III. Imaging features of invasive and noninvasive fungal sinusitis: a review. Radiographics 2007;27:1283–97.

13. Silverman CS, Mancuso AA. Periantral soft-tissue infiltration and its relevance to the early detection of invasive fungal sinusitis: CT and MR findings. AJNR Am J Neuroradiol 1998;19:321–5.

14. Sarti EJ, Blaugrund SM, Lin PT, et al. Paranasal sinus disease with intracranial extension: aspergillosis versus malignancy. Laryngoscope 1988;98:632–5.

15. Stringer SP, Ryan MW. Chronic invasive fungal rhinosinusitis. Otolaryngol Clin North Am 2000;33:375–87.

16. Manning SC, Merkel M, Kriesel K, et al. Computed tomography and magnetic resonance diagnosis of allergic fungal sinusitis. Laryngoscope 1997;107:170–6.

17. Grosjean P, Weber R. Fungus balls of the paranasal sinuses: a review. Eur Arch Otorhinolaryngol 2007;264:461–70.

18. Sodhi KS, Khandelwal N, Saxena AK, et al. Rapid lung MRI: paradigm shift in evaluation of febrile neutropenia in children with leukemia: a pilot study. Leuk Lymphoma 2016;57:70–5.

19. Attenberger UI, Morelli JN, Henzler T, et al. 3 Tesla proton MRI for the diagnosis of pneumonia/lung infiltrates in neutropenic patients with acute myeloid leukemia: initial results in comparison to HRCT. Eur J Radiol 2014;83:e61–6.

20. Kuhlman JE, Fishman EK, Siegelman SS. Invasive pulmonary aspergillosis in acute leukemia: characteristic findings on CT, the CT halo sign, and the role of CT in early diagnosis. Radiology 1985;157:611–4.

21. Aronchick JM. Pulmonary infections in cancer and bone marrow transplant patients. Semin Roentgenol 2000;35:140–51.

22. Stansell JD. Fungal disease in HIV-infected persons: cryptococcosis, histoplasmosis, and coccidioidomycosis. J Thorac Imaging 1991;6:28–35.

23. Hartman TE, Primack SL, Müller NL, et al. Diagnosis of thoracic complications in AIDS: accuracy of CT. Am J Roentgenol 1994;162:547–53.

24. McGuiness G. Changing trends in the pulmonary manifestations of AIDS. Radiol Clin North Am 1997;35:1029–82.

25. Tomas F, Nestor L, Ana G, et al. Spectrum of pulmonary aspergillosis: histologic, clinical, and radiologic findings. Radiographics 2001;21:825–37.

26. Agarwal R, Khan A, Gupta D, et al. An alternate method of classifying allergic bronchopulmonary aspergillosis based on high-attenuation mucus. PLoS One 2010;5:e15346.

27. Agarwal R, Chakrabarti A, Shah A, et al. Allergic bronchopulmonary aspergillosis: review of literature and proposal of new diagnostic and classification criteria. Clin Exp Allergy 2013;43:850–73.

28. Hruban RH, Meziane MA, Zerhouni EA, et al. Radiologic-pathologic correlation of the CT-halo sign in invasive pulmonary aspergillosis. J Comput Assist Tomogr 1987;11:534–6.

29. Kanne JP, Yandow DR, Meyer CA. Pneumocystis jiroveci pneumonia: high-resolution CT findings in patients with and without HIV infection. Am J Roentgenol 2012;198:555–61.

30. Catherinot E, Lanternier F, Bougnoux ME, et al. Pneumocystis jirovecii pneumonia. Infect Dis Clin North Am 2010;24:107–38.

31. Franquet T, Giménez A, Hidalgo A. Imaging of opportunistic fungal infections in immunocompromised patient. Eur J Radiol 2004;51:130–8.

32. Walker CM, Abbott GF, Greene RE, et al. Imaging pulmonary infection: classic signs and patterns. Am J Roentgenol 2014;202:479–92.

33. Knox KS, Hage CA. Histoplasmosis. Proc Am Thorac Soc 2010;7:169–72.

34. Sherrick AD, Brown LR, Harms GF, et al. The radiographic findings of fibrosing mediastinitis. Chest 1994;106:484–9.

35. Jude CM, Nayak NB, Patel MK, et al. Pulmonary coccidioidomycosis: pictorial review of chest radiographic and CT findings. Radiographics 2014;34:912–25.

36. Fang W, Washington L, Kumar N. Imaging manifestations of blastomycosis: a pulmonary infection with potential dissemination. Radiographics 2007;27:641–55.

37. Rebolledo M, Sarria JC. Intra-abdominal fungal infections. Curr Opin Infect Dis 2013;26:441–6.

38. Mortelé KJ, Segatto E, Ros PR. The infected liver: radiologic-pathologic correlation. Radiographics 2004;24:937–55.

39. Anttila VJ, Lamminen AE, Bondestam S, et al. Magnetic resonance imaging is superior to computed

tomography and ultrasonography in imaging infectious liver foci in acute leukaemia. Eur J Haematol 1996;56:82–7.

40. Semelka RC, Kelekis NL, Sallah S, et al. Hepatosplenic fungal disease: diagnostic accuracy and spectrum of appearances on MR imaging. Am J Roentgenol 1997;169:1311–6.

41. Domagk D, Fegeler W, Conrad B, et al. Biliary tract candidiasis: diagnostic and therapeutic approaches in a case series. Am J Gastroenterol 2006;101:2530–6.

42. Shanmugam N, Isenmann R, Barkin JS, et al. Pancreatic fungal infection. Pancreas 2003;27:133–8.

43. Paolo WF Jr, Nosanchuk JD. Adrenal infections. Int J Infect Dis 2006;10:343–53.

44. Kawashima A, Sandler CM, Fishman EK, et al. Spectrum of CT findings in nonmalignant disease of the adrenal gland. Radiographics 1998;18:393–412.

45. Hammond NA, Nikolaidis P, Miller FH. Infectious and inflammatory diseases of the kidney. Radiol Clin North Am 2012;50:259–70.

46. Symeonidou C, Standish R, Sahdev A, et al. Imaging and histopathologic features of HIV-related renal disease. Radiographics 2008;28:1339–54.

47. Keogh CF, Brown JA, Phillips P, et al. Renal mucormycosis in an AIDS patient: imaging features and pathologic correlation. Am J Roentgenol 2003;180:1278–80.

48. Domingue GJ Sr, Hellstrom WJ. Prostatitis. Clin Microbiol Rev 1998;11:604–13.

49. Roberts L Jr, Gibbons R, Gibbons G, et al. Adult esophageal candidiasis: a radiographic spectrum. Radiographics 1987;7:289–307.

50. Sinha R, Rajesh A, Rawat S, et al. Infections and infestations of the gastrointestinal tract. Part 1: bacterial, viral and fungal infections. Clin Radiol 2012;67:484–94.

51. Bariteau JT, Waryasz GR, McDonnell M, et al. Fungal osteomyelitis and septic arthritis. J Am Acad Orthop Surg 2014;22:390–401.

52. Lee SW, Lee SH, Chung HW, et al. Candida spondylitis: comparison of MRI findings with bacterial and tuberculous causes. Am J Roentgenol 2013;201:872–7.

53. Kim CW, Perry A, Currier B, et al. Fungal infections of the spine. Clin Orthop Relat Res 2006;444:92–9.

Imaging of Sarcoidosis
A Contemporary Review

Carey Guidry, MD, Robert Gaines Fricke, MD, Roopa Ram, MD,
Tarun Pandey, MD, FRCR, Kedar Jambhekar, MD*

KEYWORDS

• Sarcoidosis • Multisystem • Imaging

KEY POINTS

• Sarcoidosis is an idiopathic, chronic, multisystem disease characterized by development of noncaseating granulomas in target organs. Sarcoidosis can mimic several multisystem disorders, such as infections, lymphoma, and metastatic disease due to multiplicity of lesions.
• The most common presenting feature of sarcoidosis is thoracic lymphadenopathy and/or pulmonary nodules in a typical perilymphatic and upper lobe distribution.
• The diagnosis is often delayed by diverse and nonspecific symptoms as well as rarity of the disease. Definitive diagnosis often requires a combination of clinical, radiological, and histologic information.
• Imaging plays a crucial role in diagnosis, prognosis, and evaluating response to therapy.

INTRODUCTION

Sarcoidosis is a chronic, multisystem, inflammatory disease of unknown etiology characterized histologically by development of noncaseating granulomas.[1] Sarcoidosis is thought to result from exaggerated immune response to putative microbial antigens in genetically susceptible individuals. It affects both genders and all races, with a predilection for Swedes, Danes, and African Americans.[2] In the United States, the incidence of sarcoidosis is 5.9 per 100, 000 person-years for men and 6.3 per 100,000 person-years for women[3]; 70% of patients are aged between 25 to 45 years. Patient presentation can vary from asymptomatic with abnormal chest radiograph to nonspecific symptoms, such as fatigue and weight loss, to progressive multiorgan failure. Although there are almost always intrathoracic abnormalities seen on chest radiographs and CT, myriad extrathoracic manifestations potentially affect essentially every organ system.[4]

Sarcoidosis has been described as "the great mimicker" because its manifestations can mimic different disease processes, including metastatic disease, various primary neoplasms, vasculitis, and other granulomatous infections. For example, nodal involvement within the mediastinum can be mistaken for lymphoma, metastases, or fungal and mycobacterial infections. Similarly, within the lung parenchyma sarcoidosis may appear similar to pulmonary diseases, such as bronchiolitis, lymphangitic carcinomatosis, hypersensitivity pneumonitis, Langerhans cell histiocytosis, usual interstitial pneumonia, cryptogenic organizing pneumonia, and nonspecific interstitial pneumonia.[5]

With a wide spectrum of both radiological and clinical presentations, sarcoidosis can be a difficult diagnosis to make and hinges on 3 primary components: clinical and radiologic presentation, histologic evidence of noncaseating granulomas, and exclusion of other granulomatous entities.[2]

Disclosure Statement: The authors have nothing to disclose.
Department of Diagnostic Radiology, University of Arkansas for Medical Sciences, 4301 West Markham, Slot 556, Little Rock, AR 72205, USA
* Corresponding author.
E-mail address: Kjambhekar@uams.edu

Radiol Clin N Am 54 (2016) 519–534
http://dx.doi.org/10.1016/j.rcl.2015.12.009
0033-8389/16/$ – see front matter

radiologic.theclinics.com

Classical or compelling fulfillment of 1 or 2 of these components can obviate the others. For example, in a patient presenting with anterior uveitis, fever, and parotitis (Heerfordt syndrome), chest radiograph alone may provide the diagnosis. Alternatively (and more commonly), nonspecific clinical or imaging findings (eg, interstitial lung disease and lymphadenopathy) require histologic confirmation and exclusion of other granulomatosis syndromes.

Imaging plays a crucial role not only in making the diagnosis but also in evaluating prognosis and monitoring response to therapy. For example, chest radiograph staging at presentation is important because it portends the rate of spontaneous resolution.[6] Advanced imaging modalities like CT and PET/CT are not indicated for following uncomplicated sarcoidosis.[7] PET has been shown helpful in identifying patients with pulmonary fibrosis or those with negative serologic markers but persistent debilitating symptoms.[8,9]

A grasp of the numerous radiological appearances of sarcoidosis is essential for diagnosing and evaluating the disease. This review article describes the spectrum of imaging findings in sarcoidosis affecting various organ systems with an emphasis on the role of imaging modalities in the diagnosis and management of this elusive condition.

CARDIOTHORACIC SYSTEM

Approximately 90% of patients with sarcoidosis have pulmonary and/or intrathoracic lymphatic involvement.[10] Bilateral, symmetric mediastinal adenopathy and hilar adenopathy are the most common radiographic manifestations of the disease, present in up to 85% of patients with sarcoidosis, and are often unexpected findings on routine chest radiographs in asymptomatic patients[10] (Fig. 1).

Staging of sarcoidosis on chest radiographs is shown in Box 1.[11]

Lungs

Clinical manifestations
Among patients with sarcoidosis, 20% have lung involvement.[10] Clinically, patients may present with dyspnea and/or dry cough.

Imaging features
In patients with clinically suspected sarcoidosis, chest radiographs are often sufficient to make a diagnosis.[5] Chest CT is more sensitive in evaluating for mediastinal adenopathy. Thin-slice, high-resolution CT has higher sensitivity and specificity in the diagnosis of subtle pulmonary parenchymal

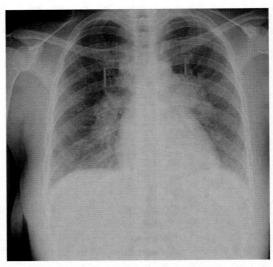

Fig. 1. Chest radiograph shows typical bilateral mediastinal and hilar lymphadenopathy (*arrows*).

disease. CT better defines disease extent and can help discriminate between reversible and irreversible lung disease.[7] Other indications for CT and PET/CT are summarized in **Box 2**.

Typical CT findings of pulmonary sarcoidosis include small (2–5 mm) granulomatous nodules in a perilymphatic distribution: along bronchovascular bundles, interlobular septae, interlobar fissures, and subpleural location (**Fig. 2**). The disease has a predilection for the upper lobes. Among patients with sarcoidosis, 20% go on to develop stage IV disease, which is irreversible and manifests as midlung and upper-lung fibrosis with linear opacities radiating from the hila, traction bronchiectasis, architectural distortion, bulla formation, honeycombing, and volume loss with posterior displacement of the main and upper lobe bronchi (**Fig. 3**).

Other findings are summarized in **Box 3**.

Alveolar sarcoid, also described as nodular sarcoidosis, is an atypical manifestation of

---

Box 1
Radiographic staging of sarcoidosis

Stage 0: normal initial chest radiograph (10%)

Stage 1: hilar/mediastinal adenopathy (50%)

Stage 2: adenopathy and pulmonary opacities (25%–30%)

Stage 3: pulmonary opacities without adenopathy

Stage 4: pulmonary fibrosis and bullous changes in the upper lobes.

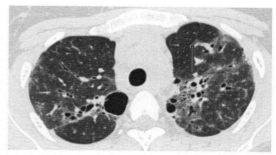

Fig. 3. CT chest in a more advanced case shows sequelae of chronic disease with honeycombing, traction bronchiectasis, and cavitary changes (*arrow*) in the upper lobes.

sarcoidosis (2.4%–4%) resulting from coalescence of multiple pulmonary interstitial granulomas.[12–14] Radiographs and CT demonstrate patchy rounded or ovoid pulmonary opacities ranging in size from 1 cm to 4 cm in diameter, most commonly located along the bronchovascular bundles or in a peripheral subpleural location. Air bronchograms may be present, and the margins of the opacities may be ill defined, helping to differentiate findings of sarcoid from metastatic lesions. Other, rare, nonspecific findings described in sarcoidosis include pleural effusion, pleural thickening, solitary pulmonary nodule/mass, and spontaneous pneumothorax.[13,15]

A few radiological signs have been described with sarcoidosis and are best seen on thoracic high-resolution CT and are shown in **Box 4** and **Fig. 4.**

Mediastinal adenopathy
Chest radiographs often demonstrate the classic triad of bilateral hilar and right paratracheal lymphadenopathy, known as Garland triad. Left paratracheal and aortopulmonary window lymph nodes may also be enlarged but are less easily distinguishable on posteroanterior chest radiographs. Unilateral or asymmetric lymphadenopathy is atypical of sarcoidosis.[12]

Mediastinal and hilar lymph nodes may calcify in chronic sarcoidosis. Amorphous or cloud-like (icing sugar) calcification is most typical for sarcoidosis because it is not associated with other forms of granulomatous disease.[7] Punctate or peripheral eggshell mediastinal calcifications, classically seen in silicosis, can also be seen but are not specific. Sarcoidosis also involves the more peripherally located bronchopulmonary lymph nodes. Frequently, there is separation between the lymph nodes and the heart, helping to distinguish sarcoidosis from other causes of lymphadenopathy, such as lymphoma.

Although nuclear medicine gallium citrate Ga 67 (gallium 67) scintigraphy and fludeoxyglucose F 18 (FDG)-PET imaging are not routinely used in the evaluation of sarcoidosis, one characteristic pattern of uptake seen with gallium 67 scintigraphy is the lambda sign, which is secondary to right paratracheal and bilateral hilar lymphadenopathy. FDG-PET can show uptake in stages II and III and

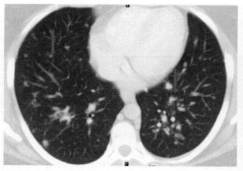
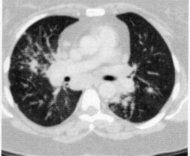

Fig. 2. Noncontiguous chest CT images (*A* and *B*) showing the characteristic perilymphatic distribution of pulmonary nodules (*arrows*).

Box 3
Pulmonary manifestations of sarcoidosis on CT

1. Upper lobe predilection with 2-mm to 5-mm granulomatous nodules in perilymphatic distribution

2. Nodular thickening of the airway wall

3. Mosaic attenuation of lungs due to air trapping, best seen on expiratory high-resolution CT

4. Upper lung and midlung fibrosis in advanced stages with sequelae of fibrosis

5. Conglomerate masses or mass-like fibrosis with irregular borders

---

lack of uptake is common in patients with stages 0, I, and IV. PET uptake may decrease with response to treatment.

Pulmonary vasculature

Pulmonary arterial hypertension is a potential complication in patients with sarcoidosis, most commonly in patients with stage IV fibrotic disease. Pulmonary hypertension is not limited, however, to stage IV sarcoidosis and can result earlier in the disease secondary to a variety of proposed pathophysiology mechanisms, shown in **Box 5**.[7]

Chest radiographs may demonstrate an enlarged pulmonary trunk and central pulmonary arteries with pruning of the more peripheral pulmonary arteries. The enlarged pulmonary trunk results in left superior mediastinal convexity on frontal chest radiograph. Cardiac silhouette is typically normal but enlargement of the right atrium and ventricle can be seen with chronic pulmonary arterial hypertension. Also, pulmonary arterial wall calcification may develop with chronic pulmonary arterial hypertension.

CT is more sensitive and specific than radiographs in detecting pulmonary arterial hypertension and manifests as dilatation of the pulmonary trunk greater than 29 mm and dilatation of the left and right pulmonary arteries. A dilated pulmonary trunk typically has a diameter greater than the adjacent ascending thoracic aorta.

Cardiac

Cardiac involvement is seen is seen in up to 25% of patients with sarcoidosis at autopsy, carries a poor prognosis, and accounts for 13% to 25% of patient deaths in the United States.[10,16] Cardiac sarcoid involvement is more common in Japan and accounts for up to 85% of patient deaths.[16]

Clinical manifestations

Cardiac sarcoidosis is often asymptomatic and, therefore, is clinically undetected. Symptomatic patients may present clinically with a variety of conduction abnormalities or arrhythmias, most commonly complete heart block and ventricular tachycardia, respectively. Sudden death from arrhythmia accounts for two-thirds of cardiac sarcoid–related deaths.[16] Congestive heart failure is the second most common cause of death and results from extensive myocardial granuloma infiltration, pulmonary hypertension, and/or arrhythmias.[16]

Imaging features

Magnetic resonance imaging (MR imaging) is the modality of choice in diagnosis and to evaluate treatment response.[17] Findings are nonspecific but include patchy areas of T2 hyperintensity within the midmyocardium or subepicardium with sparing of the endocardium, which, in the correct clinical setting, are highly suggestive. Sarcoid granulomas have a predilection for the left ventricular basal and lateral segments and the papillary muscles. Gadolinium-enhanced T1 images demonstrate a nonischemic pattern of patchy midmyocardial and subepicardial late gadolinium enhancement (**Fig. 5**). The role of MR imaging is described in **Box 6**.

Differential diagnosis includes viral myocarditis, vasculitis, Anderson-Fabry disease, and Chagas disease.

Nuclear medicine Thallium Ti 201 and FDG-PET have been used in evaluating patients with cardiac

---

Box 4
Radiologic signs associated with sarcoidosis

1. Air crescent sign—associated with mycetoma and appears as a nodule or mass within a preexisting bulla or cavity, often with fungal colonization. Adjacent pleural thickening.

2. Galaxy sign—nodular or mass-like coalescence of sarcoid granulomas surrounded by less condensed granulomas, an appearance similar to a globular galaxy[12]

3. Reverse halo or atoll sign—crescentic or ring-shaped opacity with central ground-glass attenuation. Initially described in and thought specific for cryptogenic organizing pneumonia.

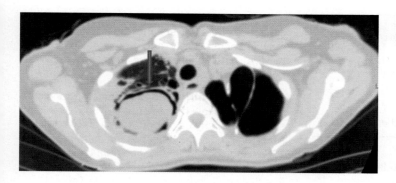

Fig. 4. CT chest showing air crescent sign (*arrow*) – secondary to fungal colonization of a sarcoid cavity.

sarcoidosis. Thallium myocardial perfusion studies demonstrate segmental areas of decreased uptake, which undergo a phenomena of reverse distribution in which the segmental defects decrease on exercise stress thallium imaging.[17] This helps differentiate from coronary artery disease–related defects. Reverse distribution is, however, not specific for cardiac sarcoid.

FDG-PET is useful in patients in whom MR imaging is contraindicated. FDG-PET shows heterogeneous areas of myocardial FDG uptake, a finding that may also be seen with idiopathic dilated cardiomyopathy.

Breast

Breast involvement with sarcoidosis is rare, reported in 1% cases, and usually occurs later in the disease course.[18]

Clinical manifestations

Breast sarcoidosis can present as a firm or hard palpable mass or enlarged axillary lymph nodes.

Imaging features

Mammographically, sarcoid breast involvement may manifest as an irregular, speculated, or circumscribed nodule or multiple masses, which are usually less than 1 cm in size. Spiculated

masses represent perigranulomatous fibrosis in chronic disease, whereas well-circumscribed nodules are seen earlier in the disease course. Concomitant intramammary and axillary lymph node involvement may be present. Axillary lymph nodes may calcify but calcification of intramammary lymph nodes is uncommon. On ultrasound, sarcoid breast granulomas are hypoechoic and may have irregular margins. Lymph nodes involved with sarcoid demonstrate thickened cortices and effaced fatty hila.

On MR imaging, sarcoid breast nodules demonstrate heterogeneous signal intensity on both T1–weighted imaging (WI) and T2-WI. Enhancement kinetics with rapid enhancement and early washout for lesions, which are more inflammatory, has been previously described. More chronic and fibrotic lesions demonstrate progressive enhancement.[19] The radiologic manifestations, described previously, of sarcoid breast involvement are nonspecific and the top differential diagnoses are

---

Box 5
Causes of pulmonary arterial hypertension in sarcoidosis

1. Extrinsic compression of the central pulmonary vessels by lymphadenopathy or mediastinal fibrosis
2. Granulomatous destruction of the pulmonary vessels
3. Vasoreactivity
4. Pulmonary veno-occlusive disease
5. Sarcoid vasculopathy

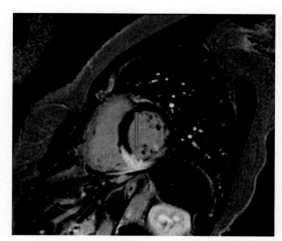

Fig. 5. Delayed hyperenhancement cardiac MR imaging in the short axis plane showing enhancement in the epicardial/midmyocardial regions (*arrow*) in a nonischemic pattern.

shown in **Box 7**. Biopsy is often prudent to exclude primary breast malignancy and confirm the diagnosis.

ABDOMINAL ORGANS

In the abdomen, sarcoidosis may involve the liver, spleen, lymph nodes, kidneys, and, rarely the gastrointestinal tract.

Liver and Spleen

Clinical manifestations

Among patients with sarcoidosis, 40% to 60% also have involvement of the liver and spleen.[20]

Isolated liver involvement without lung involvement is rare in sarcoidosis, seen in only 13% of patients.[21,22] Clinically, patients with liver involvement may be asymptomatic or manifest with fever, hepatosplenomegaly, or joint pains.[22,23] Three well-known but rare hepatic syndromes can occur secondary to hepatic sarcoid involvement, as outlined in **Box 8**.[24]

Imaging features The most common imaging finding in the abdomen is hepatosplenomegaly, which alone is a nonspecific finding. Sarcoid granulomatous involvement of the liver and spleen may also result in diffuse parenchymal heterogeneity or a multinodular pattern in either or both organs. The multinodular pattern becomes apparent with coalescence of small sarcoid granulomas into macroscopically visible lesions, more common in the spleen. Contrast-enhanced CT typically demonstrates innumerable small (<2 cm) hypoattenuating nodules throughout the liver and/or spleen (**Fig. 6**).

Box 7
Differential diagnosis for sarcoidosis of the breast

1. Breast cancer
2. Postsurgical scar
3. Fat necrosis
4. Granulomatous infection (histoplasmosis, tuberculosis)

Hepatic sarcoid nodules are most conspicuous on early post–contrast-enhanced CT because they may enhance slowly and become isodense to the liver parenchyma on the more delayed post-contrast images.

MR imaging On MR imaging, sarcoid granuloma nodules appear hypointense to the liver and splenic parenchyma on both T1-WI and T2-WI. Lesions are most conspicuous on fat-suppressed T2-WI and show mild enhancement on early post-contrast sequences[20,25] (**Figs. 7** and **8**). Other differential considerations are shown in **Table 1**.

Ultrasound Ultrasound is less sensitive in detecting sarcoid granulomas in the liver and spleen. On ultrasound, the liver and spleen may appear heterogeneous and/or have multiple small hypoechoic nodules (**Fig. 9**).

Most patients with liver or splenic involvement are asymptomatic and small hepatic granulomas may heal without significant radiographic residua. Rarely, healing of larger confluent hepatic granulomas can rarely result in extensive and irregular hepatic scarring and fibrosis giving the liver a cirrhotic appearance.

Abdominal lymph nodes

Enlarged retroperitoneal and upper abdominal lymph nodes can be seen in up to 30% of sarcoid patients; a finding that may mimic lymphoma.[20] Porta hepatis and para-aortic and celiac nodal chains are most frequently involved.[20] Unlike lymphoma, sarcoid lymph nodes are often smaller (<2 cm) and more discrete. Also, retrocrural involvement is rare in sarcoidosis and more commonly seen with non-Hodgkin lymphoma. Thus, in the presence of hepatosplenomegaly and bulky, confluent abdominal lymphadenopathy that involves the retrocrural nodes, lymphoma should be favored over sarcoidosis. Metastatic lymphadenopathy may also present with bulky nodes but is usually associated with a known primary cancer. Patient clinical history and presentation can be useful in differentiating or narrowing the differential diagnosis. Biopsy may be required for confirmation.

Gastrointestinal organs

Sarcoidosis may involve any portion of the gastrointestinal tract, but prevalence is less than 1% and most patients with gastrointestinal involvement are usually asymptomatic.[20] The stomach is the most common site of involvement with a predilection for the antrum.[10,26]

Clinical manifestations Gastric involvement may present with epigastric pain, nausea, and hematemesis and mimic symptoms of peptic ulcer

---

Box 8
Clinical syndromes associated with liver involvement in sarcoidosis

Chronic intrahepatic cholestasis syndrome

Secondary to granulomatous cholangitis-induced biliary ductopenia. These patients may present with jaundice. Enlarged lymph nodes causing compression of the extrahepatic bile ducts can also result in biliary obstruction and jaundice.[20]

Portal hypertension

Rare complication of hepatic sarcoid involvement secondary to occlusion of small intrahepatic portal vein branches via granulomatous inflammation. Cirrhosis and portal hypertension can be seen in 1% of patients with sarcoidosis.[24]

Budd-Chiari syndrome

Results from external compression or infiltration of the hepatic veins

---

disease. Confirmed gastric involvement is a rare occurrence, with only a few case reports documented in the literature. One such example of early gastric cancer secondary to chronic sarcoid involvement of the stomach has recently been reported.[27]

Imaging features Radiographically, the disease may mimic peptic ulcer disease manifesting as focal gastric ulcer due to localized mucosal infiltration. Diffuse mural infiltration by numerous sarcoid granulomas can result in fibrosis and linitis plastic-like appearance, mimicking scirrhous adenocarcinoma or gastric lymphoma. Due to chronic inflammation and fibrosis, the gastric folds may hypertrophy, resembling Ménétrier disease. Chronic inflammation has also been proposed as one of the mechanisms for carcinogenesis in sarcoid-related gastric cancer.[27] Imaging alone is not sufficient to distinguish gastric sarcoidosis from these other pathologies, and endoscopic biopsy is necessary for diagnosis.

Pancreas

Autopsy studies reveal pancreatic sarcoidosis in 1% of sarcoid patients.[20]

Clinical manifestations Patients present with nonspecific abdominal pain or jaundice. Clinical symptoms may mimic acute or chronic pancreatitis or pancreatic cancer.[28]

Imaging features Sarcoidosis of the pancreas may manifest as focal solitary ill-defined mass or multinodular diffuse parenchymal involvement. Focal lesions have a predilection for the pancreatic head and associated biliary and pancreatic ductal dilatation may be present, mimicking pancreatic adenocarcinoma. Unlike pancreatic cancer, cholangiograms typically show long, smooth, tapered narrowing of the ducts rather than abrupt termination. On MR imaging, pancreatic sarcoid masses are T1 hypointense and mildly T2 hyperintense and enhance less than the normal pancreatic parenchyma in the arterial phase after gadolinium administration. On the portal venous phase, they become isointense to the adjacent normal

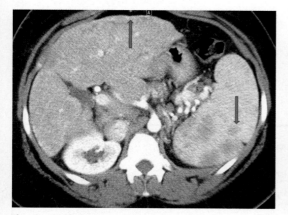

Fig. 6. CT abdomen and pelvis showing low-density lesions in the liver and spleen (*arrows*) with splenomegaly. Also note the mildly nodular contour to the liver, suggesting development of cirrhosis.

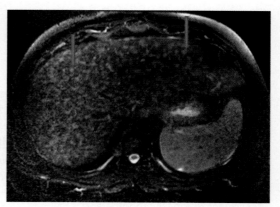

Fig. 7. Axial T2-WI of the liver showing diffusely distributed T2 hyperintense lesions in the liver.

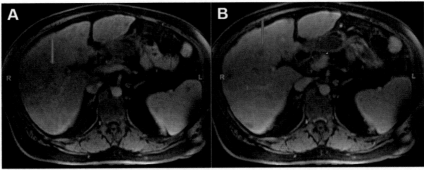

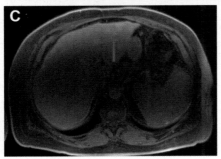

Fig. 8. (A–C) Axial postcontrast T1-WI of the liver showing T1 hypointense liver nodules (*arrows*), which do not show early enhancement but show delayed postcontrast enhancement. (*Courtesy of* Christine Menias, MD, Mayo Clinic.)

pancreatic parenchyma.[29] Solitary sarcoid granulomatous mass is often difficult to differentiate from pancreatic adenocarcinoma, which also has similar imaging findings. When the masses are multiple, other differential considerations to include are summarized in the following **Table 2**.

GENITOURINARY SYSTEM

Genitourinary involvement of sarcoidosis is exceedingly rare, occurring in less than 0.2% of patients with clinically diagnosed sarcoidosis and 5% at autopsy.[30] The disease can involve any organ of the genitourinary system, commonly masquerading as more common conditions, including malignancy and infection.

Kidneys

Clinical manifestations
Urolithiasis is the most common renal manifestation of sarcoidosis secondary to altered calcium metabolism and resultant hypercalcemia and can be seen in up to 10% of patients can present with symptoms of renal colic. Urolithiasis can lead to renal impairment even in the absence of renal granulomas. Approximately one-third of patient with renal sarcoidosis slowly develop renal insufficiency with changes of granulomatous interstitial nephritis[30] (**Fig. 10**).

Imaging features
On contrast-enhanced CT examination, interstitial nephritis characteristically appears as striated nephrogram. Rarely, renal sarcoidosis presents with multiple hypoattenuating soft tissue renal nodules or masses, which may mimic renal cell carcinoma, lymphoma, or tuberculosis.

Testis and Epididymis

The epididymis is the most frequent site of intrascrotal involvement and is bilateral in one-third of cases. Testicular involvement is less common

Table 1	
Differential diagnosis of abdominal sarcoidosis on MR imaging	
Differential Diagnosis	**MR Imaging Findings**
Infections (histoplasma, tuberculosis)	Mildly T2 hyperintense, peripheral low-grade enhancement
Benign lesions (hamartoma, hemangioma)	T2 hyperintense, significant enhancement
Malignant lesions (lymphoma and metastasis)	T1 and T2 isointense, isoenhancing on delayed images (lymphoma), peripheral enhancement (metastasis)

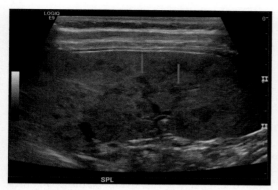

Fig. 9. Ultrasound image of the spleen (*arrows*) showing multiple rounded hypoechoic lesions in the spleen.

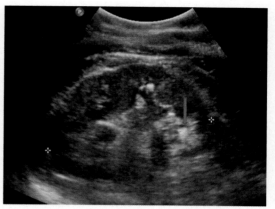

Fig. 10. Ultrasound of the kidney showing renal calculi (*arrow*) and loss of corticomedullary distinction, nonspecific feature associated with interstitial nephritis in sarcoidosis. (*Courtesy of* Neeraj Lalwani, MD, University of Washington, Seattle, WA.)

and is usually bilateral and often accompanies epididymal sarcoidosis. Unlike testicular cancers, testicular sarcoidosis is much more prevalent in African Americans than whites by a ratio of 20:1.[30]

Clinical manifestations

Patients with scrotal or epididymal involvement often present with painless unilateral or bilateral palpable scrotal mass. Tumors in the epididymis can also cause obstructive oligospermia or azoospermia and infertility; however, sarcoid lesions are often responsive to steroid therapy.[31]

Imaging features

Ultrasound of the scrotum shows diffusely enlarged, heterogeneous epididymis with or without solitary hypoechoic mass and/or multiple small distinct hypoechoic nodules. Solitary testicular mass or multiple nodules, which are usually hypoechoic and less commonly hyperechoic, are also seen (**Fig. 11**). MR imaging demonstrates enhancing lesions, which are hypointense on T2-WI.[10]

CENTRAL NERVOUS SYSTEM

Patients with sarcoidosis exhibit neurologic involvement in approximately 5% of cases, although autopsy studies have reported a histologic prevalence as high as 27%.[32,33] Neurosarcoidosis (NS) patients usually have disease evident outside the central nervous system, with isolated NS occurring in only 10% of patients. MR imaging is the most sensitive modality for diagnosis and evaluating treatment efficacy in these patients.[34]

Brain

Clinical manifestations

Because NS can affect any part of the brain, the neurologic symptoms of NS are varied. Patients may present with weakness, paresthesia, diplopia,

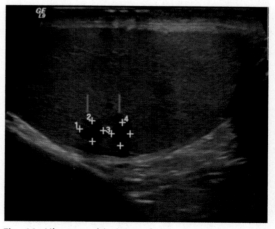

Fig. 11. Ultrasound images of the testis shows multiple well-circumscribed hypoechoic lesions (*arrows*).

Table 2 Differential diagnosis for neurosarcoidosis	
Differential Considerations	**Imaging Features**
1. Metastases	Similar to primary tumor
2. Lymphoma	Nodular form, diffuse form, and invasion by adjacent lymphadenopathy
3. Nonfunctioning neuroendocrine tumors	T2 hyperintense, enhance more than adjacent parenchyma

meningismus, seizures, psychiatric symptoms, neuroendocrine symptoms, or gait ataxia. The most common presentation is cranial neuropathy, with 7th nerve palsy seen most commonly. The initial presenting symptom of sarcoidosis is neurologic in approximately 16% of patients.[32]

Imaging features

Leptomeninges Leptomeningeal involvement is seen in approximately 31% with proclivity for the base of the brain[35] (**Fig. 12**).

Dura Dural involvement is present in approximately 34% of patients with NS.[35] **Table 3** describes the differential diagnosis and **Figs. 12** and **13** illustrate the MR imaging appearance of leptomeningeal and dural involvement with sarcoidosis.

Parenchyma Intraparenchymal findings are present in 69% of patients with NS.[34] The most common manifestation is multiple small hyperintense lesions within the periventricular white matter, seen along perivascular spaces, which may or may not enhance.[36] This appearance can mimic demyelinating lesions of MS. Other appearances include randomly distributed T2 hyperintense masses, which may or may not enhance. The commonly affected regions include the brainstem and cerebellum, with a reported frequency of 21%, with less frequent involvement of the posterior pituitary and hypothalamus.[36] Pituitary and hypothalamic involvement can manifest as diffuse glandular

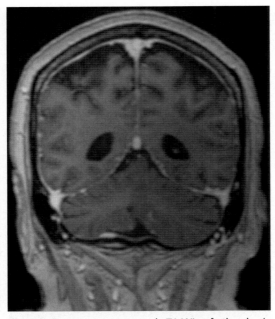

Fig. 12. Postcontrast coronal T1-WI of the brain showing nodular leptomeningeal enhancement in known case of sarcoidosis.

thickening, cystic pituitary lesions, stalk thickening, or simply postcontrast enhancement.[37] Hydrocephalus is present in approximately 6% of patients with NS.[32,34,36] This is most commonly communicating hydrocephalus, presumably secondary to granulomatous infiltration and subsequent arachnoid granulation dysfunction.[34,38] Rarely, tumefactive NS lesions may cause external compression and an obstructive type of hydrocephalus.

Cranial nerve involvement is seen in approximately 72% of patients with NS.[36] Although facial nerve palsy is the most common clinical manifestation of cranial nerve involvement, the optic nerve is the most commonly affected cranial nerve on imaging.[32,34,35] On MR imaging evaluation, involvement is usually seen as cranial nerve enhancement and swelling.

Spinal Cord

Clinical manifestations

Reported frequency of involvement ranges from 7% to 28% among various populations.[34–36] When symptomatic, patients with spinal cord involvement present with insidious paresthesia or weakness.[39]

Imaging features

Spinal cord involvement may appear as T2 hyperintense, elongated, and peripherally oriented intramedullary lesions, which enhance after contrast (**Fig. 14**). Similar findings may be seen in demyelinating disease, infection, or neoplasm.

Isolated involvement of the spinal cord is extremely rare, and, after taking into account the patient's presentation and evidence of disease outside the central nervous system, the diagnosis can usually be assumed without the need for biopsy. Intramedullary lesions are seen typically within the thoracic and cervical spine. There is often spinal cord swelling and edema, which, if long-standing, may progress to atrophy. Nodular leptomeningeal enhancement along the spinal cord is regularly seen and is thought to represent early disease. Junger and colleagues[40] have proposed a 4-stage MR imaging classification of spinal cord disease, outlined in **Box 9**, where intramedullary involvement represents invasion of initial leptomeningeal disease via perivascular spaces, with later stages progressing through spinal cord swelling and subsequent atrophy.

HEAD AND NECK
Sinonasal Cavity

Clinical manifestations

Involvement of the sinonasal cavity is rare, occurring in approximately 1% of patients with systemic sarcoidosis.[41] Common presenting symptoms

Table 3
Patterns on involvement in neurosarcoidosis

MR Imaging Findings	Type of Involvement	Differential

Hypointense on T2
May have homogenous
  or heterogeneous
  enhancement
	Diffuse	Lymphoma
		Meningiomatosis
		Pachymeningitis

	Focal	Meningioma (+/− internal calcification depending on homogeneous or heterogeneous enhancement) Focal dural metastasis

include obstruction, anosmia, epistaxis, and rhinorrhea.[42]

Imaging features

CT and MR imaging show nodular thickening of the nasal septum and turbinates. In more advanced disease, cartilaginous necrosis with accompanying lytic or sclerotic osseous lesions may be evident.[42] Definitive diagnosis is often not possible, and clinical correlation with signs of systemic sarcoidosis elsewhere is important, because these imaging findings may be seen in other granulomatous disorders, including tuberculosis, granulomatosis with polyangiitis, and Churg-Strauss syndrome.

Orbit

Clinical manifestations

Intraorbital involvement is seen in approximately 25% of sarcoidosis.[43] The most common presentation is self-limiting anterior uveitis.

Imaging features

Bilateral enlarged and homogeneously enhancing lacrimal glands are seen (**Fig. 15**). The differential for such findings should include lymphoma and Sjögren syndrome. Extraocular muscle involvement is also possible, evident on imaging as well-defined diffuse enlargement of 1, multiple, or all muscles.[44] Optic nerve involvement is common and typically manifests as nodular thickening and enhancement along the nerve sheath.

Parotid Gland

Clinical manifestations

Approximately 6% of patients with sarcoidosis exhibit parotid gland involvement; it is usually

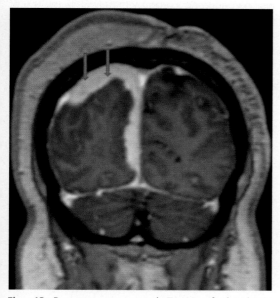

Fig. 13. Postcontrast coronal T1-WI of the brain showing thick plaque-like dural enhancement (*arrows*) in known case of sarcoidosis, mimicking other dural-based masses, such as meningioma.

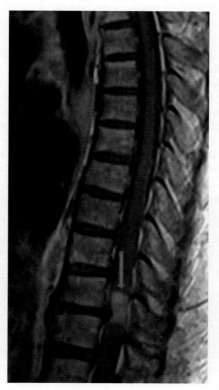

Fig. 14. Sagittal postcontrast T1-WI of the spine showing an enhancing intramedullary intradural lesion (*arrow*) in a patient with known history of sarcoidosis.

Box 9
Progression of spinal cord involvement on MR imaging as proposed by Junger and colleagues[40]

Stage 1: leptomeningeal inflammation with linear nodular enhancement along the surface of the spinal cord

Stage 2: perivascular spread with fusiform spinal cord enlargement

Stage 3: focal or diffuse intramedullary enhancement

Stage 4: spinal cord atrophy

Data from Junger SS, Stern BJ, Levine SR, et al. Intramedullary spinal sarcoidosis: clinical and magnetic resonance imaging characteristics. Neurology 1993;43(2):333–7.

bilateral and presents with painless parotid gland swelling.[2]

Imaging features

CT findings include diffuse enlargement of the glands and nodularity, potentially with a more confluent mass formation (**Fig. 16**). On MR imaging, the parotid glands appear enlarged and hyperintense on T2-WI and demonstrate diffuse postcontrast enhancement. Additionally, sarcoidosis predisposes to the formation of glandular calcifications.[45] Concomitant lacrimal gland involvement may occur, and on gallium 67 scintigraphy, the combination of physiologic nasopharyngeal uptake with bilateral lacrimal and parotid gland activity has classically been described as the panda sign.[46]

Thyroid Gland

Clinical manifestations

Involvement of the thyroid gland occurs in approximately 4% of patients with sarcoidosis.[47] Clinically, patients are asymptomatic or have subclinical thyroid dysfunction. Sarcoid involvement of the thyroid gland is usually incidentally discovered after work-up and biopsy of an enlarged thyroid gland or lesion.

Imaging features

Findings on ultrasound can mimic multinodular goiter, appearing as diffuse thyroid enlargement with heterogeneous echo texture and multiple hypoechoic nodules. On MR imaging, thyroid involvement may appear as heterogeneous signal within the thyroid with irregular nodular enhancement.

MUSCULOSKELETAL SYSTEM

Musculoskeletal manifestations of sarcoidosis are rare and can involve any component of the musculoskeletal system.

Bone Involvement

Bony involvement is rare and occurs in approximately 5% to 10% of patients with sarcoidosis.[10] It has a high association, however, with pulmonary involvement with concomitant pulmonary sarcoid lesions occurring in approximately 80% to 90% of cases.[48]

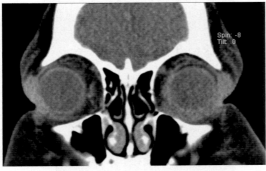

Fig. 15. Coronal reformatted CT images through the orbit showing mass-like infiltration of the lateral rectus and the right lacrimal gland, secondary to sarcoidosis. (*Courtesy of* Girish Fatterpekar, MD, NYUMC, NY.)

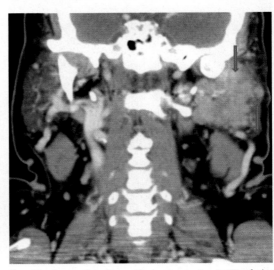

Fig. 16. Coronal reformatted postcontrast CT of the neck showing asymmetry of the parotid glands with a lobulated mass infiltrating the left gland (*arrow*) and adjacent satellite soft tissue nodules.

Clinical manifestations

Sarcoid lesions in small bones, such as phalanges, are associated with skin involvement, in particular lupus pernio. Phalanges of the hands and feet are the most common sites of involvement and these lesions may have associated soft tissue swelling.

Imaging features

Radiographs are often sufficient for detecting characteristic sarcoid lesions in the phalanges of the hands and feet. On radiographs, osseous sarcoid classically manifests as lacelike lytic bone lesions in the phalanges of the hands or feet, findings that are virtually pathognomonic in patients with clinical sarcoidosis (**Fig. 17**). The lacy appearance is secondary to cortical tunneling of the granulomas and subsequent bony remodeling. As a result, the concave shapes of the phalangeal shafts are lost and they become more tubular in appearance.

Lesions in the digits may also be purely lytic, giving a punched-out appearance and, if large enough, may cause cortical erosions or pathologic fracture. Granulomatous involvement of distal phalangeal tufts can mimic acro-osteolysis.

Sarcoid bone lesions in large bones or within the axial skeleton may not have the characteristic lacelike pattern and are often occult on radiographs and bone scintigraphy. When visible, they have variable and nonspecific lytic, sclerotic, or mixed appearance. On CT, phalangeal lesions echo the radiographic appearance described previously. Large bone lesions, as with radiographs, may not be visible on CT or they may exhibit subtle sclerosis. MR imaging may unveil more extensive involvement and is also better suited in detecting lesions within the large bones and axial skeleton, which may be occult on radiographs and bone scan. MR imaging appearance of sarcoid bone involvement is nonspecific.[49] Lesions are typically homogenously hypointense on T1-WI, are hyperintense on fluid-sensitive sequences, and demonstrate postcontrast enhancement (**Fig. 18**). Lesions may be indistinct or well marginated and are of varying sizes. Sequelae of prior lesions may demonstrate signal intensities consistent with fat or fibrosis.

Sarcoid bone lesions are often multiple and lesions have imaging features that may be identical to osseous metastatic disease or multiple myeloma. MR imaging cannot confidently differentiate sarcoid bone lesions from osseous metastatic disease or multiple myeloma. Unlike sarcoidosis, small bone acral involvement is rare with metastatic disease and multiple myeloma. Biopsy may be required for definitive differentiation of large bone or axial skeletal lesions.

Joint Involvement

Sarcoidosis-related arthropathy occurs in 10% to 38% of patients with sarcoidosis and manifests in 2 forms: acute arthropathy and chronic relapsing arthropathy.[50]

Clinical features

The 2 forms differ in their clinical course and prognosis, as described in **Table 4**.

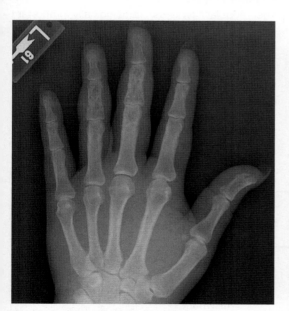

Fig. 17. Radiograph of the hand shows the characteristic bony involvement with lacelike appearance of the phalanges.

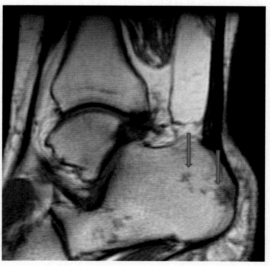

Fig. 18. Sagittal T1-WI of the ankle showing ill-defined T1 hypointense lesions in the calcaneus (arrows) in a patient with known systemic sarcoidosis.

Table 4
Sarcoid arthropathy

Acute Arthropathy	Chronic Relapsing Arthropathy
More common	Less common, occurring in only 0.2% of cases[50]
Self-limiting condition, which resolves within 4–6 wk, with disease clusters observed in spring and early summer	Relapsing and usually occurs >6 mo after sarcoidosis diagnosis Occurs later in life—in late 40s.
Involves the bilateral ankles in >90% of cases Knee, proximal interphalangeal joints, and wrists are other sites of involvement.	Knees, ankles, and/or proximal interphalangeal joints
Patients present with painful, stiff joints. Löfgren syndrome, the most common variant of acute sarcoid arthropathy, is summarized in Table 5.	Similar to acute sarcoidosis, patients may present with joint pain and stiffness in knees, ankles and/or proximal interphalangeal joints.

Imaging findings

In both acute and chronic sarcoid arthropathy, radiographs may be normal or demonstrate nonspecific soft tissue swelling, including dactylitis, and osteoporosis. Occasionally, subchondral cysts and erosions may be present, which may be more apparent on MR imaging. Joint effusion is rare. Hands and feet may demonstrate characteristic bone lesions, which can help confirm diagnosis.

Acute or chronic sarcoid arthropathy can mimic rheumatoid arthritis and is usually detected by clinical criteria, including negative serology for rheumatoid factor and antinuclear antibodies. Patients with chronic sarcoid arthropathy, however, may be rheumatoid factor positive in up to 47% of cases.[51] In such cases, synovial or soft tissue biopsy is required to establish sarcoidosis granulomatous etiology.

Muscle Involvement

Intramuscular sarcoid involvement is clinically rare, reported in less than 1.4% of patients with systemic disease.[49] Granulomatous involvement of the muscles, however, in histologic studies is reportedly present in 50% to 80% of patients.[49]

Thus, a large number of patients with muscular involvement are asymptomatic.

Clinical manifestations

The proximal muscles of the lower extremities are the most commonly affected, and palpable nodules in this area are associated with proximal muscle weakness.[52] Three types of muscular sarcoid involvement have been described: nodular type, acute myositis, and chronic myopathic/atrophic type. The nodular type can present as a palpable intramuscular mass whereas the chronic atrophic type presents with muscle weakness due to associated muscle atrophy.

Imaging features

The nodular type is radiologically important because the nodules can mimic intramuscular masses, although they demonstrate fairly distinctive findings on MR imaging evaluation. Typically, these lesions are oriented longitudinally along the myotendinous junction and demonstrate as a central, nonenhancing, fibrotic area that is hypointense on T1-WI and T2-WI and is surrounded by edematous granulomatous tissue, which is T2 hyperintense and demonstrates postcontrast enhancement.[37] This combination can produce

Table 5
Cutaneous manifestations of sarcoidosis

Erythema Nodosum	Lupus Pernio
Associated with acute sarcoid	Associated with chronic sarcoid
Nonspecific inflammation of skin and subcutaneous fat	High association with pulmonary sarcoid
Tender nodules along anterior lower extremity	Reddish-purple indurated nodules on the face/hands
Fever + arthralgia + erythema nodosum = Löfgren syndrome	Can have underlying bone involvement of phalanges

the so-called dark star appearance, which, when present, is characteristic of sarcoidosis.[52] The lesions may be elongated, and, on coronal images, the central low-intensity fibrosis flanked by high signal granulomatous tissue appears as the 3 stripes sign.[52]

Acute myositis may occur in the early inflammatory stage of the disease. Affected areas either are occult on imaging or appear as nonspecific intramuscular edema, which enhances on MR imaging. Patients with chronic myopathic involvement demonstrate muscular atrophy on MR imaging evaluation. Although this atrophy is nonspecific, it can direct biopsy for definitive diagnosis.[37]

Cutaneous Involvement

Among patients with sarcoidosis, 25% develop skin involvement, with the 2 most classically identifiable manifestations erythema nodosum and lupus pernio.[53] The distinguishing features of these 2 entities are described in **Table 5**.

REFERENCES

1. Newman LS, Rose CS, Maier LA. Sarcoidosis. N Engl J Med 1997;336(17):1224–34.
2. Statement on sarcoidosis. Joint statement of the American thoracic society (ATS), the European respiratory society (ERS) and the world association of sarcoidosis and other granulomatous disorders (WASOG) adopted by the ATS board of directors and by the ERS executive committee, 1999. Am J Respir Crit Care Med 1999;160(2):736–55.
3. Henke CE, Henke G, Elveback LR, et al. The epidemiology of sarcoidosis in Rochester, Minnesota: a population-based study of incidence and survival. Am J Epidemiol 1986;123(5):840–5.
4. Valeyre D, Prasse A, Nunes H, et al. Sarcoidosis. Lancet 2014;383(9923):1155–67.
5. Hawtin KE, Roddie ME, Mauri FA, et al. Pulmonary sarcoidosis: the 'Great Pretender'. Clin Radiol 2010;65(8):642–50.
6. Criado E, Sanchez M, Ramirez J, et al. Pulmonary sarcoidosis: typical and atypical manifestations at high-resolution CT with pathologic correlation. Radiographics 2010;30(6):1567–86.
7. Spagnolo P, Sverzellati N, Wells AU, et al. Imaging aspects of the diagnosis of sarcoidosis. Eur Radiol 2014;24(4):807–16.
8. Sobic-Saranovic D, Artiko V, Obradovic V. FDG PET imaging in sarcoidosis. Semin Nucl Med 2013;43(6):404–11.
9. Mostard RL, van Kroonenburgh MJ, Drent M. The role of the PET scan in the management of sarcoidosis. Curr Opin Pulm Med 2013;19(5):538–44.

10. Koyama T, Ueda H, Togashi K, et al. Radiologic manifestations of sarcoidosis in various organs. Radiographics 2004;24(1):87–104.
11. Siltzbach LE. Sarcoidosis: clinical features and management. Med Clin North Am 1967;51(2):483–450.
12. Al-Jahdali H, Rajiah P, Koteyar SS, et al. Atypical radiological manifestations of thoracic sarcoidosis: a review and pictorial essay. Ann Thorac Med 2013;8(4):186–96.
13. Park HJ, Jung JI, Chung MH, et al. Typical and atypical manifestations of intrathoracic sarcoidosis. Korean J Radiol 2009;10(6):623–31.
14. Malaisamy S, Dalal B, Bimenyuy C, et al. The clinical and radiologic features of nodular pulmonary sarcoidosis. Lung 2009;187(1):9–15.
15. Soskel NT, Sharma OP. Pleural involvement in sarcoidosis. Curr Opin Pulm Med 2000;6(5):455–68.
16. Doughan AR, Williams BR. Cardiac sarcoidosis. Heart 2006;92(2):282–8.
17. Dubrey SW, Falk RH. Diagnosis and management of cardiac sarcoidosis. Prog Cardiovasc Dis 2010;52(4):336–46.
18. Sabate JM, Clotet M, Gomez A, et al. Radiologic evaluation of uncommon inflammatory and reactive breast disorders. Radiographics 2005;25(2):411–24.
19. Kenzel PP, Hadijuana J, Hosten N, et al. Boeck sarcoidosis of the breast: mammographic, ultrasound, and MR findings. J Comput Assist Tomogr 1997;21(3):439–41.
20. Warshauer DM, Lee JK. Imaging manifestations of abdominal sarcoidosis. AJR Am J Roentgenol 2004;182(1):15–28.
21. Kennedy PT, Zakaria N, Modawi SB, et al. Natural history of hepatic sarcoidosis and its response to treatment. Eur J Gastroenterol Hepatol 2006;18(7):721–6.
22. Harder H, Buchler MW, Frohlich B, et al. Extrapulmonary sarcoidosis of liver and pancreas: a case report and review of literature. World J Gastroenterol 2007;13(17):2504–9.
23. Mueller S, Boehme MW, Hofmann WJ, et al. Extrapulmonary sarcoidosis primarily diagnosed in the liver. Scand J Gastroenterol 2000;35(9):1003–8.
24. Tan CB, Rashid S, Rajan D, et al. Hepatic sarcoidosis presenting as portal hypertension and liver cirrhosis: case report and review of the literature. Case Rep Gastroenterol 2012;6(1):183–9.
25. Elsayes KM, Narra VR, Mukundan G, et al. MR imaging of the spleen: spectrum of abnormalities. Radiographics 2005;25(4):967–82.
26. Gezer NS, Basara I, Altay C, et al. Abdominal sarcoidosis: cross-sectional imaging findings. Diagn Interv Radiol 2015;21(2):111–7.
27. Matsubara T, Hirahara N, Hyakudomi R, et al. Early gastric cancer associated with gastric sarcoidosis. Int Surg 2015;100(5):949–53.
28. Caceres M, Sabbaghian MS, Braud R, et al. Pancreatic sarcoidosis: unusual presentation resembling a

periampullary malignancy. Curr Surg 2006;63(3): 179–85.

29. Baroni RH, Pedrosa I, Tavernaraki E, et al. Pancreatic sarcoidosis: MRI features. J Magn Reson Imaging 2004;20(5):889–93.

30. Rao PK, Sabanegh ES. Genitourinary sarcoidosis. Rev Urol 2009;11(2):108–13.

31. Svetec DA, Waguespack RL, Sabanegh ES Jr. Intermittent azoospermia associated with epididymal sarcoidosis. Fertil Steril 1998;70(4):777–9.

32. Stern BJ, Krumholz A, Johns C, et al. Sarcoidosis and its neurological manifestations. Arch Neurol 1985;42(9):909–17.

33. Manz HJ. Pathobiology of neurosarcoidosis and clinicopathologic correlation. Can J Neurol Sci 1983;10(1):50–5.

34. Scott TF, Yandora K, Valeri A, et al. Aggressive therapy for neurosarcoidosis: long-term follow-up of 48 treated patients. Arch Neurol 2007;64(5):691–6.

35. Shah R, Roberson GH, Cure JK. Correlation of MR imaging findings and clinical manifestations in neurosarcoidosis. AJNR Am J Neuroradiol 2009;30(5): 953–61.

36. Zajicek JP, Scolding NJ, Foster O, et al. Central nervous system sarcoidosis–diagnosis and management. QJM 1999;92(2):103–17.

37. Vardhanabhuti V, Venkatanarasimha N, Bhatnagar G, et al. Extra-pulmonary manifestations of sarcoidosis. Clin Radiol 2012;67(3):263–76.

38. Scott TF. Cerebral herniation after lumbar puncture in sarcoid meningitis. Clin Neurol Neurosurg 2000; 102(1):26–8.

39. Bradley DA, Lower EE, Baughman RP. Diagnosis and management of spinal cord sarcoidosis. Sarcoidosis Vasc Diffuse Lung Dis 2006;23(1):58–65.

40. Junger SS, Stern BJ, Levine SR, et al. Intramedullary spinal sarcoidosis: clinical and magnetic resonance imaging characteristics. Neurology 1993;43(2):333–7.

41. Som PM, Brandwein-Gensler MS, Wang BY. Inflammatory Diseases of the Sinonasal Caities. In: Som PM, Curtin HD, editors. Head and Neck

Imaging. 5th edition. St Louis, MO: Mosby; 2011. p. 167–252.

42. Aubart FC, Ouayoun M, Brauner M, et al. Sinonasal involvement in sarcoidosis: a case-control study of 20 patients. Medicine (Baltimore) 2006; 85(6):365–71.

43. Som PM, Brandwein-Gensler MS, Wang BY. Pathology of the Eye and Orbit. In: Som PM, Curtin HD, editors. Head and Neck Imaging. 5th edition. St Louis, MO: Mosby; 2011. p. 591–756.

44. Mavrikakis I, Rootman J. Diverse clinical presentations of orbital sarcoid. Am J Ophthalmol 2007; 144(5):769–75.

45. Yousem DM, Kraut MA, Chalian AA. Major salivary gland imaging. Radiology 2000;216(1):19–29.

46. Kurdziel KA. The panda sign. Radiology 2000; 215(3):884–5.

47. BRANSON JH, PARK JH. Sarcoidosis hepatic involvement: presentation of a case with fatal liver involvement; including autopsy findings and review of the evidence for sarcoid involvement of the liver as found in the literature. Ann Intern Med 1954; 40(1):111–45.

48. Fisher AJ, Gilula LA, Kyriakos M, et al. MR imaging changes of lumbar vertebral sarcoidosis. AJR Am J Roentgenol 1999;173(2):354–6.

49. Moore SL, Teirstein AE. Musculoskeletal sarcoidosis: spectrum of appearances at MR imaging. Radiographics 2003;23(6):1389–99.

50. Nessrine A, Zahra AF, Taoufik H. Musculoskeletal involvement in sarcoidosis. J Bras Pneumol 2014; 40(2):175–82.

51. Chatham W. Rheumatic manifestations of systemic disease: sarcoidosis. Curr Opin Rheumatol 2010; 22(1):85–90.

52. Tohme-Noun C, Le Breton C, Sobotka A, et al. Imaging findings in three cases of the nodular type of muscular sarcoidosis. AJR Am J Roentgenol 2004; 183(4):995–9.

53. Sharma OP. Cutaneous sarcoidosis: clinical features and management. Chest 1972;61(4):320–5.

Immunoglobulin G4–Related Disease: Recent Advances in Pathogenesis and Imaging Findings

Venkata S. Katabathina, MD[a],[*], Suhare Khalil, MD[a],
Sooyoung Shin[b], Narayan Lath, MD[c], Christine O. Menias[d],
Srinivasa R. Prasad, MD[b]

KEYWORDS

- IgG4-related disease • Lymphoplasmacytic infiltration • Computed tomography
- Magnetic resonance imaging • 18FDG-PET • Autoimmune pancreatitis • IgG4 cholangitis
- Riedel thyroiditis

KEY POINTS

- IgG4-RD is a distinct, steroid responsive, idiopathic fibroinflammatory disorder characterized by lymphoplasmacytic infiltration rich in IgG4 plasma cells, obliterative phlebitis, and storiform fibrosis. The disease manifests as tumefactive lesions in multiple organs.
- Select conditions of IgG4-RD demonstrate characteristic imaging findings on cross-sectional studies that may help in diagnosis, evaluating treatment response, and surveillance. Although ultrasound, computed tomography (CT), and MR imaging are helpful in the initial diagnosis, PET/CT plays a major role in monitoring disease activity after treatment as well as in long-term surveillance.
- Although most patients with IgG4-RD have elevated serum IgG4 concentrations, they are neither sensitive nor specific for the diagnosis; up to 30% of patients with characteristic histopathological features may have normal serum IgG4 levels. However, IgG4 levels can be helpful for assessing treatment response.
- Orbital inflammation, submandibular gland disease, Riedel thyroiditis, mediastinal lymphadenopathy, type 1 autoimmune pancreatitis, IgG4 cholangitis, retroperitoneal fibrosis, and renal masses are the most common manifestations of IgG4-RD.
- Glucocorticoids are the mainstay of treatment; recently, rituximab, a select B-cell depleting agent, has been shown to provide an excellent clinical response in select patients.

INTRODUCTION

Immunoglobulin G4–related disease (IgG4-RD) is a newly characterized, fibroinflammatory disorder encompassing a wide spectrum of diseases that share characteristic clinical (multifocal tumefactive lesions), serologic (elevated serum IgG4 concentrations), and pathologic (lymphoplasmacytic infiltration rich in IgG4 plasma cells, obliterative phlebitis, and storiform fibrosis) findings.[1,2] Type 1 autoimmune pancreatitis (AIP) was the first entity to be characterized as a prototype IgG4-RD; other disparate entities were subsequently

[a] Department of Radiology, University of Texas Health Science Center at San Antonio, 7703 Floyd Curl Drive, San Antonio, TX 78229, USA; [b] Department of Radiology, The University of Texas MD Anderson Cancer Center, Houston, TX, USA; [c] Department of Radiology, Singapore General Hospital, Outram road, Singapore 169608, Singapore; [d] Department of Radiology, Mayo Clinic, Scottsdale, AZ, USA
* Corresponding author.
E-mail address: katabathina@uthscsa.edu

Radiol Clin N Am 54 (2016) 535–551
http://dx.doi.org/10.1016/j.rcl.2015.12.010

thought to show similar pathologic findings.[3–7] Consistent identification of IgG4-positive plasma cells on tissue samples, as well as raised serum IgG4 levels, led to the term "IgG4-related autoimmune disease,"[2,6,8,9] Since then, nomenclature had been evolving, with multiple new names being proposed by different investigators. The unifying standard term of "IgG4-RD" is currently recommended for the condition.[10] Specific names have been proposed to each organ system involved while also replacing the previously well-recognized entities (**Fig. 1**).[1,2,10] Recent advances in pathology have identified the seminal roles of T and B lymphocytes, and eosinophils in the pathogenesis of IgG4-RD that have opened new avenues for targeted therapeutics.[9] IgG4-RD demonstrates characteristic imaging findings on cross-sectional studies, which may help in the initial detection, treatment follow-up, and surveillance, as well as testing efficacy of novel drugs. IgG4-RD exhibits a favorable response to glucocorticoid

therapy. Given the systemic nature of IgG4-RD that may mimic many infectious, inflammatory, and neoplastic entities, improved awareness of this condition may help in avoiding unnecessary invasive procedures.[11]

In this article, we first discuss epidemiology, clinical features, pathology, and evolving concepts in the pathophysiology of IgG4-RD; we then review characteristic imaging findings of IgG4-RD in various organ systems.

EPIDEMIOLOGY AND CLINICAL FEATURES

As a relatively new clinicopathologic entity, sparse data exist on the epidemiology of IgG4-RD. The exact prevalence rates are definitely underestimated owing to poor awareness and lack of diagnostic standards until now. AIP is considered as the prototypic manifestation of IgG4-RD and is seen in up to 60% of patients with IgG4-RD. Most epidemiologic data have

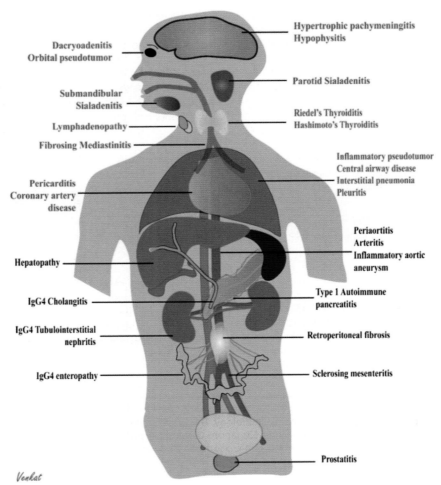

Fig. 1. Drawing shows multisystem involvement of IgG4-related disease with specific names to each organ system.

come from the studies of patients with AIP, particularly in Japan.[10,12] A Japanese study done by Umehara and colleagues[4] estimated an incidence of 0.28 to 1.08/100,000 population, with 336 to 1300 patients being diagnosed annually. Although the prevalence of IgG4-RD in North America is definitely lower than in Asian countries, the exact figures are unknown. The typical patient with IgG4-RD is a middle-aged to elderly man; more than 90% of patients are older than 50 years.[12] There is a definite male predominance with male-to-female ratio of 3.5 to 1 in most organ systems with the exception of head and neck disease (dacryoadenitis and sialadenitis), in which gender ratio may be equal or slightly female predominant.[1,13] This feature contrasts strikingly with classic autoimmune diseases such as systemic lupus erythematous, for which females outnumber males by 9 to 1. As of now, there are no reported familial cases of IgG4-RD. No clear genetic predisposition has been identified; however, there is need for more extensive studies from different geographic and ethnic backgrounds before any conclusions regarding genetic predisposition may be inferred.[1]

Most patients with IgG4-RD present in a subacute fashion without constitutional symptoms such as fever; however, fewer than 10% of patients may have dramatic presentation, with weight loss, fever, elevation of acute phase reactants, and other signs of inflammation.[1,14] Multiorgan involvement is seen in up to 90% of patients and may occur either in a synchronous or metachronous way; unexplained swelling of a single or multiple organs should raise the suspicion of IgG4-RD.[14] As clinical signs and symptoms are nonspecific, IgG4-RD is oftentimes diagnosed unexpectedly through imaging findings and/or pathologic examination.[15]

CURRENT CONCEPTS IN PATHOGENESIS

Although exact pathogenesis of IgG4-RD is not well understood, multiple immune-mediated mechanisms have been identified as contributing factors. A combination of autoimmunity and allergic phenomenon is thought to be responsible for the fibroinflammatory response in IgG4-RD.[1,16] It is proposed that an aberrant immune response to infections, commensal microbes, food and environmental allergens, or tissue damage may be the initiating event in the pathogenesis of IgG4-RD that may activate T-helper (both type 1 and 2) and T-regulatory lymphocytes.[1,13] Activated T cells may produce an inflammatory cytokine milieu that includes multiple interleukins (IL)

such as IL-4, IL-5, IL-10, and IL-13, interferon gamma (INF-γ), and transcription growth factor beta (TGF-β).[1,16]

The major function of IL-4 and IL-10 is to drive preferential class switching of autoreactive B lymphocytes to IgE and IgG4 and to promote the differentiation of IgG4-positive plasma cells.[2,13] Although IL-5, IL-13, and TGF-β play a major role in recruitment of eosinophils as well as fibroblast activation, INF-γ may contribute to activation of macrophages.[1] IgG4 and Ig-E antibodies may cross-react to self-antigens. B cells that recognize self-antigens may present them to auto-reactive T cells that perpetuate a vicious cycle of collaboration between T cells and B cells.[6,9,17] Activated fibroblasts and macrophages cause dense fibrosis and obliterative phlebitis. The tissue damage in IgG4-RD is mainly from extensive expansion of fibroblasts; the degree of fibrosis is more profound in pancreatic, biliary tract, and retroperitoneal disease, when compared with the disease of salivary glands or lymph nodes.[4,18] Activated self-reactive T cells are capable of facilitating germinal center formation and recruitment of more B lymphocytes and plasma cells into the involved organ that results in typical pathologic manifestations[8] (**Fig. 2**). Given the inability of IgG4 antibodies to cross-link antigens to form immune complexes and activate complement system, they are thought to be noninflammatory in nature; their precise role in the pathophysiology remains unclear.[1,13]

DIAGNOSIS

The definite diagnosis of IgG4-RD is primarily based on the characteristic histopathological and immunohistochemical findings that include dense lymphoplasmacytic infiltrate rich in IgG4-positive plasma cells, a storiform pattern of fibrosis, and obliterative phlebitis (**Fig. 3**).[19,20] Additional histologic findings, including a moderate amount of tissue eosinophilia, absolute IgG4-positive plasma cell count (more than 40/high-power field), and IgG4:IgG ratio greater than 40%, are also useful in select cases.[20] Although most patients with IgG4-RD have elevated serum IgG4 concentrations (>135 mg/dL), it is neither sensitive nor specific for the diagnosis; up to 30% of patients with characteristic histopathological features may have normal serum IgG4 levels.[2,13] Additionally, serum IgG4 levels are shown to be elevated in healthy volunteers, various neoplastic and inflammatory conditions including pancreatic cancer

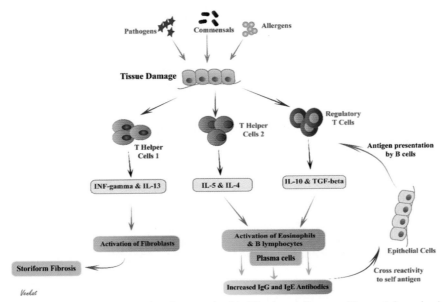

Fig. 2. Illustration demonstrates proposed pathogenesis of IgG4-related disease with special emphasis on the role of T and B lymphocytes and multiple cytokines in producing characteristic pathologic findings. (*Data from* Refs.[1,2,16])

and overreliance on these values may lead to a false-positive diagnosis of IgG4-RD.[13]

ROLE OF IMAGING

Cross-sectional imaging techniques, such as ultrasound, computed tomography (CT), and MR imaging play a pivotal role in the management of patients with IgG4-RD; in addition to timely diagnosis, these tests help to establish the extent of the disease.[11,21,22] Because IgG4-RD commonly involves multiple organs, understanding the characteristic findings for each affected organ is essential in appropriate diagnosis.[23] As most patients come to medical attention with symptoms

related to one organ system, the radiologist's role is invaluable in identifying multisystem involvement, including body systems without any appreciable symptoms.[23,24] Diffuse or focal enlargement of the organs with associated encasement by inflammatory and fibrotic tissue is commonly identified on imaging studies and may mimic malignancies.[2,23] It is crucial to differentiate IgG4-RD from malignancies in the respective organs to avoid aggressive intervention.

Involvement of the salivary and thyroid glands, as well as multiple abdominal organs, can be either diagnosed confidently or at least suspected on ultrasound examination.[23] CT of the chest, abdomen, and pelvis is recommended in all

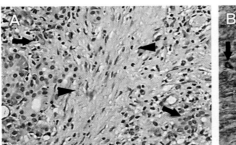 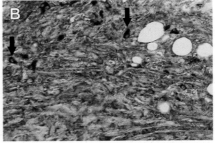

Fig. 3. Pathologic features of IgG4-related disease. (*A*) Photomicrograph (original magnification, ×100; hematoxylin-eosin stain) from a patient with type 1 autoimmune pancreatitis demonstrates lymphoplasmacytic infiltration (*arrows*), associated with storiform fibrosis (*arrowheads*). (*B*) Photomicrograph (original magnification, ×100; IgG4 immunohistochemical stain) shows multiple, intensely positive plasma cells (*arrows*) confirming the diagnosis of IgG4-related disease.

patients diagnosed with IgG4-RD, given the high frequency of pancreatic involvement (up to 60%) that shows characteristic imaging findings.[21,25,26] MR imaging of the brain and orbit is helpful in assessing the ophthalmic, pituitary, and meningeal involvement of IgG4-RD. Functional imaging with 18-fluorodeoxy glucose PET (18FDG-PET) is highly effective in establishing the extent of the disease and should be considered in all patients at the time of initial diagnosis as a baseline.[22,27] In addition, PET/CT is useful in monitoring disease activity after treatment as well as long-term surveillance given the significant relapse rates of IgG4-RD.[27]

HEAD, NECK, AND INTRACRANIAL DISEASE
Orbits

The term "IgG4-related orbital disease" refers to the inflammation involving the soft tissues of the orbital and periorbital region in patients with IgG4-RD; lacrimal glands (dacryoadenitis) are the most commonly involved organs, followed by ocular muscles, and orbital nerves.[28] Idiopathic orbital inflammatory syndrome (inflammatory pseudotumor) and lymphoid hyperplasia are now considered as part of the IgG4-RD.[1,29] Lacrimal gland involvement is commonly bilateral and often associated with parotid and submandibular gland involvement.[1] Diffuse enlargement of the lacrimal glands that demonstrate intermediate soft tissue attenuation on CT and low signal intensity on T1-weighted images (T1-WIs) and T2-WIs (secondary to increased cellularity and fibrosis) with homogeneous enhancement after contrast administration is typical for IgG4-RD (Fig. 4).[30–32]

Enlargement of the orbital nerves (optic, trigeminal, and ophthalmic) and ocular muscles can also be identified on CT/MR imaging; particularly, diffuse thickening of the infraorbital nerve is considered somewhat specific for IgG4-RD.[33] Diffuse, irregular, masslike enlargement with associated enhancement of the orbital soft tissues is the characteristic imaging appearance of orbital pseudotumors; IgG-RD may account for up to 50% of these cases (Fig. 5).[29]

Salivary Glands

Inflammation of the salivary glands is the most common presentation of IgG4-RD involving the head and neck, with the submandibular gland being the most common target.[1,28] Chronic sclerosing sialadenitis (Küttner tumor) and the Mikulicz disease are now classified in the continuum of IgG4-RD. Küttner tumor typically affects one or both submandibular glands, but it can also involve other salivary glands and clinically presents as a "hard swelling."[32] Ultrasound shows diffuse enlargement of the submandibular glands with multiple ill-defined hypoechoic foci scattered against a heterogeneous background giving to "mottled, netlike" appearance and minimally increased vascularity (Fig. 6).[30,34] Enlarged glands show homogeneous attenuation on CT and low to intermediate signal intensity on T2-WIs and intermediate signal intensity on T1-WIs on MR imaging with associated homogeneous enhancement (Fig. 7).[30,32] Multiple, enlarged lymph nodes are commonly seen in these patients with salivary gland disease. Differential considerations include malignant salivary gland tumors, lymphoma, and acute phase of Sjogren syndrome, especially if unilateral involvement is seen; whereas parotid gland involvement is more common in Sjogren syndrome, isolated submandibular gland disease favors the possibility of IgG4-RD.[32]

Mikulicz disease is defined clinically as bilateral painless swelling of the submandibular,

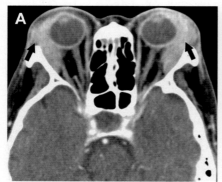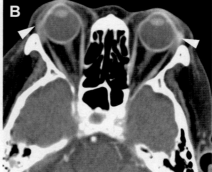

Fig. 4. IgG4-related dacryoadenitis in a 64-year-old man. (A) Axial contrast-enhanced CT at the level of orbits demonstrates diffusely enlarged, homogenous appearance of the bilateral lacrimal glands with associated proptosis (arrows). (B) Axial contrast-enhanced CT after treatment with steroids shows near-normal appearing lacrimal glands with significant improvement in proptosis (arrowheads).

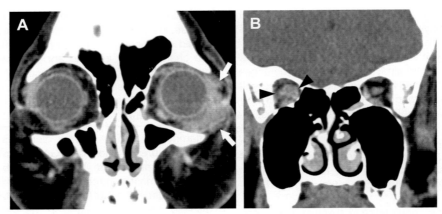

Fig. 5. IgG4-related orbital inflammatory pseudotumor and optic neuritis in a 34-year-old man. (*A, B*) Coronal contrast-enhanced CT images of the orbits show heterogeneously enhancing, soft-tissue thickening abutting the left globe (*arrows*) and irregular thickening of the right optic nerve (*arrowheads*). Both findings were completely resolved after steroid treatment.

sublingual, parotid, and lacrimal glands for the duration of at least 3 months.[1,28] Although CT demonstrates homogeneous attenuation and enhancement of the involved glands, MR shows homogeneous low to intermediate signal intensity on T2-WIs and low signal intensity on T1-WIs, with homogeneous enhancement on post gadolinium T1-WI.[30–32] Differential considerations to consider include acute phase of Sjogren, lymphoma, sarcoidosis, and mumps.[32]

Thyroid

"IgG4-related thyroiditis" is the new name given to the thyroid lesions associated with hypothyroidism in patients with IgG4-RD; an association between IgG4-RD and Riedel and Hashimotos thyroiditis has been confirmed recently on multiple studies.[1,28,35] Currently, a significant proportion of Hashimoto thyroiditis cases and almost all cases of Riedel thyroiditis are considered as part of the IgG4-RD.[28,36] Riedel thyroiditis may affect one or both thyroid lobes; unlike most of the other IgG4-RD, female predominance is identified in most cases.[35] On CT, IgG4-related thyroiditis may appear as focal or diffuse hypoattenuation of the thyroid gland; on MR imaging, homogeneous low signal intensity of the thyroid tissue on T2WIs with delayed enhancement after contrast administration is commonly seen, indicating the presence of profound fibrosis (**Fig. 8**).[31,32] Fibrosis of the thyroid gland may extend into adjacent structures with possible encasement of the parathyroid glands, nerves, muscles, and trachea.[8,36] Early diagnosis may lead to timely intervention that can prevent destruction of the thyroid gland and associated hypothyroidism.

Intracranial Disease

Hypertrophic pachymeningitis and hypophysitis are 2 principal intracranial manifestations of IgG4-RD; brain parenchymal involvement is exceedingly rare.[37,38] Headache, visual field

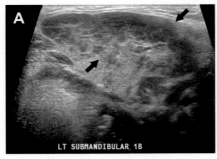
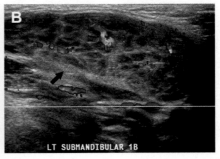

Fig. 6. IgG4-related sialadenitis of the submandibular glands in a 46-year-old man. Axial ultrasound (*A*) and color Doppler (*B*) images of the left submandibular gland shows diffusely enlarged gland that shows multiple ill-defined hypoechoic lesions and increased vascularity (*arrows*). The right submandibular gland also shows similar findings (not shown here).

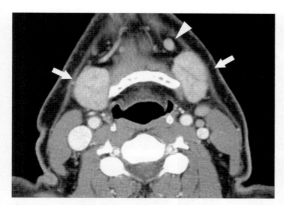

Fig. 7. IgG4-related sialadenitis of the submandibular glands in a 59-year-old man. Axial contrast-enhanced CT of the neck demonstrates diffusely enlarged, homogeneous appearance of the bilateral submandibular glands (*arrows*) consistent with Küttner tumor. Also note few enlarged lymph nodes (*arrowhead*).

defects, and lactation abnormalities are common clinical features in hypophysitis; diffuse thickening and mass formation within the pituitary stalk that shows diffuse contrast enhancement is the common MR imaging finding (**Fig. 9**).[30,31] Diffuse enlargement and/or mass formation also may be seen in the pituitary gland.[30] Pachymeningitis tends to involve both intraspinal and intracranial meninges; chronic headache, cranial nerve palsies, radiculopathy, and signs of spinal cord compression are common clinical findings.[37] On MR, diffuse nodular thickening of the meninges that show homogeneous and gradual enhancement is the characteristic feature; associated meningeal masses mimicking meningiomas also maybe identified (see **Fig. 9**).[31,38] Diffuse wall

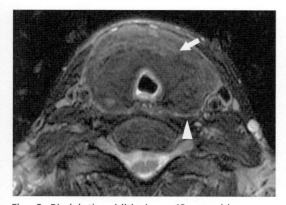

Fig. 8. Riedel thyroiditis in a 42-year-old woman. Axial T2-weighted MR image of the neck shows diffusely hypointense thyroid gland (*arrow*) with hyperintense capsule (*arrowhead*), which was proven to be Riedel thyroiditis on pathology.

thickening and enhancement of the carotid and vertebral arteries without vascular occlusion also may be seen (see **Fig. 9**).[30]

THORAX
Lung Parenchymal, Airway, and Pleural Disease

"IgG4-related pulmonary disease" can be identified in up to 15% of patients with autoimmune pancreatitis and can present as one of the following pulmonary syndromes: central airway disease, inflammatory pseudotumor, localized or diffuse interstitial pneumonia, and pleuritis.[1,39,40] Depending on the type and extent of involvement, clinical presentation varies with cough, dyspnea, pleural effusion, and chest pain being the common symptoms.[39,40] On pathology, obliterative arteritis and obliterative phlebitis, and neutrophilic infiltration are more common in lung disease compared with other organs.[1,40]

On CT, 4 major categories of lung involvement have been described: solid nodular type (single or multiple nodules), ground-glass opacity type (round ground-glass opacities), alveolar interstitial type (diffuse ground-glass and reticular opacities, and honeycombing), and bronchovascular type (thickening of the bronchovascular bundles and interlobular septa) (**Fig. 10**).[39,41,42] These CT findings are often nonspecific and can mimic lung malignancy, idiopathic interstitial pneumonias, cryptogenic organizing pneumonia, and sarcoidosis.[42] Although solid-appearing masses with spiculated margins mimic small cell/squamous carcinoma, ground-glass opacities may simulate bronchoalveolar carcinoma. Awareness of these findings, along with identification of systemic involvement, may avert unnecessary lung surgery.[42]

On imaging, pleural disease appears as marked, nodular thickening of the visceral and parietal pleura with associated masses, mimicking mesothelioma; pleural effusions are rare.[39,43] Although uncommon, airway disease appears as irregular wall thickening of the trachea and major bronchi, bronchiectasis, or extrinsic compression of the central airways secondary to mediastinal fibrosis.[41]

Mediastinal Disease

The most common intrathoracic manifestation of IgG4-RD is mediastinal and/or hilar lymphadenopathy, which can be seen in up to 90% of the patients and is often associated with unilateral or bilateral soft tissue thickening on CT/MR imaging (see **Fig. 10**).[39] Fibrosing mediastinitis is a rare mediastinal manifestation of IgG4-RD,

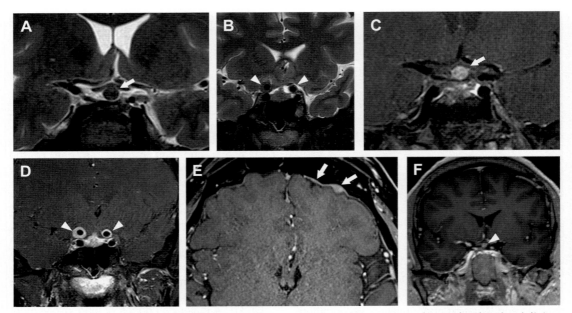

Fig. 9. Intracranial manifestations of IgG4-related disease in a 38-year-old man. Coronal T2-WI (*A, B*) and gadolinium-enhanced T1-WIs (*C, D*) of the brain demonstrate an enhancing mass of the pituitary stalk (*arrows*) consistent with pituitary hypophysitis; irregular wall thickening and enhancement of the bilateral internal carotid arteries, right more than left (*arrowheads*) suggestive of vasculitis. (*E*) Axial contrast-enhanced MR image of the brain shows nodular thickening of the meninges with associated mass (*arrows*) concerning for hypertrophic pachymeningitis. (*F*) Gadolinium-enhanced T1-weighted image of the brain shows complete resolution of the pituitary stalk mass (*arrow*).

characterized by an aggressive fibroinflammatory process that results in significant fibrosis; it has been shown that at least some cases appear to fall within the spectrum of IgG4-RD.[1,44] On imaging, diffuse, masslike soft tissue thickening in mediastinum that demonstrates delayed contrast enhancement indicating the fibrous nature of the disease is the characteristic feature of fibrosing mediastinitis; this can invade into adjacent structures, exerting significant mass effect with resultant organ dysfunction (**Fig. 11**).[39] Thoracic paravertebral space is commonly involved in IgG4-RD and appears as diffuse soft tissue thickening with multiple prominent bands in adjacent thoracic paravertebral space that shows increased metabolic activity on 18FDG-PET, particularly during the phase of active inflammation (**Fig. 12**).[45]

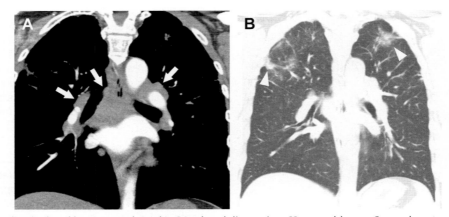

Fig. 10. Mediastinal and lung parenchymal IgG4-related disease in a 62-year-old man. Coronal contrast-enhanced chest CT images in mediastinal (*A*) and lung windows (*B*) shows bilateral hilar and subcarinal lymphadenopathy with associated soft tissue thickening (*arrows*) and ill-defined alveolar and interstitial opacities involving the bilateral upper lobe lung parenchyma (*arrowheads*) consistent with IgG4-related pulmonary and mediastinal disease.

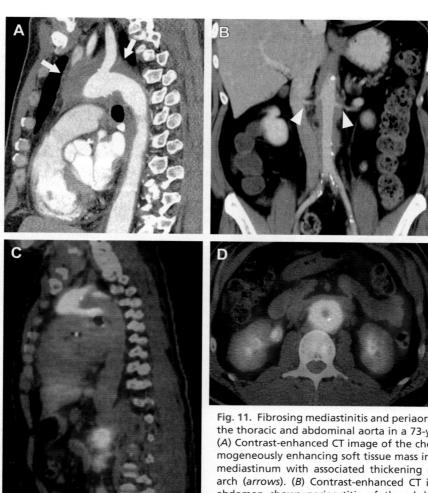

Fig. 11. Fibrosing mediastinitis and periaortitis involving the thoracic and abdominal aorta in a 73-year-old man. (*A*) Contrast-enhanced CT image of the chest shows homogeneously enhancing soft tissue mass in the anterior mediastinum with associated thickening of the aortic arch (*arrows*). (*B*) Contrast-enhanced CT image of the abdomen shows periaortitis of the abdominal aorta with involvement of the bilateral main renal arteries (*arrowheads*). (*C, D*) 18FDG-PET/CT images show increased metabolic activity in the mediastinum and periaortic region indicating active inflammation.

Cardiovascular Disease

IgG4-related cardiovascular disease mainly involves the aorta and its major branches, including coronary arteries, and pericardium in the form of aortitis/periaortitis, arteritis/periarteritis, inflammatory aneurysm, pericarditis, and coronary artery lesions.[46,47] The abdominal aorta is the most commonly involved segment in IgG4-related periaortitis/periarteritis; on CT/MR imaging, the characteristic findings include arterial wall thickening with relatively clear circumscription, associated luminal changes (mostly dilated and rarely stenotic), exaggerated atherosclerotic changes, and homogeneous enhancement of the thickened arterial wall on delayed phase, which corresponds to sclerosing inflammation, predominantly located in the adventitia (see **Figs. 11** and **12**).[48] Approximately 50% of inflammatory abdominal aortic

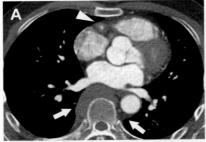

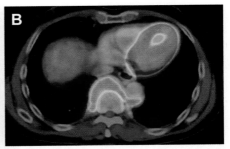

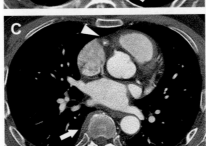

Fig. 12. IgG4-related disease involving thoracic paravertebral space and right coronary artery in a 54-year-old man. (*A*) Contrast-enhanced CT image of the chest shows diffuse soft tissue thickening in the thoracic paravertebral space (*arrows*) abutting the descending thoracic aorta and circumferential, irregular wall thickening of the right coronary artery consistent with coronary pseudotumor (*arrowhead*). (*B*) 18FDG-PET/CT image shows increased metabolic activity of the paravertebral space. (*C*) Contrast-enhanced CT image of the chest after steroid treatment shows significant improvement of paravertebral soft tissue thickening (*arrow*) and moderate improvement of right coronary artery wall thickening (*arrowhead*).

aneurysms are estimated to be IgG4-related that can rupture spontaneously or during/after corticosteroid treatment, likely secondary to weakening of the aneurysmal wall.[46]

IgG4-RD pericarditis appears as irregular thickening and nodularity of the pericardium with associated pericardial effusion on echocardiogram and CT; significant mass effect on the underlying cardiac chambers may result in constrictive cardiomyopathy and right heart failure.[46,47] Coronary artery lesions include pseudotumors, aneurysms, wall calcifications, and intimal thickening; on CT, irregular, nodular soft tissue thickening around coronary arteries with relatively well-preserved lumens is somewhat characteristic of IgG4-related coronary pseudotumors (see **Fig. 12**).[46,49]

ABDOMEN AND PELVIS
Pancreas

Type 1 AIP is the first recognized and prototypical manifestation of IgG4-RD that can be seen in more than 60% patients.[1,23] Given the complete reversal of pancreatic morphology and function following steroid treatment in patients with AIP, it is important to differentiate this condition from chronic alcoholic pancreatitis; typical imaging findings of AIP are an important part of most of the criteria used in the diagnosis of IgG4-RD.[23,25] Additionally, initial diagnosis of AIP will alert clinicians

and radiologists to search for extrapancreatic manifestations that lead to the diagnosis of IgG4-RD in most cases. At histology, IgG4-positive plasma cells are predominantly seen around the pancreatic duct with associated periductal fibrosis, narrowing of main pancreatic duct, and acinar atrophy.[50] Depending on extent of involvement, 3 morphologic patterns of AIP have been described that include diffuse, focal, and multifocal; among them, the diffuse form is the most common.[23]

On ultrasound, the involved pancreas appears bulky and hypoechoic; a diffusely enlarged, sausage-shaped pancreas that demonstrate peripheral hypodense rim of soft tissue is a characteristic finding on CT (**Fig. 13**).[23,26] At MR imaging, the involved parenchyma is hypointense on T1-WI and mildly hyperintense on T2-WI; peripancreatic soft tissue rim is typically hypointense on T2-WI; on contrast administration, parenchyma as well as peripheral rim show progressive enhancement indicating fibrosis (**Fig. 14**).[11,21,51] Associated enlarged lymph nodes in the retroperitoneum and mesentery are common. On magnetic resonance cholangiopancreatography (MRCP), the affected segments of the main pancreatic duct are irregularly narrowed with normal-appearing adjacent duct.[51] A less common, focal form of disease usually involves the pancreatic head and results in upstream dilatation of the main pancreatic duct and may mimic malignancy.[23] However, in

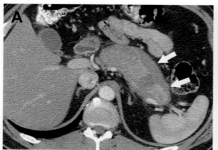
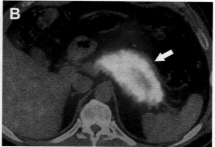

Fig. 13. Type 1 AIP in a 72-year-old man. (*A*) Axial contrast-enhanced CT image shows diffusely, enlarged pancreas with peripancreatic soft tissue rim (*arrows*) consistent with type 1 AIP. (*B*) Axial 18FDG-PET/CT image shows increased metabolic activity of the pancreas (*arrow*) and peripancreatic soft tissue.

pancreatic malignancy, the pancreatic duct distal to the mass is commonly dilated with associated parenchymal atrophy.[23] Increased activity in the pancreatic parenchyma and peripancreatic fibrosis is common on 18FDG-PET examination and is found to be useful in diagnosis and monitoring of AIP (see **Fig. 13**).[27]

Hepatobiliary System

Also known as IgG4 cholangiopathy, IgG4-related sclerosing cholangitis (IgG4-SC) is the most common extrapancreatic manifestation of type 1 AIP (more than 80% patients) and is the biliary manifestation of IgG4-RD.[1,13,50] Massive infiltration of IgG-positive plasma cells with associated fibrosis within the bile duct walls resulting in focal wall thickening and stenosis may lead to multiple strictures of the intrahepatic and extrahepatic biliary system.[52] IgG4-SC is responsible for a minority of the patients who had been previously diagnosed to have primary sclerosing cholangitis (PSC); contrast-enhanced MR with MRCP is

helpful in differentiating select cases of IgG4-SC from PSC and cholangiocarcinoma.[1,53]

On MRCP, 4 different patterns of biliary strictures have been described in IgG4-SC that include stricture of the distal common bile duct, diffuse strictures of the intrahepatic and extrahepatic bile ducts, hilar as well as distal common bile duct stricture, and isolated hilar stricture (**Fig. 15**).[54] Although tissue biopsy is the gold standard in differentiating IgG4-SC from PSC, multifocal strictures are long and continuous, and are associated with prestenotic dilation in IgG4-SC when compared with PSC.[53]

IgG4-RD involving the hepatic parenchyma resulting in the liver dysfunction is termed "IgG4-related hepatopathy"; diffuse infiltration of IgG4-positive plasma cells with portal inflammation, fibrosis, and lobular hepatitis is seen on pathology.[50,55] A single or multiple hepatic masses that show characteristic delayed enhancement may be seen on CT/MR and these masses can involve hilar and perihilar bile ducts resembling cholangiocarcinoma (**Fig. 16**).[1,21,56]

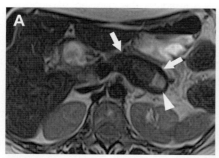
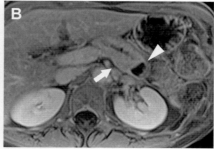

Fig. 14. MR findings of type 1 AIP in a 47-year-old man. Axial T2-weighted (*A*) and gadolinium-enhanced T1-weighted (*B*) MR images show decrease in size of the pancreas with T2 hypointense, peripancreatic halo that shows enhancement after contrast administration (*arrows*). Also note a pseudocyst in the pancreatic tail region (*arrowhead*).

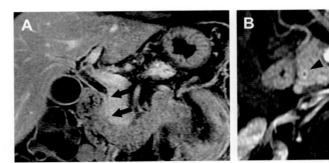

Fig. 15. IgG4-related cholangitis in a 53-year-old man. Gadolinium-enhanced coronal (*A*) and axial (*B*) T1-WIs show a long segment stricture involving the distal common bile duct (*arrows*) that shows enhancing, thickened wall (*arrowhead*).

Retroperitoneal Fibrosis

Retroperitoneal fibrosis (RPF) can be of 2 types: idiopathic and secondary. Up to two-thirds of idiopathic RPF cases, popularly known as Ormond disease, are now confirmed to be a part of IgG4-RD.[57] Idiopathic RPF is now classified within a larger disease group, "chronic periaortitis" that includes 3 major components: IgG4-related RPF, IgG4-related abdominal aortitis, and IgG4-related perianeurysmal fibrosis.[13] Up to 20% of patients with type 1 AIP may develop IgG4-related RPF and present with poorly localized pain in the back and pelvis, lower extremity edema, and hydronephrosis.[23] Increased ratio of IgG4-positive plasma cells to total number of plasma cells in tissues with associated storiform-type fibrosis and obliterative phlebitis help in differentiating IgG4-related RPF from other causes.[1]

Based on the location of fibrosis, IgG4-related RPF can be divided into 3 subtypes: (1) periaortic/arterial regions involving connective tissue of the abdominal aorta and its first branches, (2) periureteral areas causing hydronephrosis, and (3) plaquelike masses that involve the retroperitoneum.[1] It is difficult to differentiate IgG4-related RPF from other causes. On ultrasound, it appears as diffusely, hypoechoic soft tissue surrounding the aorta and its major branches.[11,21] CT and MR findings may vary depending on the degree of active inflammation and fibrosis. Although a homogeneous retroperitoneal soft tissue mass typically has the same attenuation as that of muscle on CT, intermediate to low signal intensity on T1-WIs and T2-WIs is a characteristic finding on MR (see **Figs. 11** and **20**).[21,23] Contrast enhancement may vary depending on the maturity of the fibrous tissue.[23]

Kidney

Tubulointerstitial nephritis (TIN) is the most common renal manifestation of IgG4-RD. Membranous glomerulonephropathy, other glomerular lesions, and pyelitis are uncommon. All these lesions are collectively referred to as "IgG4-related kidney disease."[58,59] Approximately one-third of patients with type 1 AIP may develop renal disease and present with hematuria, proteinuria, decreased kidney function, and hypocomplementemia.[59]

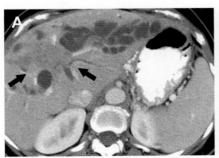
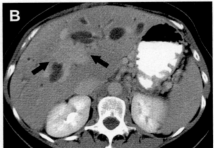

Fig. 16. IgG4-related hepatopathy in a 63-year-old man. Contrast-enhanced CT images of the liver during portal venous (*A*) and delayed (*B*) phases show a heterogeneously enhancing hepatic mass that shows progressive enhancement on the delayed phase (*arrows*) with associated intrahepatic biliary dilatation.

In addition to fibrosis and lymphoplasmacytic infiltrate, histopathology may show IgG and C3 granular deposits on the basement membranes of tubules, raising the possibility of immune complexes in the pathogenesis of IgG4-related TIN.[1,58,60]

Four types of disease patterns can be identified on cross-sectional imaging that include round or wedge-shaped cortical masses, peripheral cortical nodules, ill-defined, masslike lesions, and renal sinus/pelvic involvement (**Figs. 17–19**).[11,23] Renal lesions are typically hypodense on noncontrast CT; isointense on T1-WI, hypointense on T2-WI, and hyperintense on diffusion-WI; after contrast administration, they are hypointense on arterial phase and show progressive contrast enhancement (see **Figs. 17–19**).[61] Diffusion-WIs are more sensitive than T2-WIs for detecting renal lesions.[61]

Sclerosing Mesenteritis

Sclerosing mesenteritis is a chronic fibroinflammatory disease that commonly involves the small bowel mesentery. IgG4-positive plasma cell infiltration with associated fibrosis has been reported in select cases, suggesting the possibility of IgG4-RD.[62–64] On imaging, heterogeneously enhancing, soft-tissue attenuating mass encasing mesenteric vessels is the typical feature of sclerosing mesenteritis; this mass may encase vital organs that can interfere with surgical resection.[64]

Gastrointestinal Tract

IgG4-RD affecting the gastrointestinal tract is uncommon, with few cases reported in the literature, especially involving the stomach and small bowel loops.[65,66] On imaging, irregular bowel wall thickening with associated fat stranding, aneurysmal dilation, loss of mural stratifications, and interloop adhesions may be seen (**Fig. 20**).[67]

Prostate

A rare association exists between IgG4-related prostatitis and type 1 AIP; patients may have an enlarged prostate and lower urinary tract symptoms.[68] Prostate-specific antigen levels may be elevated in patients with IgG4-related disease involving the prostate, almost similar to prostate cancer; some patients have shown dramatic improvement in their urinary stream after treatment for IgG4-RD.[68] Diffuse enlargement of the prostate gland with or without focal mass/masses is the common imaging finding that cannot be differentiated from the more common prostate cancer.

MANAGEMENT

Glucocorticoids are the mainstay of treatment for remission induction in all patients with active, untreated IgG4-RD.[1,13,69] There have been some documented cases of complete resolution of lesions; however, relapse rates are high.[13] Continued surveillance with imaging and serum IgG4 levels is currently the standard of care. Apart from steroids, increasing evidence has shown rituximab, a select B-cell depleting agent, provides an excellent clinical response. B-cell depletion will target those plasma cells involved in producing IgG4 and prevent the reactivation of T-helper cells, through the lack of antigen-presenting cells.[2,69–71] Other steroid-sparing drugs have been implicated, including azathioprine, mycophenolate mofetil, and methotrexate, to protect patients from the serious side effects of long-term steroid use.[54]

The natural history of IgG4-RD has not been well-defined; spontaneous improvement can be seen in some, but most patients have chronic disease that progresses at variable rates.[1] There are mixed data regarding increased risk of malignancy in patients with IgG4-RD and this requires further study.[72,73]

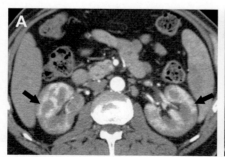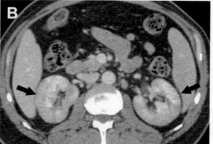

Fig. 17. IgG-4 related kidney disease in a 77-year-old man. Contrast-enhanced CT images of the kidneys during cortico-medullary (*A*) and nephrographic (*B*) phases show multiple ill-defined hypodense masses involving bilateral renal parenchyma that demonstrate progressive enhancement (*arrows*).

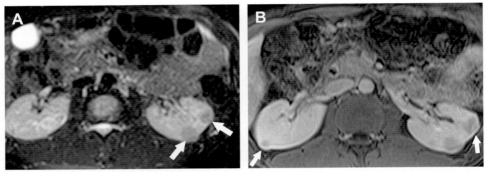

Fig. 18. MR findings of IgG-4 related kidney disease in a 37-year-old man. Axial T2-WIs (*A*) and gadolinium-enhanced T1-WIs (*B*) of the kidneys demonstrate ill-defined hypoenhancing, T2 hypointense focal lesions in the bilateral kidneys (*arrows*).

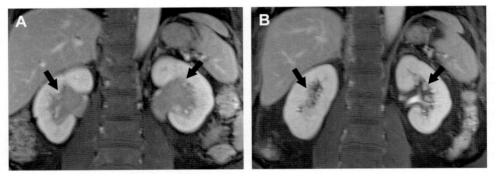

Fig. 19. MR findings of IgG-4 related renal sinus/pelvic disease in a 53-year-old man. (*A*) Gadolinium-enhanced coronal T1-WI of the kidneys shows homogeneously enhancing soft tissue masses involving bilateral renal sinuses (*arrows*). (*B*) Posttreatment scan demonstrates complete resolution of these masses (*arrows*).

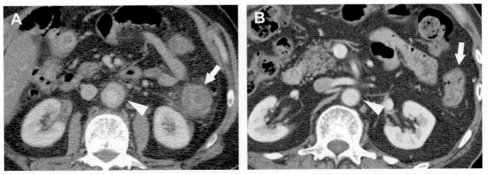

Fig. 20. IgG4-related colopathy in a 43-year-old man. (*A*) Axial contrast-enhanced CT of the abdomen shows irregular wall thickening of a segment of descending colon with associated fat stranding (*arrow*). Also note peri-aortitis of the abdominal aorta (*arrowhead*). (*B*) After treatment with steroids, there is complete resolution of colonic wall thickening and periaortitis (*arrowhead*).

SUMMARY

IgG4-RD is a fibroinflammatory disorder that can affect any organ in the body and cause tumefactive lesions that are often mistaken for malignancies. Recent advances in pathology have allowed better understanding of the underlying pathophysiologic mechanisms potentially leading to development of targeted therapeutic drugs. Improved awareness of this condition will help in avoiding aggressive management, as this condition usually demonstrates a favorable response to steroid therapy. The role of imaging allows for the differentiation of IgG4-RD from malignancy, as well as documenting response to therapy. Imaging also plays a major role in long-term surveillance, as IgG4-RD is associated with high rates of disease relapse.

REFERENCES

1. Mahajan VS, Mattoo H, Deshpande V, et al. IgG4-related disease. Annu Rev Pathol 2014;9:315–47.
2. Stone JH, Zen Y, Deshpande V. IgG4-related disease. N Engl J Med 2012;366(6):539–51.
3. Yoshida K, Toki F, Takeuchi T, et al. Chronic pancreatitis caused by an autoimmune abnormality. Proposal of the concept of autoimmune pancreatitis. Dig Dis Sci 1995;40(7):1561–8.
4. Umehara H, Okazaki K, Masaki Y, et al. A novel clinical entity, IgG4-related disease (IgG4RD): general concept and details. Mod Rheumatology 2012; 22(1):1–14.
5. Masaki Y, Dong L, Kurose N, et al. Proposal for a new clinical entity, IgG4-positive multiorgan lymphoproliferative syndrome: analysis of 64 cases of IgG4-related disorders. Ann Rheum Dis 2009;68(8):1310–5.
6. Kamisawa T, Funata N, Hayashi Y, et al. A new clinicopathological entity of IgG4-related autoimmune disease. J Gastroenterol 2003;38(10):982–4.
7. Hamano H, Kawa S, Horiuchi A, et al. High serum IgG4 concentrations in patients with sclerosing pancreatitis. N Engl J Med 2001;344(10):732–8.
8. Pieringer H, Parzer I, Wohrer A, et al. IgG4- related disease: an orphan disease with many faces. Orphanet J Rare Dis 2014;9:110.
9. Yamamoto M, Takahashi H, Shinomura Y. Mechanisms and assessment of IgG4-related disease: lessons for the rheumatologist. Nat Rev Rheumatol 2014;10(3):148–59.
10. Stone JH, Khosroshahi A, Deshpande V, et al. Recommendations for the nomenclature of IgG4-related disease and its individual organ system manifestations. Arthritis Rheum 2012;64(10):3061–7.
11. Al Zahrani H, Kyoung Kim T, Khalili K, et al. IgG4-related disease in the abdomen: a great mimicker. Semin Ultrasound CT MR 2014;35(3):240–54.
12. Inoue D, Yoshida K, Yoneda N, et al. IgG4-related disease: dataset of 235 consecutive patients. Medicine 2015;94(15):e680.
13. Kamisawa T, Zen Y, Pillai S, et al. IgG4-related disease. Lancet 2015;385(9976):1460–71.
14. Brito-Zeron P, Ramos-Casals M, Bosch X, et al. The clinical spectrum of IgG4-related disease. Autoimmun Rev 2014;13(12):1203–10.
15. Okazaki K, Uchida K, Miyoshi H, et al. Recent concepts of autoimmune pancreatitis and IgG4-related disease. Clin Rev Allergy Immunol 2011;41(2):126–38.
16. Della-Torre E, Lanzillotta M, Doglioni C. Immunology of IgG4-related disease. Clin Exp Immunol 2015; 181(2):191–206.
17. Kleger A, Seufferlein T, Wagner M, et al. IgG4-related autoimmune diseases: Polymorphous presentation complicates diagnosis and treatment. Dtsch Arztebl Int 2015;112(8):128–35.
18. Zen Y, Nakanuma Y. Pathogenesis of IgG4-related disease. Curr Opin Rheumatol 2011;23(1):114–8.
19. Umehara H, Okazaki K, Masaki Y, et al. Comprehensive diagnostic criteria for IgG4-related disease (IgG4-RD), 2011. Mod Rheumatol 2012;22(1):21–30.
20. Deshpande V, Zen Y, Chan JK, et al. Consensus statement on the pathology of IgG4-related disease. Mod Pathol 2012;25(9):1181–92.
21. Horger M, Lamprecht HG, Bares R, et al. Systemic IgG4-related sclerosing disease: spectrum of imaging findings and differential diagnosis. AJR Am J Roentgenol 2012;199(3):W276–82.
22. Takahashi H, Yamashita H, Morooka M, et al. The utility of FDG-PET/CT and other imaging techniques in the evaluation of IgG4-related disease. Joint Bone Spine 2014;81(4):331–6.
23. Vlachou PA, Khalili K, Jang HJ, et al. IgG4-related sclerosing disease: autoimmune pancreatitis and extrapancreatic manifestations. Radiographics 2011;31(5):1379–402.
24. Tan TJ, Ng YL, Tan D, et al. Extrapancreatic findings of IgG4-related disease. Clin Radiol 2014;69(2):209–18.
25. Lee LK, Sahani DV. Autoimmune pancreatitis in the context of IgG4-related disease: review of imaging findings. World J Gastroenterol 2014;20(41):15177–89.
26. George V, Tammisetti VS, Surabhi VR, et al. Chronic fibrosing conditions in abdominal imaging. Radiographics 2013;33(4):1053–80.
27. Ebbo M, Grados A, Guedj E, et al. Usefulness of 2-[18F]-fluoro-2-deoxy-D-glucose-positron emission tomography/computed tomography for staging and evaluation of treatment response in IgG4-related disease: a retrospective multicenter study. Arthritis Care Res 2014;66(1):86–96.
28. Deshpande V. IgG4 related disease of the head and neck. Head Neck Pathol 2015;9(1):24–31.

29. Lee CS, Harocopos GJ, Kraus CL, et al. IgG4-associated orbital and ocular inflammation. J Ophthalmic Inflamm Infect 2015;5:15.

30. Katsura M, Mori H, Kunimatsu A, et al. Radiological features of IgG4-related disease in the head, neck, and brain. Neuroradiology 2012;54(8):873–82.

31. Toyoda K, Oba H, Kutomi K, et al. MR imaging of IgG4-related disease in the head and neck and brain. AJNR Am J Neuroradiol 2012;33(11):2136–9.

32. Fujita A, Sakai O, Chapman MN, et al. IgG4-related disease of the head and neck: CT and MR imaging manifestations. Radiographics 2012;32(7):1945–58.

33. Ohshima K, Sogabe Y, Sato Y. The usefulness of infraorbital nerve enlargement on MRI imaging in clinical diagnosis of IgG4-related orbital disease. Jpn J Ophthalmol 2012;56(4):380–2.

34. Asai S, Okami K, Nakamura N, et al. Sonographic appearance of the submandibular glands in patients with immunoglobulin G4-related disease. J Ultrasound Med 2012;31(3):489–93.

35. Watanabe T, Maruyama M, Ito T, et al. Clinical features of a new disease concept, IgG4-related thyroiditis. Scand J Rheumatol 2013;42(4):325–30.

36. Dahlgren M, Khosroshahi A, Nielsen GP, et al. Riedel's thyroiditis and multifocal fibrosclerosis are part of the IgG4-related systemic disease spectrum. Arthritis Care Res 2010;62(9):1312–8.

37. Lu LX, Della-Torre E, Stone JH, et al. IgG4-related hypertrophic pachymeningitis: clinical features, diagnostic criteria, and treatment. JAMA Neurol 2014;71(6):785–93.

38. Wallace ZS, Carruthers MN, Khosroshahi A, et al. IgG4-related disease and hypertrophic pachymeningitis. Medicine 2013;92(4):206–16.

39. Ryu JH, Sekiguchi H, Yi ES. Pulmonary manifestations of immunoglobulin G4-related sclerosing disease. Eur Respir J 2012;39(1):180–6.

40. Zen Y, Inoue D, Kitao A, et al. IgG4-related lung and pleural disease: a clinicopathologic study of 21 cases. Am J Surg Pathol 2009;33(12):1886–93.

41. Inoue D, Zen Y, Abo H, et al. Immunoglobulin G4-related lung disease: CT findings with pathologic correlations. Radiology 2009;251(1):260–70.

42. Matsui S, Hebisawa A, Sakai F, et al. Immunoglobulin G4-related lung disease: clinicoradiological and pathological features. Respirology 2013;18(3):480–7.

43. Choi IH, Jang SH, Lee S, et al. A case report of IgG4-related disease clinically mimicking pleural mesothelioma. Tuberc Respir Dis 2014;76(1):42–5.

44. Peikert T, Shrestha B, Aubry MC, et al. Histopathologic overlap between fibrosing mediastinitis and IgG4-related disease. Int J Rheumatol 2012;2012:207056.

45. Fu L, Yang B, Xian J, et al. Computed tomograph findings of tissue adjacent to thoracic vertebrae involved by IgG4-related disease. Zhonghua Yi Xue Za Zhi 2014;94(41):3262–4 [in Chinese].

46. Tajima M, Nagai R, Hiroi Y. IgG4-related cardiovascular disorders. Int Heart J 2014;55(4):287–95.

47. Carbajal H, Waters L, Popovich J, et al. IgG4 related cardiac disease. Methodist DeBakey Cardiovasc J 2013;9(4):230–2.

48. Inoue D, Zen Y, Abo H, et al. Immunoglobulin G4-related periaortitis and periarteritis: CT findings in 17 patients. Radiology 2011;261(2):625–33.

49. Ishizaka N. IgG4-related disease underlying the pathogenesis of coronary artery disease. Clin Chim Acta 2013;415:220–5.

50. Okazaki K, Yanagawa M, Mitsuyama T, et al. Recent advances in the concept and pathogenesis of IgG4-related disease in the hepato-bilio-pancreatic system. Gut Liver 2014;8(5):462–70.

51. Sahani DV, Kalva SP, Farrell J, et al. Autoimmune pancreatitis: imaging features. Radiology 2004;233(2):345–52.

52. Okazaki K. Current concept, diagnosis and pathogenesis of autoimmune pancreatitis as IgG4-related disease. Minerva Med 2014;105(2):109–19.

53. Katabathina VS, Dasyam AK, Dasyam N, et al. Adult bile duct strictures: role of MR imaging and MR cholangiopancreatography in characterization. Radiographics 2014;34(3):565–86.

54. Nakazawa T, Ohara H, Sano H, et al. Schematic classification of sclerosing cholangitis with autoimmune pancreatitis by cholangiography. Pancreas 2006;32(2):229.

55. Joshi D, Webster GJ. Biliary and hepatic involvement in IgG4-related disease. Aliment Pharmacol Ther 2014;40(11–12):1251–61.

56. Kim JH, Byun JH, Lee SS, et al. Atypical manifestations of IgG4-related sclerosing disease in the abdomen: imaging findings and pathologic correlations. AJR Am J Roentgenol 2013;200(1):102–12.

57. Wang WH, Chou CT, Chang PM, et al. Retroperitoneal fibrosis in IgG4-related disease. J Clin Rheumatol 2014;20(3):175–6.

58. Kawano M, Saeki T. IgG4-related kidney disease–an update. Curr Opin Nephrol Hypertens 2015;24(2):193–201.

59. Cortazar FB, Stone JH. IgG4-related disease and the kidney. Nat Rev Nephrol 2015;11(10):599–609.

60. Kuroda N, Nao T, Fukuhara H, et al. IgG4-related renal disease: clinical and pathological characteristics. Int J Clin Exp Pathol 2014;7(9):6379–85.

61. Kim B, Kim JH, Byun JH, et al. IgG4-related kidney disease: MRI findings with emphasis on the usefulness of diffusion-weighted imaging. Eur J Radiol 2014;83(7):1057–62.

62. Nomura Y, Naito Y, Eriguchi N, et al. A case of IgG4-related sclerosing mesenteritis. Pathol Res Pract 2011;207(8):518–21.

63. Minato H, Shimizu J, Arano Y, et al. IgG4-related sclerosing mesenteritis: a rare mesenteric disease of unknown etiology. Pathol Int 2012;62(4):281–6.

64. Akram S, Pardi DS, Schaffner JA, et al. Sclerosing mesenteritis: clinical features, treatment, and outcome in ninety-two patients. Clin Gastroenterol Hepatol 2007;5(5):589–96 [quiz: 23–4].

65. Uehara T, Hamano H, Kawa S, et al. Chronic gastritis in the setting of autoimmune pancreatitis. Am J Surg Pathol 2010;34(9):1241–9.

66. Deshpande V. IgG4-related disease of the gastrointestinal tract: a 21st century chameleon. Arch Pathol Lab Med 2015;139(6):742–9.

67. Ko Y, Woo JY, Kim JW, et al. An immunoglobulin G4-related sclerosing disease of the small bowel: CT and small bowel series findings. Korean J Radiol 2013;14(5):776–80.

68. Hart PA, Smyrk TC, Chari ST. IgG4-related prostatitis: a rare cause of steroid-responsive obstructive urinary symptoms. Int J Urol 2013;20(1):132–4.

69. Khosroshahi A, Wallace ZS, Crowe JL, et al. International consensus guidance statement on the management and treatment of IgG4-related disease. Arthritis Rheumatol 2015;67(7):1688–99.

70. Khosroshahi A, Bloch DB, Deshpande V, et al. Rituximab therapy leads to rapid decline of serum IgG4 levels and prompt clinical improvement in IgG4-related systemic disease. Arthritis Rheum 2010;62(6):1755–62.

71. Yamamoto M, Awakawa T, Takahashi H. Is rituximab effective for IgG4-related disease in the long term? Experience of cases treated with rituximab for 4 years. Ann Rheum Dis 2015;74(8):e46.

72. Hirano K, Tada M, Sasahira N, et al. Incidence of malignancies in patients with IgG4-related disease. Intern Med 2014;53(3):171–6.

73. Yamamoto M, Takahashi H, Shinomura Y. IgG4-related disease and malignancy. Intern Med 2012;51(4):349–50.

Inflammatory Myofibroblastic Tumors
Current Update

Venkateswar R. Surabhi, MD[a],*, Steven Chua, MD[a], Rajan P. Patel, MD[a],
Naoki Takahashi, MD[b], Neeraj Lalwani, MD[c], Srinivasa R. Prasad, MD[d]

KEYWORDS

- Inflammatory myofibroblastic tumors • Mesenchymal neoplasms • Local recurrence
- Inflammatory pseudotumor • Imaging findings

KEY POINTS

- Inflammatory myofibroblastic tumor (IMT) is a mesenchymal neoplasm of intermediate biological potential with a predilection for the lung and abdominopelvic region.
- IMT represents the neoplastic subset of the family of inflammatory pseudotumors, an umbrella term for spindle cell proliferations of uncertain histogenesis with a variable inflammatory component.
- IMTs show characteristic fasciitis-like, compact spindle cell and hypocellular fibrous histologic patterns and distinctive molecular features.
- Characteristic translocations resulting in the overexpression of anaplastic lymphoma kinase are seen in 50% of IMTs and may be a favorable prognostic factor.
- Imaging findings reflect pathologic features and vary from an ill-defined, infiltrating lesion to a well-circumscribed, soft tissue mass owing to variable inflammatory, stromal, and myofibroblastic components.

INTRODUCTION

Inflammatory pseudotumor (IPT) encompasses a wide spectrum of nonneoplastic and neoplastic entities, including inflammatory myofibroblastic tumor (IMT), pseudosarcomatous myofibroblastic proliferations (PMPs) of the genitourinary tract, postinfectious/reparative disorders, and IPTs of the lymph node, spleen, and orbit. IPTs are characterized by an inflammatory infiltrate consisting of lymphocytes, plasma cells, and histiocytes admixed with a variable proportion of fibroblasts and myofibroblasts.[1] There is an overlap of clinical and histologic features between IPTs and select fibroinflammatory conditions such as

immunoglobulin (IgG)-4–related disorders as well. IPTs have been associated with a wide spectrum of different etiologies ranging from trauma, inflammatory, and postoperative conditions, as well as infection.[2] A small subset of IPTs of the lymph node, liver, and spleen demonstrate Epstein–Barr virus.[2] Although initially described in the lung, extrapulmonary IPTs have been described in many somatic and visceral sites.[1]

IMT has emerged as a distinct pathologic entity from within the broad category of IPTs. Both pulmonary and extrapulmonary IMTs are characterized by rearrangements involving the ALK (anaplastic lymphoma kinase) gene locus on 2p23 in 50% of cases leading to constitutive activation

[a] Department of Diagnostic and Interventional Imaging, The University of Texas Health Science Center at Houston, 6431 Fannin Street, MSB 2.130, Houston, TX 77030, USA; [b] Department of Radiology, Mayo Clinic, 200 First Street SW, Rochester, MN 55905, USA; [c] Department of Radiology, University of Washington, 1959 NE Pacific Street, Seattle, WA 98195-7117, USA; [d] Department of Radiology, The University of Texas MD Anderson Cancer Center, 1400 Pressler Street, Unit 1473, Houston, TX 77030, USA
* Corresponding author.
E-mail address: Venkateswar.R.Surabhi@uth.tmc.edu

Radiol Clin N Am 54 (2016) 553–563
http://dx.doi.org/10.1016/j.rcl.2015.12.005
0033-8389/16/$ – see front matter © 2016 Elsevier Inc. All rights reserved.

of the tyrosine kinase. The fusion partners identified thus far include *TPM3/4*, *CLTC*, and *RANBP2* genes (tropomyosin [TPM]; clathrin heavy chain [CLTC]; RAN-binding protein 2 [RANBP2]). A subset of ALK-negative IMTs demonstrates *ROS-1* gene fusions. The imaging features of IMTs are protean and are likely related to inflammatory cell infiltration, degree of stromal fibrosis, and tumor location within different sites of the body.[3,4] Based on understanding of ALK-related tumor pathways, specific tyrosine kinase inhibitors such as crizotinib are being used to treat advanced or unresectable IMTs.[5] The objective of this review is to discuss the imaging manifestations of IMTs in the thorax, abdomen, pelvis, and head/neck region and to familiarize the reader with recognizing this unique, diverse group of tumors. IPTs of the lymph node, spleen, and orbit are distinct clinicopathologic entities that are distinguishable from IMTs[2] and hence are not discussed in this article.

EPIDEMIOLOGY, ETIOPATHOGENESIS, AND CLINICAL MANIFESTATIONS

IMTs are indolent mesenchymal tumors that typically affect children and young adults. A wide spectrum of tumors, including inflammatory fibrosarcomas comprises, the entity of IMTs.[6] The true incidence and prevalence of IMTs is difficult to estimate as the definition and nomenclature of fibroinflammatory conditions are still evolving. Until now, IMTs were described under a broad rubric of entities including plasma cell granuloma, inflammatory myofibrohistiocytic proliferation, fibrous histiocytoma, plasma cell–histiocytoma complex, and inflammatory fibrosarcoma.[3] IMT typically shows benign clinical behavior, although aggressive behavior and recurrences have been described in the literature.[1] Recurrence rates vary between 2% and 25% for pulmonary and extrapulmonary IMTs, respectively; distant metastasis occur in less than 5% of cases.[2] The diagnosis of IMTs may be delayed owing to nonspecific presenting symptoms. Site-specific symptoms such as abdominal pain or gastrointestinal symptoms for intraabdominal lesions, and cough or chest pain for pulmonary tumors[2] may be seen. An 'inflammatory syndrome' consisting of fever, weight loss, and malaise is seen in 15% to 30% of patients; laboratory evaluation in these patients may reveal microcytic anemia, an increased erythrocyte sedimentation rate, thrombocytosis, and/or polyclonal hypergammaglobulinemia, likely related to overproduction of interleukin (IL)-6.[1]

Grossly, IMTs may be firm, fleshy, or gelatinous, with a white or tan cut surface. Calcification, hemorrhage, and necrosis are rare. Histologically, IMTs are characterized by a spindle cell proliferation in a myxoid to collagenous stroma with a prominent plasma cell and lymphocyte infiltration.[2] IMTs demonstrate characteristic fasciitis-like, compact spindle cell, and hypocellular fibrous histologic patterns. There is no consensus about reliable pathologic predictors of biology of IMTs, although the presence of ganglion-like cells, p53 expression, and aneuploidy has been associated with a more aggressive behavior.[7] Approximately one-half of IMTs harbor a cytogenetic translocation that activates the anaplastic lymphoma kinase receptor tyrosine kinase gene located at 2p23 locus resulting in overexpression of ALK protein.[8] The pathogenesis of the remaining one-half of IMTs lacking ALK expression is not clear. However, in a recent study using next-generation sequencing, 6 of 9 ALK-negative IMT tumors showed the presence of fusions involving *ROS-1* or *PDGFRβ* genes (platelet-derived growth factor [PDGFR]), suggesting that IMT is largely a kinase fusion–driven neoplasm.[9]

IMAGING FEATURES OF INFLAMMATORY MYOFIBROBLASTIC TUMOR

IMTs are found most frequently in the lungs, abdomen, and pelvis of children and adolescents but can also occur in many other sites throughout the body.[2] These sites include the central nervous system, head and neck region, larynx, uterus, somatic soft tissues, and bones.[1,2] The imaging features of IMTs are heterogeneous and reflect histopathologic findings. IMTs within the abdomen may present as multiple, discrete masses in the same anatomic region.[2] Imaging appearances vary from an ill-defined, infiltrating lesion to a well-circumscribed, soft tissue mass corresponding with differing proportions of inflammatory and fibrotic components within the mass.[3,10] Variable attenuation and echogenicity are noted at CT and ultrasonography, respectively. Delayed and persistent contrast enhancement is seen within fibrotic component of IMTs. Calcifications are better depicted on CT. Variable contrast enhancement and Doppler flow patterns are also noted. MR imaging may show low signal intensity on T1- and T2-weighted images owing to fibrosis, along with restricted diffusion. In general, hepatic, retroperitoneal, and genitourinary lesions are well-circumscribed, whereas those involving the gastrointestinal tract and biliary system are ill-defined and infiltrating.[3,11]

Inflammatory Myofibroblastic Tumor of the Lung

Pulmonary IPTs are associated with lower respiratory tract infection in 20% to 30% of cases. Other risk factors include history of pulmonary infarcts or prior radiation therapy. Some IPTs demonstrate increased IgG4-positive plasma cells and obliterative phlebitis indicative of an autoimmune etiology and form the spectrum of the IgG4-related sclerosing disease. Many cases of pulmonary IPTs show granulomatous inflammation, abscess formation, and lymphoid follicles with germinal centers unlike IMTs.[2] A subset of pulmonary IPTs is neoplastic with classic ALK-positive immunocytochemistry. The lungs are the most frequent site for IMTs accounting for about 0.04% to 1% of all lung lesions.[12] In children, pulmonary IMTs make up about 50% of benign lesions and are the most common primary lung lesions.[13,14] Pulmonary IMTs occur more frequently in the lower lobes with a predilection for peripheral lung parenchyma and subpleural locations.[13] Patients with pulmonary IMTs may manifest chest pain, cough, hemoptysis, and shortness of breath.[13] Pulmonary IMTs may invade locally to involve the bronchi, mediastinum, chest wall, and the diaphragm.[15] Surgical treatment is the mainstay of therapy.[3] On chest radiographs, pulmonary IMTs appear as solitary, circumscribed, lobulated lesions preferentially localized to the lower lobes. On CT, these lesions show heterogeneous enhancement (**Fig. 1**) and may be associated with atelectasis and/or pleural effusions. Amorphous or dystrophic calcifications in pulmonary IMTs occur more frequently in children than adults.[3,13,14] Pulmonary IMTs may also be fludeoxyglucose avid.[16] PET/CT may be used to monitor response to therapy.[17]

Tracheobronchial Inflammatory Myofibroblastic Tumor

Tracheobronchial IMTs are rare and are commonly seen in children and young adults. Airway IMTs may be asymptomatic, or cause dyspnea, wheezing, hemoptysis, and postobstructive pneumonia.[18,19] Tracheobronchial IMTs may present as a well-defined, endoluminal mass or a heterogeneous mass with exophytic component.[18,19] Associated lymphadenopathy is reported.[20]

Mediastinal Inflammatory Myofibroblastic Tumor

Mediastinal localization of IMT is rare. The clinical presentation is variable and may be secondary to mass effect on adjacent structures and include dyspnea, dysphagia, or hemoptysis.[17,21] CT may show a heterogeneously enhancing soft tissue mass that may encase or invade adjacent structures (**Fig. 2**). Dystrophic calcifications may be seen in large tumors. It is difficult to differentiate IMTs from the more common malignant mediastinal tumors based on imaging findings alone.[3] Treatment is surgical resection.[17,21]

Cardiac Inflammatory Myofibroblastic Tumor

Cardiac involvement by IMT is rare; as with thoracic IMTs, children and young adults are commonly affected. The clinical manifestations of cardiac IMT may include constitutional symptoms such as fever, weight loss, anemia, thrombocytopenia, and cardiovascular symptoms such as chest pain, syncope, transient ischemic attack, and arrhythmias.[22,23] Cardiac IMTs often occur in the right atrium and right ventricle. The MR imaging findings are nonspecific and are similar to those of other tumors. IMTs show heterogeneous enhancement following administration of gadolinium (**Fig. 3**).[3]

Inflammatory Myofibroblastic Tumor of the Hepatobiliary System

Pack and Baker[24] first described hepatic IPTs. Hepatic IPTs represent a diverse group of lesions

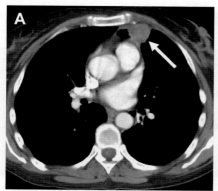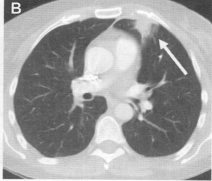

Fig. 1. Pulmonary inflammatory myofibroblastic tumor. (*A*) Axial contrast-enhanced computed tomography (CT; soft tissue window) and (*B*) axial CT (lung window) images of the chest show a heterogeneous mass in the lingula (*white arrows*) with perilesional ground glass haze.

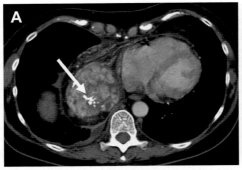
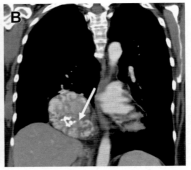

Fig. 2. Mediastinal inflammatory myofibroblastic tumor. (*A*) Axial and (*B*) coronal contrast-enhanced computed tomography images show a lobulated mediastinal mass exhibiting heterogeneous enhancement. Associated coarse calcifications are demonstrated (*white arrows*).

similar to pulmonary IPTs with infectious, autoimmune, and neoplastic etiologies.[25,26] Prior reports of Epstein–Barr virus–induced hepatic IPTs are now believed primarily to represent IPT-like follicular dendritic cell sarcomas.[2] Hepatic IPTs may exhibit symptoms of abdominal pain, fever, biliary obstruction, and/or portal hypertension related to obliterative phlebitis. Histologically, hepatic IPTs can be divided into 2 types: fibrohistiocytic and lymphoplasmacytic.[27] The fibrohistiocytic type is characterized by exuberant xanthogranulomatous inflammatory cells in the background of abundant fibrosis. The lymphoplasmacytic type shows predominant plasma cells and lymphocytes in variable stroma. The lymphoplasmacytic type of hepatic IPT consistently shows increased IgG4-positive plasma cells, obliterative phlebitis, and periductal inflammation with concentric fibrosis suggesting a manifestation of the systemic IgG4-related sclerosing disease.[2,27] Hepatic IPTs of the lymphoplasmacytic type tend to affect the hepatic hilum with distribution along bile ducts mimicking periductal, infiltrating type of hilar cholangiocarcinoma whereas fibrohistiocytic type resembles mass forming type of intrahepatic cholangiocarcinoma[27–29] (**Fig. 4**).

Hepatic IMTs are distinct tumors that commonly occur as solitary masses. Multiple lesions are seen in 20% of patients. The imaging findings of hepatic IMTs are variable and nonspecific. On ultrasonography, IMTs can present as hypoechoic or hyperechoic lesions. CT findings include delayed enhancement related to desmoplasia to heterogeneous enhancement with central necrosis.[30] On MR imaging, hepatic IMTs are typically T1 hypointense and T2 intermediate signal intensity with variable enhancement after contrast administration[31] (**Fig. 5**). Nodular extensions at the lesion boundary during hepatobiliary phase on gadoxetic acid MR imaging is reported in a recent case report of hepatic IMT.[32] Gallbladder may also be involved similar to biliary system with diffuse infiltration of the gallbladder wall (**Fig. 6**) and/or intraluminal polypoid masses.

Pancreatic Inflammatory Myofibroblastic Tumor

IMTs in the pancreas are rare, with only about 25 cases reported by 2004.[33] These lesions are seen in all age groups (between 2.5 and 70 years) and with a female preponderance. Patients with

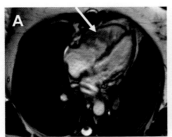
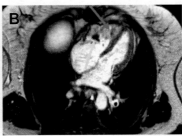
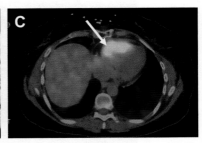

Fig. 3. Cardiac inflammatory myofibroblastic tumor. (*A*) Axial balanced turbo field echo MR image, (*B*) axial contrast-enhanced MR image, and (*C*) axial PET-computed tomography fusion images show a right ventricular mass (*white arrow*) with heterogeneous enhancement after contrast (*red arrow*) along with associated bland, nonenhancing thrombus (*yellow arrow*). The mass is fludeoxyglucose avid (*white arrow*).

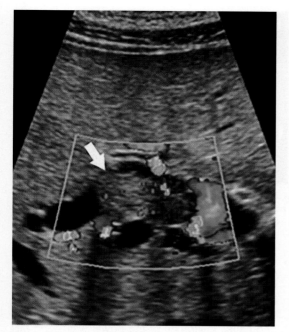

Fig. 4. Biliary tract inflammatory myofibroblastic tumor. Transverse Doppler sonogram image shows an expansile soft tissue mass (*white arrow*) within a dilated intrahepatic bile duct.

pancreatic IMTs present with nonspecific abdominal symptoms, back pain, and vomiting.[33] IMTs commonly involve the head of the pancreas; they may cause obstructive jaundice owing to extrinsic compression of the biliary system. CT features of pancreatic IMTs include a hypoattenuating mass with delayed enhancement after contrast administration (**Fig. 7**). Calcifications may be seen. Pancreatic IMT appears as a hypointense mass (to the pancreas) that demonstrates delayed enhancement on MR imaging. Treatment of choice is surgical resection with distal pancreatectomy for body and tail lesions and a Whipple procedure for pancreatic head IMTs.[33–36]

Gastrointestinal Tract Inflammatory Myofibroblastic Tumor

IMTs of the gastrointestinal tract can occur anywhere and are seen most frequently in the stomach, followed by the small intestine, colon, and rarely esophagus.[3] Presenting symptoms include abdominal pain, dysphagia, intestinal obstruction, and iron deficiency anemia. Imaging features of gastrointestinal IMTs resemble malignant lesions and present either as polypoid intraluminal lesions or infiltrative mural lesions (**Fig. 8**)

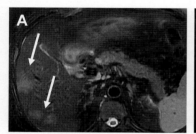
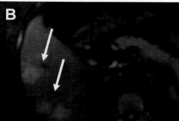
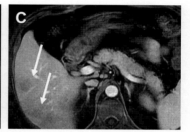

Fig. 5. Hepatic inflammatory myofibroblastic tumor. (*A*) Axial T2-weighted fat saturated, (*B*) axial diffusion-weighted image obtained at b 1000, and (*C*) axial portal venous phase post contrast images show multifocal nodular focal lesions (*white arrows*) within the right hepatic lobe that demonstrate intermediate T2 signal, restricted diffusion and faint enhancement after administration of contrast.

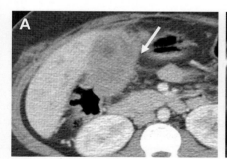
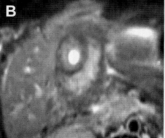
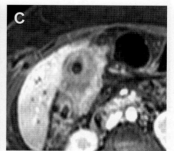

Fig. 6. Gallbladder inflammatory myofibroblastic tumor. (*A*) Axial contrast-enhanced computed tomography image (*B*) T2-weighted MR image, and (*C*) contrast-enhanced MR image show diffuse gall bladder wall thickening and enhancement (*white arrow*). Histopathology after cholecystectomy confirmed the diagnosis of inflammatory myofibroblastic tumor.

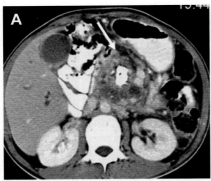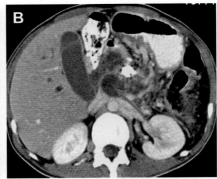

Fig. 7. Pancreatic inflammatory myofibroblastic tumor. (*A, B*) Axial contrast-enhanced computed tomography images of the abdomen show a heterogeneous mass in the pancreatic head (*white arrows*) with central dense calcification (*red arrowheads*), and dilated common bile duct (*red arrow*).

with possible exophytic growth.[37,38] IMTs involving the stomach and duodenum show homogenous low attenuation on CT scans (**Fig. 9**) and as hypoechoic lesions on ultrasonongraphy.[38] Because of their close association with the pancreatic head, it is difficult to distinguish duodenal IMTs from pancreatic head lesions.[39] Surgical resection of the mass is usually curative. The recurrence rate of gastrointestinal pseudotumors is 18% to 40%.[3]

Mesenteric Inflammatory Myofibroblastic Tumor

Mesenteric IMTs may manifest with nonspecific abdominal pain and mass. If large enough to cause mass effect on the bowel, they may present with obstruction. It is difficult to distinguish mesenteric IMTs from other mesenteric masses.[40] Mesenteric

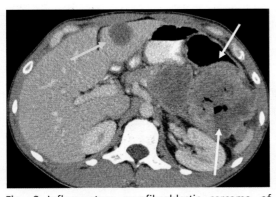

Fig. 8. Inflammatory myofibroblastic sarcoma of the gastrointestinal tract. Axial contrast-enhanced computed tomography image of the abdomen shows a heterogeneous mass involving the splenic flexure (*white arrows*) with extension to the pancreatic tail. Note the associated hepatic hypoattenuating metastasis (*yellow arrow*).

IMTs present as well-circumscribed masses and demonstrate variable enhancement patterns, from no enhancement to heterogeneous and peripheral enhancement on CT (**Fig. 10**).[41] Mesenteric IMTs may also extend to the adjacent bowel and cause infiltration of the bowel wall.[40] On MR imaging, mesenteric IMTs show intermediate signal on T1-weighted imaging and heterogeneous signal, on T2-weighted imaging with variable contrast enhancement.[42] Similar to IMTs of the gastrointestinal tract, the recurrence rates are high after surgery mainly owing to incomplete resection.[40]

Retroperitoneal Inflammatory Myofibroblastic Tumor

Retroperitoneal IMTs manifest as large soft tissue masses with variable contrast enhancement and mass effect on adjacent structures. IMTs of the abdomen and pelvis can demonstrate multifocal involvement within the same anatomic region (**Fig. 11**). On MR imaging, retroperitoneal IMTs show hyperintense signal on T2-weighted imaging and isointense to slightly hyperintense signal on T1-weighted imaging with heterogeneous enhancement.

Renal Inflammatory Myofibroblastic Tumor

Renal IMTs are extremely rare. Presenting symptoms and signs may include flank pain, hydronephrosis, and hematuria. The imaging characteristics are nonspecific.[11] On ultrasound imaging, renal IMTs range from hypoechoic to heterogeneous echogenic masses with increased Doppler vascularity. On MR/CT imaging, renal lesions show heterogeneous density/signal with patchy to uniform enhancement (**Fig. 12**). Heterogeneity may be owing to necrosis or intratumoral bleeding; renal IMTs may extend to the adjacent ureter.[11,43]

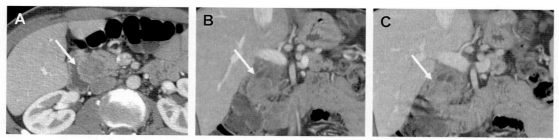

Fig. 9. Duodenal inflammatory myofibroblastic tumor. (*A*) Axial contrast-enhanced computed tomography (CT) image and (*B*, *C*) coronal contrast-enhanced CT images show a well-circumscribed mass involving the pancreaticoduodenal groove (*white arrows*) with heterogeneous enhancement.

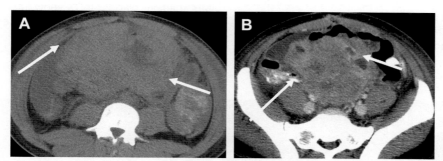

Fig. 10. Mesenteric inflammatory myofibroblastic tumor. (*A*) Axial noncontrast and (*B*) axial contrast-enhanced computed tomography images of the abdomen show a large, heterogeneous, expansile mass in the mesentery (*arrows*) with heterogeneous enhancement.

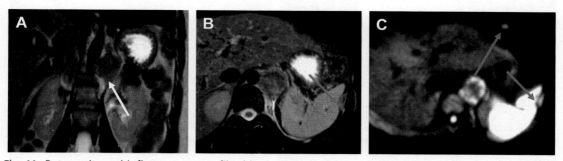

Fig. 11. Retroperitoneal inflammatory myofibroblastic sarcoma. (*A*) Coronal single shot fast spin echo, (*B*) axial T2-weighted fat saturated, and (*C*) diffusion-weighted image obtained at b 1000 images show an ill-defined, retrocrural mass (*white arrow*) that demonstrates low T2 signal indicative of predominant fibrous component with associated perisplenic and pericardial metastatic deposits (*red arrows*).

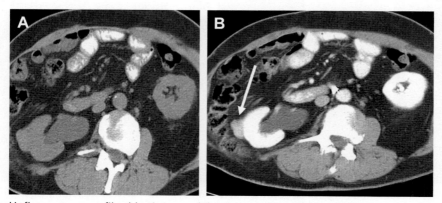

Fig. 12. Renal inflammatory myofibroblastic tumor. (*A*) Axial noncontrast computed tomography (CT) and (*B*) axial contrast-enhanced CT images of the abdomen at the level of the kidneys, show a noncalcified, high-density, soft tissue mass arising from the right kidney, which demonstrates diffuse, uniform enhancement (*arrow*).

Urinary Bladder Inflammatory Myofibroblastic Tumor

Pseudosarcomatous spindle cell lesions in the genitourinary tract is an umbrella term for spindle cell proliferations that include pseudosarcomatous fibromyxoid tumor, IPT, PMP, pseudomalignant spindle cell proliferation, and postoperative spindle cell nodule.[2] Bladder PMPs are more frequently found in young women than in men and are rare in children.[11] PMP is not associated with systemic symptoms, and may recur locally in 10% to 20% of cases. Urinary bladder PMPs manifest with hematuria, frequency–dysuria syndrome, and bladder outlet obstruction.

The urinary bladder IMT is very rare. The relationship of PMP to IMT remains controversial. However, there are certainly rare examples of "true" IMTs that arise in the urinary bladder.[2] On CT scans, a bladder PMP may present as a variable density, intraluminal polypoid or submucosal mass with or without perivesicular fat stranding. The urinary bladder trigone is usually spared. On MR imaging, bladder IMTs show intermediate T1 signal and high T2 signal with heterogeneous contrast enhancement (**Fig. 13**).[44]

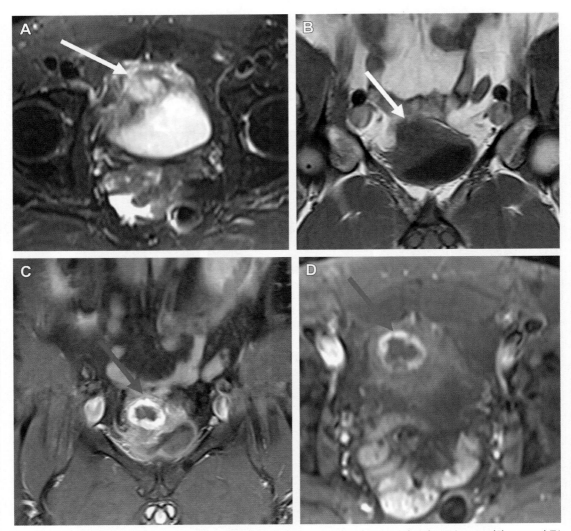

Fig. 13. Urinary bladder inflammatory myofibroblastic tumor. (*A*) Axial T2-weighted MR image, (*B*) coronal T1-weighted MR image, and (*C, D*) coronal and axial T1 postcontrast images at the level of the urinary bladder show focal wall thickening involving the anterior wall and dome of the bladder (*white arrows*), which exhibits peripheral rim enhancement after contrast administration (*red arrows*).

Inflammatory Myofibroblastic Tumor in the Head and Neck, Central Nervous System, and Bone

IMTs in the head and neck and the central nervous system are rare. The symptomatology depends on the involved site. IMTs can involve virtually any of the facial and skull base bones, neck spaces, nasopharynx, oropharynx, infratemporal fossa, pterygopalatine fossa, and salivary glands.[4] Sinonasal IMTs can erode and remodel

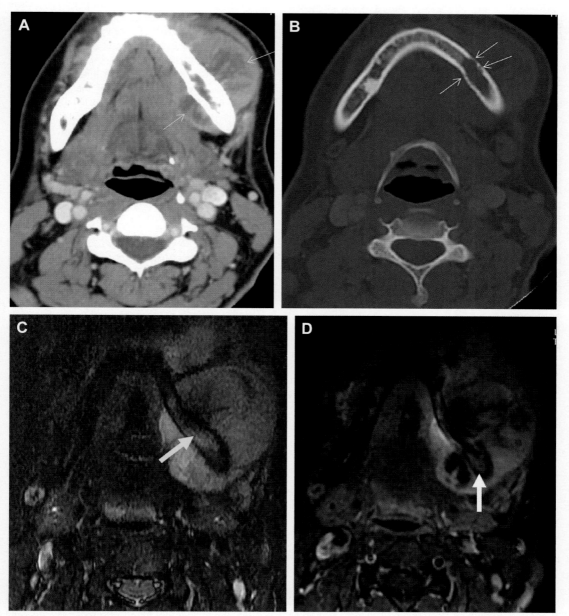

Fig. 14. Mandibular inflammatory myofibroblastic tumor. (*A*) Axial contrast-enhanced computed tomography (CT) image, soft tissue window, (*B*) axial contrast-enhanced CT image, bone window show heterogeneously enhancing mass (*thin yellow arrows*) on either side of the left mandibular ramus with associated lytic changes and medullary expansion as well as few areas of cortical breakthrough (*thin white arrows*). (*C*) Axial T2 short T1 inversion recovery MR image (*D*) Axial postcontrast T1-weighted fat saturation MR image show T2 hyperintense, heterogeneously enhancing mass on either side of the left mandibular ramus with associated bone marrow edema (*thick yellow arrow*) and mild expansion as well as postcontrast enhancement (*thick white arrow*).

bone and present with an aggressive appearance on CT.[45] Primary IMT of the bone has been reported in the temporal bone, mandible, ilium, sacrum, spine, and long bones.[46] Imaging findings include expansile osteolytic lesion with associated soft tissue component mimicking other aggressive bone tumors. Imaging features also include predominant soft tissue component adjacent to an ill-defined cortical bone erosion or destruction (Fig. 14).

SUMMARY

IMT is a distinctive myofibroblastic neoplasm characterized by chromosomal translocations leading to activation of the ALK tyrosine kinase in approximately one-half of the cases. IMT has a predilection for the lung, abdomen, and pelvis of children and young adults, and shows increased tendency for local recurrence. Metastasis is rare. IMTs should be distinguished from a wide spectrum of neoplastic and nonneoplastic masses that are included under the umbrella term "inflammatory pseudotumor." Imaging findings reflect pathologic features and vary from an ill-defined, infiltrating lesion to a well-circumscribed, soft tissue mass owing to variable inflammatory, stromal, and myofibroblastic components.

REFERENCES

1. Coffin CM, Humphrey PA, Dehner LP. Extrapulmonary inflammatory myofibroblastic tumor: a clinical and pathological survey. Semin Diagn Pathol 1998; 15:85–101.
2. Gleason BC, Hornick JL. Inflammatory myofibroblastic tumours: where are we now? J Clin Pathol 2008;61:428–37.
3. Patnana M, Sevrukov AB, Elsayes KM, et al. Inflammatory pseudotumor: the great mimicker. AJR Am J Roentgenol 2012;198:W217–27.
4. Park SB, Lee JH, Weon YC. Imaging findings of head and neck inflammatory pseudotumor. AJR Am J Roentgenol 2009;193:1180–6.
5. Butrynski JE, D'Adamo DR, Hornick JL, et al. Crizotinib in ALK-rearranged inflammatory myofibroblastic tumor. N Engl J Med 2010;363:1727–33.
6. Meis JM, Enzinger FM. Inflammatory fibrosarcoma of the mesentery and retroperitoneum. A tumor closely simulating inflammatory pseudotumor. Am J Surg Pathol 1991;15:1146–56.
7. Hussong JW, Brown M, Perkins SL, et al. Comparison of DNA ploidy, histologic, and immunohistochemical findings with clinical outcome in inflammatory myofibroblastic tumors. Mod Pathol 1999;12:279–86.

8. Coffin CM, Hornick JL, Fletcher CD. Inflammatory myofibroblastic tumor: comparison of clinicopathologic, histologic, and immunohistochemical features including ALK expression in atypical and aggressive cases. Am J Surg Pathol 2007;31:509–20.
9. Lovly CM, Gupta A, Lipson D, et al. Inflammatory myofibroblastic tumors harbor multiple potentially actionable kinase fusions. Cancer Discov 2014;4:889–95.
10. George V, Tammisetti VS, Surabhi VR, et al. Chronic fibrosing conditions in abdominal imaging. Radiographics 2013;33:1053–80.
11. Park SB, Cho KS, Kim JK, et al. Inflammatory pseudotumor (myoblastic tumor) of the genitourinary tract. AJR Am J Roentgenol 2008;191:1255–62.
12. Sakurai H, Hasegawa T, Watanabe S, et al. Inflammatory myofibroblastic tumor of the lung. Eur J Cardiothorac Surg 2004;25:155–9.
13. Agrons GA, Rosado-de-Christenson ML, Kirejczyk WM, et al. Pulmonary inflammatory pseudotumor: radiologic features. Radiology 1998;206:511–8.
14. Patankar T, Prasad S, Shenoy A, et al. Pulmonary inflammatory pseudotumour in children. Australas Radiol 2000;44:318–20.
15. Hedlund GL, Navoy JF, Galliani CA, et al. Aggressive manifestations of inflammatory pulmonary pseudotumor in children. Pediatr Radiol 1999;29:112–6.
16. Oguz B, Ozcan HN, Omay B, et al. Imaging of childhood inflammatory myofibroblastic tumor. Pediatr Radiol 2015;45(11):1672–81.
17. Alongi F, Bolognesi A, Samanes Gajate AM, et al. Inflammatory pseudotumor of mediastinum treated with tomotherapy and monitored with FDG-PET/CT: case report and literature review. Tumori 2010;96: 322–6.
18. Bumber Z, Jurlina M, Manojlovic S, et al. Inflammatory pseudotumor of the trachea. J Pediatr Surg 2001;36:631–4.
19. Andrade FM, Abou-Mourad OM, Judice LF, et al. Endotracheal inflammatory pseudotumor: the role of interventional bronchoscopy. Ann Thorac Surg 2010;90:e36–7.
20. Restrepo S, Mastrogiovanni LP, Palacios E. Inflammatory pseudotumor of the trachea. Ear Nose Throat J 2003;82:510–2.
21. Sugiyama K, Nakajima Y. Inflammatory myofibroblastic tumor in the mediastinum mimicking a malignant tumor. Diagn Interv Radiol 2008;14:197–9.
22. Li L, Burke A, He J, et al. Sudden unexpected death due to inflammatory myofibroblastic tumor of the heart: a case report and review of the literature. Int J Legal Med 2011;125:81–5.
23. Obikane H, Ariizumi K, Yutani C, et al. Inflammatory pseudotumor (inflammatory myofibroblastic tumor) of the mitral valve of the heart. Pathol Int 2010;60: 533–7.
24. Pack GT, Baker HW. Total right hepatic lobectomy; report of a case. Ann Surg 1953;138:253–8.

25. Goldsmith PJ, Loganathan A, Jacob M, et al. Inflammatory pseudotumours of the liver: a spectrum of presentation and management options. Eur J Surg Oncol 2009;35:1295–8.

26. Horiuchi R, Uchida T, Kojima T, et al. Inflammatory pseudotumor of the liver. Clinicopathologic study and review of the literature. Cancer 1990;65:1583–90.

27. Zen Y, Fujii T, Sato Y, et al. Pathological classification of hepatic inflammatory pseudotumor with respect to IgG4-related disease. Mod Pathol 2007;20:884–94.

28. Menias CO, Surabhi VR, Prasad SR, et al. Mimics of cholangiocarcinoma: spectrum of disease. Radiographics 2008;28:1115–29.

29. Tublin ME, Moser AJ, Marsh JW, et al. Biliary inflammatory pseudotumor: imaging features in seven patients. AJR Am J Roentgenol 2007;188:W44–8.

30. Nam KJ, Kang HK, Lim JH. Inflammatory pseudotumor of the liver: CT and sonographic findings. AJR Am J Roentgenol 1996;167:485–7.

31. Lee NK, Kim S, Kim DU, et al. Diffusion-weighted magnetic resonance imaging for non-neoplastic conditions in the hepatobiliary and pancreatic regions: pearls and potential pitfalls in imaging interpretation. Abdom Imaging 2015;40:643–62.

32. Durmus T, Kamphues C, Blaeker H, et al. Inflammatory myofibroblastic tumor of the liver mimicking an infiltrative malignancy in computed tomography and magnetic resonance imaging with Gd-EOB. Acta Radiol short Rep 2014;3. 2047981614544404.

33. Pungpapong S, Geiger XJ, Raimondo M. Inflammatory myofibroblastic tumor presenting as a pancreatic mass: a case report and review of the literature. JOP 2004;5:360–7.

34. McClain MB, Burton EM, Day DS. Pancreatic pseudotumor in an 11-year-old child: imaging findings. Pediatr Radiol 2000;30:610–3.

35. Wreesmann V, van Eijck CH, Naus DC, et al. Inflammatory pseudotumour (inflammatory myofibroblastic tumour) of the pancreas: a report of six cases associated with obliterative phlebitis. Histopathology 2001;38:105–10.

36. Yamamoto H, Watanabe K, Nagata M, et al. Inflammatory myofibroblastic tumor (IMT) of the pancreas. J Hepatobiliary Pancreat Surg 2002;9:116–9.

37. Estevao-Costa J, Correia-Pinto J, Rodrigues FC, et al. Gastric inflammatory myofibroblastic proliferation in children. Pediatr Surg Int 1998;13:95–9.

38. Kim SJ, Kim WS, Cheon JE, et al. Inflammatory myofibroblastic tumors of the abdomen as mimickers of malignancy: imaging features in nine children. AJR Am J Roentgenol 2009;193:1419–24.

39. Fong SS, Zhao C, Yap WM, et al. Inflammatory myofibroblastic tumour of the duodenum. Singapore Med J 2012;53:e28–31.

40. Chaudhary P. Mesenteric inflammatory myofibroblastic tumors. Ann Gastroenterol 2015;28:49–54.

41. Uysal S, Tuncbilek I, Unlubay D, et al. Inflammatory pseudotumor of the sigmoid colon mesentery: US and CT findings (2004:12b). Eur Radiol 2005;15:633–5.

42. Ko SW, Shin SS, Jeong YY. Mesenteric inflammatory myofibroblastic tumor mimicking a necrotized malignant mass in an adult: case report with MR findings. Abdom Imaging 2005;30:616–9.

43. Selvan DR, Philip J, Manikandan R, et al. Inflammatory pseudotumor of the Kidney. World J Surg Oncol 2007;5:106.

44. Fujiwara T, Sugimura K, Imaoka I, et al. Inflammatory pseudotumor of the bladder: MR findings. J Comput Assist Tomogr 1999;23:558–61.

45. De Vuysere S, Hermans R, Sciot R, et al. Extraorbital inflammatory pseudotumor of the head and neck: CT and MR findings in three patients. AJNR Am J Neuroradiol 1999;20:1133–9.

46. Inarejos Clemente EJ, Vilanova JC, Riaza Martin L, et al. A primary inflammatory myofibroblastic tumor of the scapula in a child: imaging findings. Skeletal Radiol 2015;44:733–7.

Solitary Fibrous Tumors
2016 Imaging Update

Abhishek R. Keraliya, MD[a,b,*], Sree Harsha Tirumani, MD[a,b], Atul B. Shinagare, MD[a,b], Atif Zaheer, MD[c], Nikhil H. Ramaiya, MD[a,b]

KEYWORDS

- Solitary fibrous tumor • CT • MR imaging • Molecular targeted therapies

KEY POINTS

- The revised 2013 World Health Organization classification schemata do not differentiate between hemangiopericytomas and solitary fibrous tumors (SFTs) but now group these tumors together as SFTs under the category of fibroblastic/myofibroblastic tumors.
- Most SFTs are benign; however, approximately 20% of the tumors exhibit malignant behavior.
- Computed tomography (CT) remains the mainstay for evaluation of thoracic SFTs. MR imaging is useful for the delineation of tumor and evaluation for invasion into adjacent organs such as the diaphragm, chest wall, and nerves.
- Imaging findings of SFTs are variable and nonspecific. However, a well-circumscribed ovoid or rounded mass with characteristic hypointensity on T2-weighted MR imaging and avid enhancement on CT and MR images may suggest the diagnosis of SFTs.
- Surgical excision is the treatment of choice for localized SFTs. Novel targeted therapies with antiangiogenic action have shown therapeutic efficacy in patients with advanced/metastatic SFTs.

INTRODUCTION

Solitary fibrous tumors (SFTs) are uncommon, distinctive soft tissue neoplasms of pluripotent fibroblastic or myofibroblastic origin that may be benign or malignant. First described as a primary spindle-cell tumor of the pleura by Klemperer and Rabin in 1931,[1] most SFTs are benign. Approximately 10% to 20% of SFTs exhibit malignant behavior, including local invasion, recurrence, and metastases. Although they frequently arise in the thorax, SFTs have been reported in many organ systems. Within the thorax, they may involve the pleura, lung, or mediastinum, depending on their site of origin.

SFTs present as slow-growing masses, often with local compressive symptoms.[2] More than 50% of patients have large tumors, measuring greater than 10 cm in maximum dimension. Up to 90% of patients with extrathoracic SFTs are symptomatic at initial evaluation.[3] Various paraneoplastic syndromes, such as hypoglycemia with or without finger-clubbing[4] and hypertrophic pulmonary osteoarthropathy (Pierre Marie-Bamberger syndrome), have been described in patients with SFTs.[5] Malignant SFTs have been shown to overexpress insulinlike growth factor 2, which may result in decreased hepatic gluconeogenesis and hypoglycemia (Doege-Potter syndrome).[6] General imaging characteristics of SFTs

Disclosures: A.B. Shinagare is supported by an RSNA research grant (#RSCH1422). No disclosures for the remaining authors.
[a] Department of Imaging, Dana Farber Cancer Institute, Harvard Medical School, 450 Brookline Avenue, Boston, MA 02215, USA; [b] Department of Radiology, Brigham and Women's Hospital, Harvard Medical School, 75 Francis Street, Boston, MA 02115, USA; [c] The Russell H. Morgan Department of Radiology and Radiological Science, Johns Hopkins Medical Institutions, Baltimore, MD 21231, USA
* Corresponding author. Department of Imaging, Dana Farber Cancer Institute, Harvard Medical School, 450 Brookline Avenue, Boston, MA 02215.
E-mail address: akeraliya@partners.org

Radiol Clin N Am 54 (2016) 565–579
http://dx.doi.org/10.1016/j.rcl.2015.12.006

radiologic.theclinics.com

are summarized in **Table 1**. The differential diagnoses of SFTs according to locations are summarized in **Table 2**.

EPIDEMIOLOGY, PATHOLOGY, AND REVISED WORLD HEALTH ORGANIZATION CLASSIFICATION

SFTs typically affect older patients with a mean age at presentation between 55 and 65 years and no sex predilection.[7] Thoracic and extrathoracic SFTs have similar clinical and pathologic features, although extrathoracic tumors are more likely to be symptomatic at the time of diagnosis.[3,8]

Because of clinical and histopathological similarity between SFTs and hemangiopericytomas (HPCs), it has been proposed that HPCs and SFTs represent different entities of a wide morphologic spectrum.[9,10] Recent genetic studies have demonstrated driver, recurrent somatic mutations in most SFTs; they are characterized by distinctive somatic fusions of 2 genes: NAB2 (NGFI-A-binding protein 2) and Signal transducer and activator of transcription 6 (STAT6). The 2 genes located on the long arm of chromosome 12 undergo fusion likely due to inversion; the fusion product is thought to modulate STAT6-dependent gene expression.[11,12] Different types of gene fusions are associated with development of SFTs in specific locations with distinct pathologic features and biological behaviors. Tumors with the most common fusion variant (NAB2ex4-STAT6ex2/3) correspond to classic pleuropulmonary SFTs with diffuse fibrosis, often occur in older patients, and usually show benign behavior. In contrast, tumors with the second most common fusion variant (NAB2ex6-STAT6ex16/17) are seen in younger patients and originate from deep soft tissue with a more aggressive phenotype and clinical behavior.[13] Recent studies have also demonstrated the role of secondary genetic alterations in the biological behavior and malignant potential of these tumors. TT53 (tumor protein p53) positivity is associated with higher mitotic rate (mitosis >4/high-power-field) and nuclear atypia/pleomorphism and implies poor disease-free survival rates.[14] The revised 2013 World Health Organization classification of tumors of soft tissue and bone no longer differentiates between HPCs and SFTs but now groups these tumors together as SFTs under the category of fibroblastic/myofibroblastic tumors. Lipomatous HPCs are regarded as fat-forming variants of SFTs.[15,16]

On gross examination, SFTs are typically well-circumscribed masses with lobular or smooth external surfaces that tend to cause displacement of adjacent structures rather than invasion. They are highly vascular tumors that often have hypertrophied feeding vessels.[3] Calcification is seen in

---

Table 1
General imaging characteristics of solitary fibrous tumors

Imaging Modality	Findings
Radiography	• Well-defined lobular masses involving the pleural surfaces or fissures • Frequently located within the inferior portions of the thorax • Pedunculated lesions are mobile with change in location and shape on sequential imaging
CT	• Well marginated and generally isodense compared with adjacent muscles on unenhanced images. Tumor heterogeneity is more common in malignant variety. • Usually avid but heterogeneous enhancement following intravenous (IV) contrast administration. • Highly vascular and often demonstrates collateral feeding vessels.
MR imaging	• *T1:* Homogeneous low-to-intermediate signal intensity. • *T2:* Variable and inhomogeneous signal intensity. Areas of T2 hyperintensity correspond with hemorrhage, myxoid, and cystic degeneration, particularly in large tumors. Areas of T2 hypointensity corresponding to collagen stroma and fibrosis. • *Postcontrast T1:* Marked heterogeneous enhancement after IV gadolinium administration.
Ultrasound	Typically hypoechoic, larger may have heterogeneous appearance due to necrosis and cystic degeneration.
FDG-PET	• Benign SFTs are non-FDG-avid. • Malignant SFTs are usually FDG-avid.

Table 2
Differential diagnoses of solitary fibrous tumors according to location

Location of SFT	Differential Diagnoses
Intracranial	Fibrous meningioma, schwannoma
Orbital	Capillary hemangioma, cavernous hemangioma, orbital varix, schwannoma, giant cell angiofibroma
Pleural	Mesothelioma, lymphoma, pleural metastases
Mediastinal	Lymphoma, thymic tumors, neurogenic tumors, pericardial mesothelioma, sarcoma
Hepatic	Intrahepatic cholangiocarcinoma, sclerosing and fibrolamellar hepatocellular carcinoma, sclerosing hemangioma, metastasis
Renal	Renal cell carcinoma, oncocytoma, metastasis
Retroperitoneal	Lymphoma, neurogenic tumor, leiomyosarcoma, metastasis
Pelvic	Malignant fibrous histiocytoma, desmoid tumor, mesothelioma, uterine leiomyoma, ovarian fibroma or fibrothecoma
Soft tissues	Schwannoma, synovial sarcoma, hemangioma, fibrosarcoma, angiosarcoma, fibrous histiocytoma, desmoid tumor, dermatofibrosarcoma protuberans, peripheral nerve sheath tumors

less than 10% of tumors. Areas of myxoid or cystic degeneration and hemorrhage are often seen, particularly in large and malignant tumors.[17] Invasion of local structures is rare; local or distant lymphadenopathy is usually absent.[3] Microscopically, SFTs are well-circumscribed, unencapsulated tumors that are known to have a characteristic patternless arrangement of alternating hypercellular and hypocellular regions of spindle cells against a collagenous background and fibrous stroma. Metastatic tumors are generally hypercellular with moderate to severe nuclear atypia, infiltration of surrounding tissues, necrosis, and 4 mitoses or more per 10 high-power-fields.[18,19]

IMMUNOHISTOCHEMICAL ANALYSIS

CD34, the hematopoietic progenitor cell antigen, is the most important marker to diagnose SFT. Positivity to CD34 is seen in 80% to 100% of SFTs[20] and helps in differentiation from other spindle cell tumors. More than 80% of SFTs have positivity for B-cell lymphoma 2 protein, a marker of terminal differentiation.[21] Nearly 75% of the tumors are reactive for CD99.[22] SFTs are usually negative for epithelial, vascular, neural, and muscle markers, including cytokeratin, antiendomysial antibody, S-100 protein, desmin, and smooth muscle actin.[23] STAT6 is a highly sensitive and specific immunohistochemical marker for SFT and can be helpful to distinguish SFTs from histologic mimics.[24] Occasionally, malignant SFTs may be CD34-negative. Loss of CD34 expression and cytokeratin positivity usually correlate with high-grade tumor and unfavorable outcome in pleural SFTs.[25–27] Also, positivity for Ki67, a marker of cellular proliferation, is greater in malignant than in benign tumors.[25]

SOLITARY FIBROUS TUMORS BY LOCATION
Head and Neck Solitary Fibrous Tumors

Intracranial solitary fibrous tumors
Intracranial SFTs are rare, dural-based mesenchymal neoplasms that originate in the meninges and commonly involve the parasagittal region, tentorium, and cerebellopontine angle. Intracranial SFTs may present with a multitude of symptoms, including headache, sensory and motor weakness, seizures, and visual and memory disturbances depending on the location of the tumor.[20,28–30] According to Carneiro and colleagues,[31] intracranial SFTs may be distinguished from fibrous meningioma based on morphologic and immunohistochemical features. SFTs are Periodic acid–Schiff-negative and show strong immunoreactivity for vimentin and CD34. Approximately 6% of the central nervous system SFTs are malignant.[28]

On imaging, intracranial SFTs appear as solid, discrete, extra-axial masses. Rarely, they are intra-axial or intraventricular in location.[29] SFTs are typically hyperattenuating on unenhanced computed tomographic (CT) images with marked heterogeneous enhancement after contrast administration.[30] Intratumoral calcification is rare. On MR imaging, the lesions are usually isointense on T1-weighted image (T1WI) (**Fig. 1**). On T2-weighted image (T2WI), SFTs show heterogeneous appearance with areas of both low- and high-signal intensity and prominent vascular flow voids. The characteristic T2 hypointensity of

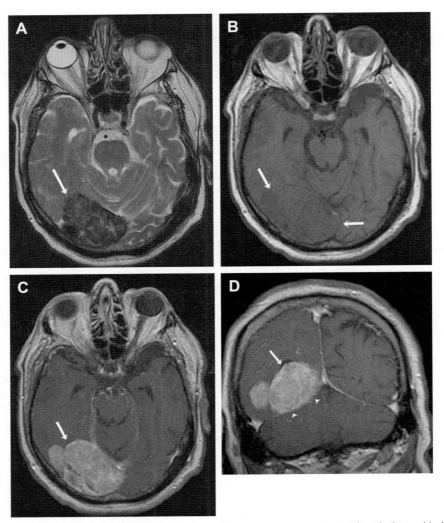

Fig. 1. Intracranial SFT. An 80-year-old man presented with progressively worsening headache and imbalance. (*A*) Axial T2WI MR image shows a lobulated hypointense dural-based mass along the right occipital convexity (*arrow*). (*B*) The mass is isointense to adjacent brain parenchyma on the corresponding axial T1WI MR image (*arrows*). (*C*, *D*) Axial (*C*) and coronal (*D*) contrast-enhanced T1WIs demonstrate marked and heterogeneous enhancement of the mass (*arrows*) abutting the tentorium (*arrowheads* in *D*).

SFTs seen on MR imaging corresponds to collagenous stroma and fibrosis on microscopic examination.[32] SFTs are hypervascular and show marked heterogeneous enhancement after gadolinium administration.[30] On diffusion-weighted imaging, intracranial SFTs have restricted diffusion with low apparent diffusion coefficient values due to cellular components of the tumor. On perfusion MR imaging, they show increased relative cerebral blood volume compared with control, cerebral white matter.[29] Intracranial SFTs typically show thickening of the adjacent meninges (dural tail) or tentorium. The main differential diagnosis of intracranial SFTs includes fibrous meningioma. In contrast to the classical bone thickening adjacent to meningiomas, intracranial SFTs show erosion of the adjacent skull. They can also mimic schwannoma when located in the cerebellopontine angle cistern. Schwannoma shows more cystic degeneration and resultant T2 hyperintensity compared with SFTs.

Extracranial solitary fibrous tumors
Most of the extracranial SFTs in the head and neck region present as a slow-growing, painless masses. Common locations for head and neck SFTs include the orbit, parotid glands, oral cavity, cheek, masticator space, parapharyngeal space, infratemporal fossa, paranasal sinuses, submandibular space, and the thyroid gland. Clinically,

the symptoms and signs of head and neck SFTs depend on the location of the tumor and the involved organs and include proptosis, palpable mass, swelling, bleeding, and facial palsy.[33] Orbital SFTs commonly present with slowly progressive painless proptosis, decreased visual acuity, restricted mobility, or palpable mass of the eyelid or orbit.[34,35]

The imaging findings of SFTs in the head and neck region are nonspecific. Similar to other organs, head and neck SFTs are mostly homogeneously isointense or mildly hypointense to the muscle on the T1WI and heterogeneously hyperintense on the T2WI with variable hypointense components (**Fig. 2**). Moderate to marked enhancement is seen on postcontrast images. On imaging, it is difficult to differentiate between benign and malignant SFTs. Certain imaging characteristics such as frank bone destruction, necrosis, or cystic degeneration is indicative of borderline or malignant tumors.[33]

Orbital SFTs are ovoid in configuration with well-defined margins. About two-thirds of the lesions are located in the extraconal space; the remainder involves the intraconal space.[35] On MR imaging, they appear homogeneously isointense to gray matter on T1WI (**Fig. 3**). The signal intensity on T2WI is variable and inhomogeneous with both hypointense and hyperintense components. The areas of T2 hyperintensity on MR imaging corresponds to hemorrhage, myxoid, and cystic degeneration on histopathological examination.[36,37] The tumor shows marked heterogeneous enhancement and delayed washout pattern on the dynamic contrast-enhanced T1WI.[35] Because of excellent contrast resolution, MR imaging is also helpful in exact delineation of the lesion and its relation to adjacent orbital structures, including the optic nerve, extraocular muscles, lacrimal gland, and orbital wall. The differential diagnosis for hypervascular orbital tumor includes capillary hemangioma, cavernous hemangioma, orbital varix, SFT, schwannoma, and giant cell angiofibroma.[38,39] Capillary hemangiomas are typically seen in infants and show involution after 6 months of age. Cavernous hemangiomas are markedly hyperintense on T2WIs and often have phleboliths. The characteristic imaging finding of orbital varices is increased in size with Valsalva maneuver. Schwannoma and giant cell angiofibroma are usually indistinguishable from SFTs on imaging alone.

Thoracic solitary fibrous tumors

SFTs account for less than 5% of primary pleural tumors. Approximately 80% of SFTs of the pleura arise from the visceral and 20% arise from the parietal pleura.[40] About 10% to 15% of intrathoracic SFTs are histologically or clinically malignant. However, according to a single-center study of 157 patients with pleural SFTs, malignant changes may be seen in up to 43% of patients.[27] Factors predicting malignancy include large tumor size at presentation, symptomatic patients, sessile morphology, and multifocality. Most patients with pleural SFTs are asymptomatic; tumors are detected as incidental findings on radiographs and CT scans. When symptomatic, most common symptoms are cough, dyspnea, and chest pain. Chest pain occurs more commonly in patients with tumor arising from the parietal pleura. As opposed to other common thoracic neoplasms, no known association with tobacco or asbestos exposure is reported.[41]

On plain radiographs, thoracic SFTs appear as well-defined lobular masses involving the pleural surfaces or fissures frequently located within the inferior portions of the thorax.[42] Pleural SFTs are often pedunculated with a fibrovascular stalk. They are usually located near the lung periphery and have well-circumscribed margins. As most thoracic SFTs are extrapulmonary, they often show indistinct borders along at least a portion

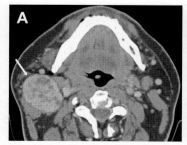
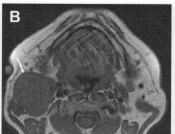
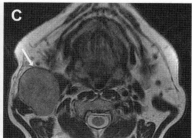

Fig. 2. Parotid SFT. A 47-year-old man with slowly enlarging right-sided cheek swelling. (*A*) Axial contrast-enhanced CT image reveals a well-defined heterogeneously enhancing mass in the right parotid gland (*arrow*). (*B*) On axial T1WI, the mass is isointense to muscles (*arrow*). (*C*) The mass is hyperintense to adjacent muscles and parotid parenchyma on the corresponding axial T2WI MR image (*arrow*).

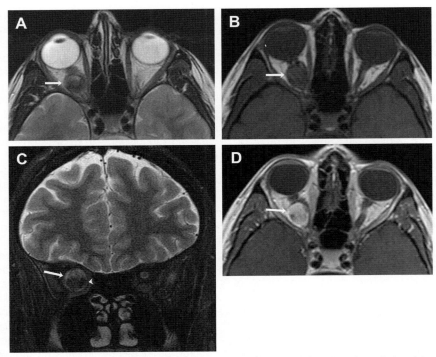

Fig. 3. Orbital SFT. A 27-year-old woman presented with gradual visual deterioration of the vision in the right eye. (*A*) Axial T2WI MR image shows a well-defined heterogeneous retro-ocular mass involving the intraconal compartment of the right orbit (*arrow*). (*B*) The mass is isointense to the cerebral parenchyma on T1WI (*arrow*). (*C*) Coronal fat-saturated T2WI MR image showing heterogeneous signal intensity of the mass with both hypointense (*arrowhead*) and hyperintense (*arrow*) components. (*D*) On corresponding contrast-enhanced fat-saturated T1WI MR image, there is intense enhancement of the superior component of the mass, which corresponds to cellular hyperintense component seen on T2WI (*arrow*).

of their margins on chest radiographs and are termed the "incomplete border sign" (**Fig. 4**).[43] They often abut the ipsilateral hemidiaphragm, conforming to its shape, and can simulate diaphragmatic elevation or eventration.[42] Approximately 25% of tumors have an associated ipsilateral pleural effusion.

Pleural origin of the tumors is better demonstrated on CT compared with radiographs. On unenhanced CT, SFTs are well-defined and usually homogenous masses abutting the pleural surface. Approximately one-third of the tumors form an obtuse or right angle against adjacent pleura. Tumor heterogeneity is more common in malignant subtypes seen as geographic or rounded areas of low attenuation.[42] The CT attenuation of the tumor also depends on the collagen content, with hyperdense lesions showing abundant collagen. Low-attenuation areas within the tumor represent central necrosis or areas of myxoid or cystic degeneration. Large lesions often have lobulated margins.[17] After contrast administration, smaller lesions typically enhance homogenously, whereas larger lesions usually demonstrate heterogeneous enhancement.

Pedunculated pleural SFTs may change position with respiration and/or posture of the patient.[44] Malignant pleural SFTs are more commonly associated with chest wall and diaphragmatic invasion and pleural effusions. Nearly 50% of the SFTs are pedunculated.[42] The pedunculated visceral pleural-based tumors can be effectively treated with a wedge resection of lung, whereas sessile SFTs often require wide local excision, often with chest wall resection because of their propensity for local recurrence.[45] The imaging differential diagnosis of pleural SFT includes mesothelioma, lymphoma, peripheral nerve sheath tumors, and other soft tissue sarcomas and metastasis. Therefore, confirmatory pathologic correlation via biopsy or resection is necessary for definite management. A staging system for thoracic SFTs based on type of attachment (pedunculated vs sessile) and histology (malignant vs benign) has been proposed to predict recurrence after resection.[46]

Because of its excellent soft tissue resolution, MR imaging is useful to differentiate tumor from surrounding structures as well as to demonstrate chest wall or diaphragmatic involvement. MR

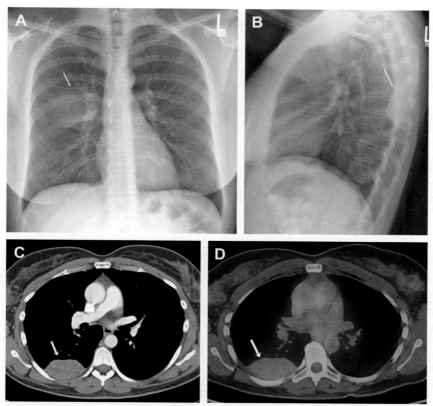

Fig. 4. Pleural SFT. A 49-year-old woman with incidental detection of chest mass on radiograph. (*A*, *B*) Posteroan-terior (*A*) and lateral (*B*) chest radiograph showing a mass in the right mid zone shows "incomplete border" sign (*arrow* in *A*) and forms obtuse angles with the adjacent pleural surface (*arrow* in *B*) suggesting pleural or extrap-leural origin. (*C*) Axial contrast-enhanced CT image in soft tissue window settings showing pleural-based mass in the right hemithorax (*arrow*). (*D*) Axial fused FDG-PET/CT (*D*) image showing FDG avidity within the mass is similar to mediastinal blood pool (*arrow*). Mass was removed via thoracotomy, and histopathology was consistent with benign SFT of pleura.

imaging is also useful for evaluation of vertebral or foraminal involvement in thoracic SFTs (**Fig. 5**). Thoracic SFTs typically have intermediate signal intensity on T1WI and heterogeneous low signal intensity on T2WI. Mature fibrous tissue containing few cells and abundant collagen stroma shows low intensity on T2WI. Hyperintensity on T2WI is related to increased cellularity, edema, cystic

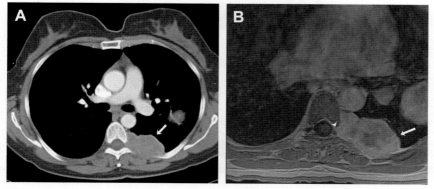

Fig. 5. Pleural SFT. A 53-year-old woman presented with gradual onset chest discomfort and back pain. (*A*) Axial contrast-enhanced CT image in soft tissue window settings showing pleural-based mass in the left hemithorax (*arrow*). (*B*) Axial contrast-enhanced T1WI demonstrating the heterogeneous enhancement of the mass (*arrow*) and neural foraminal extension (*arrowhead*).

degeneration, and hemorrhage. After gadolinium administration, avid heterogeneous enhancement is seen.

PET with fludeoxyglucose F 18 (18F-FDG-PET)/CT has shown usefulness in differentiating benign pleural SFTs from other malignant pleural-based neoplasms.[47] Benign SFTs are generally not avid on 18F-FDG-PET/CT (see **Fig. 4**).[48] Large SFTs with increased FDG uptake have a higher likelihood for malignancy (**Fig. 6**).[49] Intense FDG avidity should raise the suspicion of alternate diagnosis, including lymphoma, mesothelioma, and metastatic disease. As some centers apply a strategy of watchful waiting in asymptomatic SFTs, 18F-FDG-PET/CT positivity in this subgroup of patients may indicate a malignant phenotype, and surgical excision should be considered in these patients.[49]

Abdominal and Pelvic Solitary Fibrous Tumors

Most patients with abdominopelvic SFTs present with pain, palpable mass, and abdominal distension. Other symptoms due to local pressure effects include change in bowel habits and lower urinary tract symptoms.[3]

Hepatic solitary fibrous tumors

Hepatic SFTs are rare tumors with fewer than 60 reported cases in literature[50] and are more common in women.[51] SFTs of the liver typically manifest as a large, well-defined mass with heterogeneous appearance and high vascularity.[52] On unenhanced CT, hepatic SFT appears as well-defined low-attenuation mass. On T2WI, the lesion is heterogeneously hyperintense with areas of low signal intensity, which correspond to the fibrosis (**Fig. 7**). Hepatic SFTs are highly vascular lesions showing heterogeneous enhancement after contrast administration, which often persists on venous and delayed phases. From imaging findings, the main differential diagnoses for the hepatic SFTs include intrahepatic cholangiocarcinoma, sclerosing/fibrolamellar hepatocellular carcinoma, sclerosing hemangioma, or metastasis. Intrahepatic cholangiocarcinoma usually demonstrates peripheral enhancement in the arterial and portal phases with persistent and moderate delayed enhancement. Sclerosing hepatocellular carcinoma is extremely rare and mimics cholangiocarcinoma on imaging. Fibrolamellar hepatocellular carcinomas occur in young adults and typically have a large central scar, which is hypointense

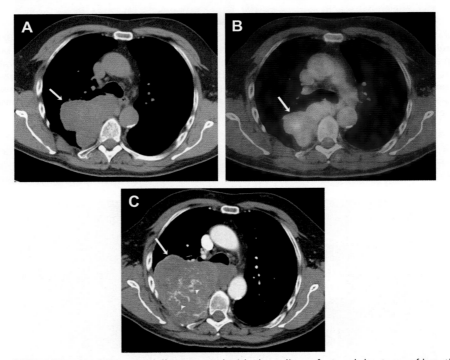

Fig. 6. Pleural SFT. A 72-year-old man initially presented with chest discomfort and shortness of breath. (*A*) Axial unenhanced CT image in soft tissue window settings showing lobulated mass in the right thorax abutting the mediastinal pleura (*arrow*). (*B*) Axial fused FDG-PET/CT image showing heterogeneous FDG avidity within the mass (*arrow*). Biopsy was consistent with malignant fibrous tumor of pleura. (*C*) Follow-up contrast-enhanced CT image showing marked interval increase in the size of the mass (*arrow*) with prominent vascular channels within (*arrowheads*).

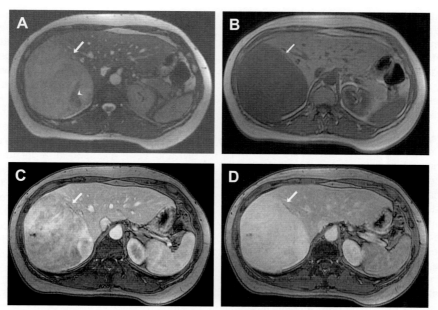

Fig. 7. Hepatic SFT. A 56-year-old woman with gradual onset heaviness in right upper abdomen. (*A*) Axial T2WI MR image shows a large, well-defined, predominantly hyperintense mass in the right lobe of liver (*arrow*) with internal hypointense components (*arrowhead*). (*B*) On corresponding axial T1WI MR image, the mass is hypointense to the adjacent hepatic parenchyma (*arrow*). (*C*, *D*) Axial gadolinium-enhanced T1WI MR images in arterial (*C*) and venous (*D*) phase demonstrating heterogeneous progressive enhancement of the tumor (*arrows*).

on T2WIs and shows delayed enhancement.[53] Sometimes, hepatic hemangiomas can undergo degeneration and fibrous replacement (sclerosing hemangioma) and can then demonstrate variable T2 hypointensity on MR imaging. However, unlike SFTs, these lesions show either the absence of enhancement or the presence of patchy internal nodular enhancement on arterial phase dynamic contrast-enhanced images with progressive filling on portal and delayed phase images.[54–56]

Renal and retroperitoneal solitary fibrous tumor

SFTs involving the kidneys and retroperitoneum are rare. Clinical features of renal SFTs resemble those of renal cell carcinoma and include hematuria, abdominal pain, and palpable mass.[57] The tumor is usually well-circumscribed and can involve the renal cortex, pelvis, renal capsule, or extrarenal soft tissue. Imaging features of renal SFTs are similar to those in other locations.[58] Ultrasound is well-suited for evaluating SFTs of the abdomen, pelvis, and extremities. On ultrasound, SFT are usually hypoechoic, but may have heterogeneous components corresponding to cystic or myxoid degeneration (**Fig. 8**). On MR imaging, they show hypointensity on T2WI with avid heterogeneous enhancement on postcontrast T1WI. The differential diagnosis on imaging includes renal cell carcinoma, angiomyolipoma, oncocytoma,

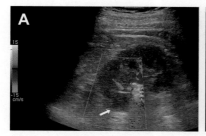
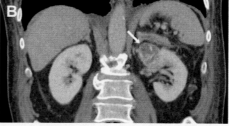

Fig. 8. Renal SFT. A 76-year-old man with incidental detection of renal mass on ultrasonogram. (*A*) Duplex Doppler ultrasound image shows hypoechoic mass at upper pole of the left kidney without internal vascularity (*arrow*). (*B*) Coronal contrast-enhanced CT image showing heterogeneously enhancing mass at upper pole of the left kidney (*arrow*). Because of suspicion of renal cell carcinoma, partial left nephrectomy was performed and histopathology was consistent with benign SFT.

and metastases. Retroperitoneal SFTs are also rare and are seen as heterogeneous hypervascular masses with cystic or necrotic changes on imaging. The differential diagnoses for retroperitoneal SFTs include primary renal tumors, lymphoma, metastasis, and other mesenchymal neoplasms, like neurogenic tumor, desmoid, leiomyosarcoma, or mesothelioma.

Pelvic solitary fibrous tumors

In the pelvis, SFTs can involve urinary bladder, uterus, ovaries, prostate, seminal vesicle, and spermatic cord.[59–61] These SFTs are often asymptomatic because of their slow growth and are usually large at presentation. Symptomatic patients may present with abdominal pain, hematuria, or urinary retention, which is due to displacement and compression of neighboring viscera, such as the intestine, urinary bladder, and uterus.[62] Radiological findings of pelvic SFTs are nonspecific. The tumor is heterogeneous on unenhanced CT images with areas of necrosis (**Fig. 9**). Calcification is rare. They often show marked heterogeneous enhancement on contrast-enhanced CT and MR imaging.

Solitary Fibrous Tumors of the Soft Tissues

Less than 10% of SFTs arise in the soft tissues of the trunk and extremities.[8] Most extremity SFTs occur in the proximal lower extremities. Other common locations include the popliteal fossa, flank, neck, shoulder, deep groin, and gluteal regions. They can be subclassified into fibrous and cellular variants on histopathology based on the amount and distribution of the organized fibrous stroma.[63]

Ultrasound and MR imaging are particularly useful imaging modalities for evaluation of soft tissue SFTs (**Fig. 10**). On MR imaging, soft tissue SFT is typically seen as a well-circumscribed mass with smooth margins showing focal or diffuse T2 hypointensity due to collagen content. The cellular SFT variants have intermediate to hyperintense signal on T2WI with only scant areas of fibrosis showing T2 hypointensity (**Fig. 11**). Heterogeneous T2 hyperintensity due to hemorrhage, cystic degeneration, or necrosis occurs in less than 5% of cases, commonly in larger and malignant tumors.[63] Most tumors are hypointense or isointense relative to muscle on T1WI. Areas of low signal intensity on T1WI and T2WI are seen in larger tumors corresponding to flow voids from prominent intralesional vessels. Few tumors show high signal intensity on T1WI due to the presence of macroscopic fat.[3] Smaller lesions usually show intense homogenous enhancement on postcontrast images, whereas larger lesions typically demonstrate heterogeneous enhancement due to necrosis, hemorrhage, and cystic degeneration.

Metastatic Disease

Approximately 20% of SFTs show malignant histologic features and propensity for local recurrence and/or metastasis. According to a retrospective analysis of 33 patients, Cranshaw and colleagues[64] found histologic features of malignancy in 54% of extrathoracic SFTs and rate of metastasis of 39%. Various sites of metastasis have been described in literature and include lungs, mediastinum, liver, bone, pancreas, kidney, mesentery, and retroperitoneum (**Fig. 12**). Assessment of metastatic disease in SFTs is primarily done with CT, MR imaging, and PET/CT. Malignant SFTs generally have a poor prognosis.[65]

MANAGEMENT OF SOLITARY FIBROUS TUMOR: ROLE OF SYSTEMIC THERAPY

Surgical excision is the treatment of choice for SFTs.[41] Surgical resection of benign SFTs is

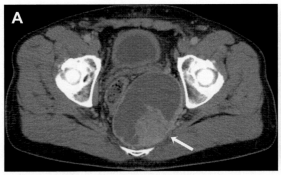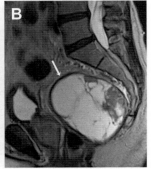

Fig. 9. Pelvic SFT. A 65-year-old man presented with constipation and pelvic discomfort. (*A*) Axial contrast-enhanced CT image showing well-defined predominantly cystic presacral mass with internal solid component (*arrow*). (*B*) Sagittal T2WI MR image demonstrating the heterogeneous T2 signal intensity within the mass (*arrow*) with solid component posteriorly.

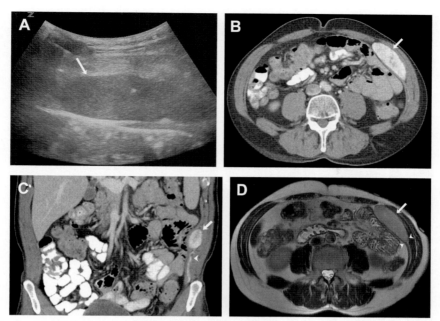

Fig. 10. Abdominal wall SFT. A 58-year-old man presented with palpable painless lump in the left flank. (*A*) Ultrasound image shows a well-defined hypoechoic lesion in the anterior abdominal wall muscles (*arrow*). (*B*) Axial contrast-enhanced CT image showing well-defined intramuscular lesion with marked predominantly homogeneous enhancement (*arrow*). (*C*) Coronal contrast-enhanced CT image demonstrating hypertrophied feeding vessel (*arrowhead*) supplying the mass (*arrow*). (*D*) Axial T2WI MR image demonstrating the well-defined hyperintense mass (*arrow*) in the intermuscular plane between the internal oblique and the transverse abdominis muscles (*arrowheads*).

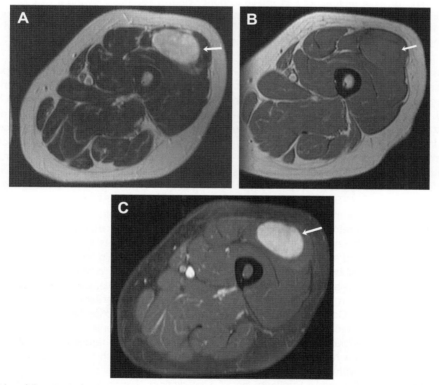

Fig. 11. SFT involving anterior compartment of left thigh. A 48-year-old woman with complaints of painless palpable lump in left thigh. (*A*) Axial T2WI MR image showing a well-defined homogeneously hyperintense mass involving the vastus lateralis muscle (*arrow*). (*B*) On corresponding T1WI, the mass is nearly isointense to adjacent muscles (*arrow*). (*C*) On contrast-enhanced fat-saturated T1WI MR image, the mass shows intense homogenous enhancement (*arrow*).

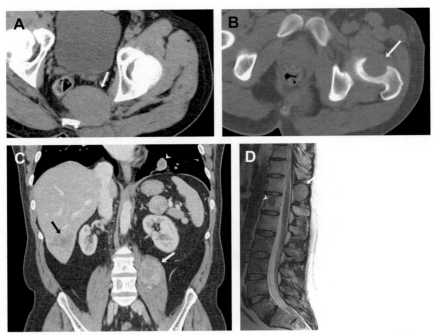

Fig. 12. Pelvic SFT and metastases. A 43-year-old man presented with pain the left hip and gluteal region. (*A*) Axial unenhanced CT image showing a well-defined mass lesion in the presacral space extending into left sciatic foramina (*arrow*). (*B*) Axial unenhanced CT image in bone window settings showing a lytic lesion in the left femoral neck suggestive of metastasis (*arrow*). (*C*) Coronal contrast-enhanced CT image showing hepatic (*black arrow*), pulmonary (*arrowhead*), and intramuscular (*white arrow*) metastases. (*D*) Sagittal T1WI of the lumbar spine showing vertebral metastases (*arrow* and *arrowhead*).

usually curative, but local recurrences can occur years after seemingly adequate surgical treatment. Positive surgical margins, tumor size greater than 10 cm, and the presence of a malignant component on histopathological examination are adverse prognostic factors.[8] Local recurrence after resection is common in tumors with malignant characteristics on histopathology. Close surveillance is recommended for these patients after surgical resection.[66] Extrathoracic SFTs have an increased risk of local recurrence compared with thoracic SFTs.[8] Patients with unresectable, recurrent, or metastatic SFTs/HPCs have worse prognosis with no established standard systemic therapy.

With recent advances and better understanding of the molecular pathogenesis and aberrations of HPCs/SFTs, many novel targeted therapies are currently in development. Combination therapy with bevacizumab and temozolomide is well tolerated and a clinically beneficial regimen for HPC/SFT patients according to a recent retrospective analysis of 14 patients with locally advanced, recurrent, or metastatic disease.[67] Sunitinib malate is a multitarget, tyrosine kinase inhibitor with activity against vascular endothelial growth factor receptors, which has been found useful in patients with progressive advanced SFTs.[68] According to a

multicenter phase II trial of sunitinib in patients with advanced nongastrointestinal stromal tumor (GIST) sarcomas, the drug has shown therapeutic benefit in patients with SFTs.[69] Dysregulation of insulinlike growth factor-1 receptor (IGF-1R) signaling and the phosphatidylinositol 3-kinase/Protein kinase B (PKB)/mammalian target of rapamycin (mTOR) signaling pathways have been implicated in pathogenesis of many soft tissue sarcomas, including SFTs. Combination everolimus (mTOR inhibitor) plus figitumumab (a fully human IgG2 anti-IGF-1R monoclonal antibody) is well tolerated in patients with metastatic SFTs.[70] Regorafenib, sorafenib, and bevacizumab are also found to be useful for metastatic SFTs.

The Response Evaluation Criteria in Solid Tumors (RECIST) is the most widely used measurement system in clinical practice for evaluation of treatment response in patients with sarcomas, including SFTs. Many new targeted therapies can cause tumor necrosis with a decrease in tumor density without a marked decrease in tumor size due to distinct biological mechanisms. Treatment-induced necrosis is not included as a part of RECIST and may even mimic progressive disease if only size criteria are used. Originally developed to assess treatment response in GISTs, Choi criteria, which

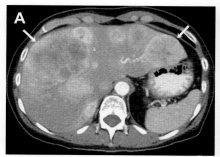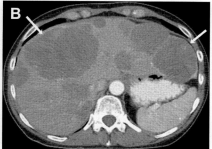

Fig. 13. A 57-year-old woman with hepatic metastases from primary intracranial SFT on treatment with sunitinib. (*A*) Axial contrast-enhanced CT image before the start of treatment showing multiple hypervascular metastatic lesions in both lobes of liver (*arrows*). (*B*) Axial contrast-enhanced CT image 2 months after completion of treatment shows a marked decrease enhancement of the metastases (*arrows*); however, the size of the lesions is mildly increased.

involves tumor size and density measurement, is useful to evaluate response to treatment in patients with SFTs and can be easily applied on contrast-enhanced CT scans to assess treatment response (**Fig. 13**).[71]

SUMMARY

SFTs are ubiquitous mesenchymal neoplasms that most commonly involve the pleura. Extrathoracic SFTs commonly occur in the head and neck region, abdomen, pelvis, and extremities. Although some imaging findings are characteristic of SFTs, histologic and immunohistochemical studies are mandatory for confirmatory diagnosis of SFTs. Surgical excision is the treatment of choice for localized tumors. There is no established standard systemic therapy for metastatic disease; however, many novel targeted therapies, in particular tyrosine kinase inhibitors and antiangiogenic agents, have shown therapeutic efficacy in patients with advanced/metastatic SFTs.

REFERENCES

1. Klemperer P, Rabin CB. Primary neoplasms of the pleura: a report of five cases. Arch Pathol 1931;11: 385–412.
2. Kunzel J, Hainz M, Ziebart T, et al. Head and neck solitary fibrous tumors: a rare and challenging entity. Eur Arch oto-rhino-laryngology 2015;1–10.
3. Wignall OJ, Moskovic EC, Thway K, et al. Solitary fibrous tumors of the soft tissues: review of the imaging and clinical features with histopathologic correlation. AJR Am J Roentgenol 2010;195(1):W55–62.
4. Kalebi AY, Hale MJ, Wong ML, et al. Surgically cured hypoglycemia secondary to pleural solitary fibrous tumour: case report and update review on the Doege-Potter syndrome. J Cardiothorac Surg 2009;4:45.
5. Fridlington J, Weaver J, Kelly B, et al. Secondary hypertrophic osteoarthropathy associated with solitary fibrous tumor of the lung. J Am Acad Dermatol 2007; 57(5 Suppl):S106–10.
6. Li Y, Chang Q, Rubin BP, et al. Insulin receptor activation in solitary fibrous tumours. J Pathol 2007; 211(5):550–4.
7. Cardillo G, Facciolo F, Cavazzana AO, et al. Localized (solitary) fibrous tumors of the pleura: an analysis of 55 patients. Ann Thorac Surg 2000;70(6): 1808–12.
8. Gold JS, Antonescu CR, Hajdu C, et al. Clinicopathologic correlates of solitary fibrous tumors. Cancer 2002;94(4):1057–68.
9. Gengler C, Guillou L. Solitary fibrous tumour and haemangiopericytoma: evolution of a concept. Histopathology 2006;48(1):63–74.
10. Park MS, Araujo DM. New insights into the hemangiopericytoma/solitary fibrous tumor spectrum of tumors. Curr Opin Oncol 2009;21(4):327–31.
11. Robinson DR, Wu YM, Kalyana-Sundaram S, et al. Identification of recurrent NAB2-STAT6 gene fusions in solitary fibrous tumor by integrative sequencing. Nat Genet 2013;45(2):180–5.
12. Schweizer L, Koelsche C, Sahm F, et al. Meningeal hemangiopericytoma and solitary fibrous tumors carry the NAB2-STAT6 fusion and can be diagnosed by nuclear expression of STAT6 protein. Acta Neuropathol 2013;125(5):651–8.
13. Barthelmess S, Geddert H, Boltze C, et al. Solitary fibrous tumors/hemangiopericytomas with different variants of the NAB2-STAT6 gene fusion are characterized by specific histomorphology and distinct clinicopathological features. Am J Pathol 2014; 184(4):1209–18.
14. Akaike K, Kurisaki-Arakawa A, Hara K, et al. Distinct clinicopathological features of NAB2-STAT6 fusion gene variants in solitary fibrous tumor with emphasis on the acquisition of highly malignant potential. Hum Pathol 2015;46(3):347–56.

15. Fletcher C, Bridge J, Hogendoorn P, et al. WHO classification of tumours of soft tissue and bone: pathology and genetics of tumours of soft tissue and bone. 4th edition. Lyon(France): IARC Press; 2013.

16. Fletcher CD. The evolving classification of soft tissue tumours—an update based on the new 2013 WHO classification. Histopathology 2014;64(1):2–11.

17. Lee KS, Im JG, Choe KO, et al. CT findings in benign fibrous mesothelioma of the pleura: pathologic correlation in nine patients. AJR Am J Roentgenol 1992;158(5):983–6.

18. Hasegawa T, Matsuno Y, Shimoda T, et al. Extrathoracic solitary fibrous tumors: their histological variability and potentially aggressive behavior. Hum Pathol 1999;30(12):1464–73.

19. Vallat-Decouvelaere AV, Dry SM, Fletcher CD. Atypical and malignant solitary fibrous tumors in extrathoracic locations: evidence of their comparability to intra-thoracic tumors. Am J Surg Pathol 1998;22(12):1501–11.

20. Chan JK. Solitary fibrous tumour–everywhere, and a diagnosis in vogue. Histopathology 1997;31(6): 568–76.

21. Hasegawa T, Matsuno Y, Shimoda T, et al. Frequent expression of bcl-2 protein in solitary fibrous tumors. Jpn J Clin Oncol 1998;28(2):86–91.

22. Alawi F, Stratton D, Freedman PD. Solitary fibrous tumor of the oral soft tissues: a clinicopathologic and immunohistochemical study of 16 cases. Am J Surg Pathol 2001;25(7):900–10.

23. Liu Y, Tao X, Shi H, et al. MRI findings of solitary fibrous tumours in the head and neck region. Dento maxillo Facial Radiol 2014;43(3):20130415.

24. Doyle LA, Vivero M, Fletcher CD, et al. Nuclear expression of STAT6 distinguishes solitary fibrous tumor from histologic mimics. Mod Pathol 2014;27(3):390–5.

25. Yokoi T, Tsuzuki T, Yatabe Y, et al. Solitary fibrous tumour: significance of p53 and CD34 immunoreactivity in its malignant transformation. Histopathology 1998;32(5):423–32.

26. Yan B, Raju GC, Salto-Tellez M. Epithelioid, cytokeratin expressing malignant solitary fibrous tumour of the pleura. Pathology 2008;40(1):98–9.

27. Lahon B, Mercier O, Fadel E, et al. Solitary fibrous tumor of the pleura: outcomes of 157 complete resections in a single center. Ann Thorac Surg 2012; 94(2):394–400.

28. Fargen KM, Opalach KJ, Wakefield D, et al. The central nervous system solitary fibrous tumor: a review of clinical, imaging and pathologic findings among all reported cases from 1996 to 2010. Clin Neurol Neurosurg 2011;113(9):703–10.

29. Clarencon F, Bonneville F, Rousseau A, et al. Intracranial solitary fibrous tumor: imaging findings. Eur J Radiol 2011;80(2):387–94.

30. Weon YC, Kim EY, Kim HJ, et al. Intracranial solitary fibrous tumors: imaging findings in 6 consecutive patients. AJNR Am J Neuroradiol 2007;28(8):1466–9.

31. Carneiro SS, Scheithauer BW, Nascimento AG, et al. Solitary fibrous tumor of the meninges: a lesion distinct from fibrous meningioma. A clinicopathologic and immunohistochemical study. Am J Clin Pathol 1996;106(2):217–24.

32. Kim HJ, Lee HK, Seo JJ, et al. MR imaging of solitary fibrous tumors in the head and neck. Korean J Radiol 2005;6(3):136–42.

33. Liu Y, Li K, Shi H, et al. Solitary fibrous tumours in the extracranial head and neck region: correlation of CT and MR features with pathologic findings. Radiol Med 2014;119(12):910–9.

34. Chen H, Xiao CW, Wang T, et al. Orbital solitary fibrous tumor: a clinicopathologic study of ten cases with long-term follow-up. Acta Neurochir 2012; 154(2):249–55 [discussion: 255].

35. Yang BT, Wang YZ, Dong JY, et al. MRI study of solitary fibrous tumor in the orbit. AJR Am J Roentgenol 2012;199(4):W506–11.

36. Krishnakumar S, Subramanian N, Mohan ER, et al. Solitary fibrous tumor of the orbit: a clinicopathologic study of six cases with review of the literature. Surv Ophthalmol 2003;48(5):544–54.

37. Gigantelli JW, Kincaid MC, Soparkar CN, et al. Orbital solitary fibrous tumor: radiographic and histopathologic correlations. Ophthal Plast Reconstr Surg 2001;17(3):207–14.

38. Tailor TD, Gupta D, Dalley RW, et al. Orbital neoplasms in adults: clinical, radiologic, and pathologic review. Radiographics 2013;33(6):1739–58.

39. Meltzer DE. Orbital imaging: a pattern-based approach. Radiol Clin North Am 2015;53(1):37–80.

40. Briselli M, Mark EJ, Dickersin GR. Solitary fibrous tumors of the pleura: eight new cases and review of 360 cases in the literature. Cancer 1981;47(11): 2678–89.

41. Enon S, Kilic D, Yuksel C, et al. Benign localized fibrous tumor of the pleura: report of 25 new cases. Thorac Cardiovasc Surg 2012;60(7):468–73.

42. Rosado-de-Christenson ML, Abbott GF, McAdams HP, et al. From the archives of the AFIP: localized fibrous tumor of the pleura. Radiographics 2003;23(3):759–83.

43. Hsu CC, Henry TS, Chung JH, et al. The incomplete border sign. J Thorac Imaging 2014;29(4):W48.

44. Akman C, Cetinkaya S, Ulus S, et al. Pedunculated localized fibrous tumor of the pleura presenting as a moving chest mass. South Med J 2005;98(4):486–8.

45. Robinson LA. Solitary fibrous tumor of the pleura. Cancer control 2006;13(4):264–9.

46. de Perrot M, Fischer S, Brundler MA, et al. Solitary fibrous tumors of the pleura. Ann Thorac Surg 2002;74(1):285–93.

47. Kruse M, Sherry SJ, Paidpally V, et al. FDG PET/CT in the management of primary pleural tumors and pleural metastases. AJR Am J Roentgenol 2013; 201(2):W215–26.

48. Cortes J, Rodriguez J, Garcia-Velloso MJ, et al. [(18) F]-FDG PET and localized fibrous mesothelioma. Lung 2003;181(1):49–54.

49. Kohler M, Clarenbach CF, Kestenholz P, et al. Diagnosis, treatment and long-term outcome of solitary fibrous tumours of the pleura. Eur J cardio-thoracic Surg 2007;32(3):403–8.

50. Debs T, Kassir R, Amor IB, et al. Solitary fibrous tumor of the liver: report of two cases and review of the literature. Int J Surg 2014;12(12):1291–4.

51. Changku J, Shaohua S, Zhicheng Z, et al. Solitary fibrous tumor of the liver: retrospective study of reported cases. Cancer Invest 2006;24(2):132–5.

52. Fuksbrumer MS, Klimstra D, Panicek DM. Solitary fibrous tumor of the liver: imaging findings. AJR Am J Roentgenol 2000;175(6):1683–7.

53. McLarney JK, Rucker PT, Bender GN, et al. Fibrolamellar carcinoma of the liver: radiologic-pathologic correlation. Radiographics 1999;19(2):453–71.

54. Ridge CA, Shia J, Gerst SR, et al. Sclerosed hemangioma of the liver: concordance of MRI features with histologic characteristics. J Magn Reson Imaging 2014;39(4):812–8.

55. Doyle DJ, Khalili K, Guindi M, et al. Imaging features of sclerosed hemangioma. AJR Am J Roentgenol 2007;189(1):67–72.

56. Vilgrain V, Boulos L, Vullierme MP, et al. Imaging of atypical hemangiomas of the liver with pathologic correlation. Radiographics 2000;20(2):379–97.

57. Kuroda N, Ohe C, Sakaida N, et al. Solitary fibrous tumor of the kidney with focus on clinical and pathobiological aspects. Int J Clin Exp Pathol 2014; 7(6):2737–42.

58. Yoneyama T, Koie T, Yamamoto H, et al. Solitary fibrous tumor of the kidney: a case report. Hinyokika kiyo 2009;55(8):479–81 [in Japanese].

59. Khandelwal A, Virmani V, Amin MS, et al. Radiology-pathology conference: malignant solitary fibrous tumor of the seminal vesicle. Clin Imaging 2013; 37(2):409–13.

60. Dozier J, Jameel Z, McCain DA, et al. Massive malignant solitary fibrous tumor arising from the bladder serosa: a case report. J Med case Rep 2015;9:46.

61. Strickland KC, Nucci MR, Esselen KM, et al. Solitary fibrous tumor of the uterus presenting with lung metastases: a case report. Int J Gynecol Pathol 2015;35(1):25–9.

62. Zhang WD, Chen JY, Cao Y, et al. Computed tomography and magnetic resonance imaging findings of solitary fibrous tumors in the pelvis: correlation with histopathological findings. Eur J Radiol 2011;78(1): 65–70.

63. Musyoki FN, Nahal A, Powell TI. Solitary fibrous tumor: an update on the spectrum of extrapleural manifestations. Skeletal Radiol 2012;41(1):5–13.

64. Cranshaw IM, Gikas PD, Fisher C, et al. Clinical outcomes of extra-thoracic solitary fibrous tumours. Eur J Surg Oncol 2009;35(9):994–8.

65. Rena O, Filosso PL, Papalia E, et al. Solitary fibrous tumour of the pleura: surgical treatment. Eur J cardio-thoracic Surg 2001;19(2):185–9.

66. Santos RS, Haddad R, Lima CE, et al. Patterns of recurrence and long-term survival after curative resection of localized fibrous tumors of the pleura. Clin Lung Cancer 2005;7(3):197–201.

67. Park MS, Patel SR, Ludwig JA, et al. Activity of temozolomide and bevacizumab in the treatment of locally advanced, recurrent, and metastatic hemangiopericytoma and malignant solitary fibrous tumor. Cancer 2011;117(21):4939–47.

68. Stacchiotti S, Negri T, Libertini M, et al. Sunitinib malate in solitary fibrous tumor (SFT). Ann Oncol 2012; 23(12):3171–9.

69. George S, Merriam P, Maki RG, et al. Multicenter phase II trial of sunitinib in the treatment of nongastrointestinal stromal tumor sarcomas. J Clin Oncol 2009;27(19):3154–60.

70. Quek R, Wang Q, Morgan JA, et al. Combination mTOR and IGF-1R inhibition: phase I trial of everolimus and figitumumab in patients with advanced sarcomas and other solid tumors. Clin Cancer Res 2011;17(4):871–9.

71. Choi H, Charnsangavej C, Faria SC, et al. Correlation of computed tomography and positron emission tomography in patients with metastatic gastrointestinal stromal tumor treated at a single institution with imatinib mesylate: proposal of new computed tomography response criteria. J Clin Oncol 2007; 25(13):1753–9.

State-of-the-Art Imaging and Staging of Plasma Cell Dyscrasias

 CrossMark

Behrang Amini, MD, PhD[a], Sarvari Yellapragada, MD[b],
Shetal Shah, MD[c], Eric Rohren, MD, PhD[d],
Raghunandan Vikram, MD[e],*

KEYWORDS

- Plasma cell dyscrasias • Monoclonal gammopathy of unknown clinical significance
- Smoldering myeloma • Multiple myeloma • Solitary plasmacytoma • Imaging

KEY POINTS

- Monoclonal gammopathy of unknown significance (MGUS) is a clinically asymptomatic premalignant clonal plasma cell or lymphoplasmacytic proliferative disorder.
- Smoldering multiple myeloma (SMM), also called asymptomatic multiple myeloma (MM), is an intermediate stage between MGUS and symptomatic MM.
- As the name implies, extraosseous or extramedullary myeloma refers to the presence of myeloma deposits outside the skeletal system.
- Waldenström macroglobulinemia (WM) is a distinct subtype of plasma cell dyscrasia characterized by lymphoplasmacytic lymphoma (LPL) in the bone marrow with an associated IgM monoclonal gammopathy.
- Amyloidosis is a condition characterized by extracellular deposition of fibrils composed of a variety of normal serum proteins.

INTRODUCTION

Plasma cell neoplasms, characterized by clonal proliferation of plasma cells in the bone marrow, comprise a wide spectrum of tumors of variable clinicobiological behavior. They are typically associated with secretion of monoclonal immunoglobulins or immunoglobulin fragments (M-protein, myeloma protein, or paraprotein).[1] These M proteins classically consist of 2 heavy polypeptide chains of the same class (IgG, IgA, and less commonly IgD, IgE, and IgM) and 2 light polypeptide chains of the same type (kappa and lambda).

Plasma cell neoplasms have been challenging to classify in a way that is both biologically correct and clinically useful.[2] The current World Health Organization (WHO) classification places plasma cell neoplasms under the broad category of mature B-cell neoplasms and includes MGUS, solitary plasmacytoma of bone (SPB), plasma cell myeloma (PCM) or multiple myeloma (MM), extraosseous plasmacytoma, and monoclonal immunoglobulin deposition diseases as subcategories.[3]

[a] Musculoskeletal Imaging, Diagnostic Radiology, The University of Texas MD Anderson Cancer Center, 1515 Holcombe Boulevard, Houston, TX 77030, USA; [b] Hematology & Oncology, Medicine, Michael E DeBakey VA Medical Center, Baylor College of Medicine, 2002 Holcombe Boulevard, Houston, TX 77030, USA; [c] Diagnostic Radiology, Cleveland Clinic, 9500 Euclid Avenue, Cleveland, OH 44195, USA; [d] Nuclear Medicine, The University of Texas MD Anderson Cancer Center, 1515 Holcombe Boulevard, Houston, TX 77030, USA; [e] Abdominal Imaging, Diagnostic Radiology, The University of Texas MD Anderson Cancer Center, 1515 Holcombe Boulevard, Houston, TX 77030, USA
* Corresponding author.
E-mail address: rvikram@mdanderson.org

Radiol Clin N Am 54 (2016) 581–596
http://dx.doi.org/10.1016/j.rcl.2015.12.008
0033-8389/16/$ – see front matter © 2016 Elsevier Inc. All rights reserved.

From a clinical perspective, classification aims to separate patients who do not require systemic therapy (those with MGUS, asymptomatic PCM, and SPB) from those who do (those with symptomatic PCM and MM). This classification is predominantly laboratory based (**Box 1**); however, imaging plays an important role in evaluating the disease burden as well as its complications. Performance of laboratory tests, such as total serum protein, serum albumin, serum and urine protein electrophoresis, quantitative immunoglobulins, immunofixation in serum and urine, and for detection of immunoglobulin free light chains, allows accurate diagnosis of patients with suspected plasma cell dyscrasias. In addition, complete blood cell count, serum creatinine, and electrolytes, including calcium, lactate dehydrogenase, and β_2-microglobulin are obtained. In a patient with suspected MM, a bone marrow aspirate and biopsy should be obtained to determine the percentage of plasma cells and for prognostic studies, such as fluorescence in situ hybridization (FISH).

Once a diagnosis of symptomatic MM is made, its staging under the International Staging System is entirely laboratory based, which relies on serum β_2-microglobulin and serum albumin to classify the disease into a 3-stage system to indicate different levels of projected survival rates and point to increasingly aggressive treatment strategies.[4] Recently, the revised ISS has also been published, which incorporates the FISH data and lactate dehydrogenase level creating a more robust prognostic model.[5]

An important point is that the number of bone lesions on skeletal survey is not included in the current diagnostic or prognostic models. A minimum of 2 or 3 lytic bone lesions has been erroneously propagated in radiology literature as required for the diagnosis of symptomatic PCM; however, as noted by other investigators,[6] cutoffs for bone lesions on skeletal survey do not appear in the myeloma literature. As evident in **Box 1**, a single bone lesion in the setting of the appropriate laboratory findings is sufficient for a diagnosis of MM. A more recent staging system, the Durie/Salmon PLUS staging system,[7] uses the number of bone lesions on PET-CT and MR imaging in categorizing the severity of disease; however, this system has failed to gain widespread acceptance.

MONOCLONAL GAMMOPATHY OF UNKNOWN SIGNIFICANCE

MGUS is a clinically asymptomatic premalignant clonal plasma cell or lymphoplasmacytic proliferative disorder. It is the most common type of plasma cell dyscrasia and is seen in more than 3% of the general population aged 50 years or older.[8] It is 2 to 3 times more common in Africans and African Americans compared with whites and the incidence increases with age. It is clinically important because it is considered a premalignant condition, a precursor to MM. Patients with MGUS are associated with an overall 1% per year risk of progression to MM (**Fig. 1**). MGUS can further be stratified into risk categories based on the type and quantity of the M protein and the serum free light chain, helping define the risk of evolution per year into symptomatic MM. MGUS, by definition, should have no symptoms that can be attributable to the underlying plasma cell disorder

---

Box 1
Diagnostic criteria for plasma cell myeloma and related disorders

Monoclonal gammopathy of undetermined significance

M protein in serum <30 g/L

Bone marrow clonal plasma cells <10% and low level of plasma cell infiltration in a trephine biopsy (if done)

No evidence of other B-cell proliferative disorders

No related organ or tissue impairment (see **Box 2**)

Asymptomatic (smoldering) myeloma

M protein in serum ≥30 g/L and/or ≥10% clonal plasma cells in bone marrow

No related organ or tissue impairment (see **Box 2**)

Solitary plasmacytoma (solitary plasmacytoma of bone; solitary extraosseous plasmacytoma)

Single area of bone destruction due to clonal plasma cells or single extraosseous deposit

No M protein in serum and/or urine

Bone marrow not consistent with MM

Normal skeletal survey (and MR imaging of spine and pelvis if done)

No related organ or tissue impairment (see **Box 2**)

Symptomatic multiple myeloma

M protein in serum or urine (no levels specified)

Clonal plasma cells in bone marrow or plasmacytoma (>60%)

Related organ or tissue impairment heavy chain disease

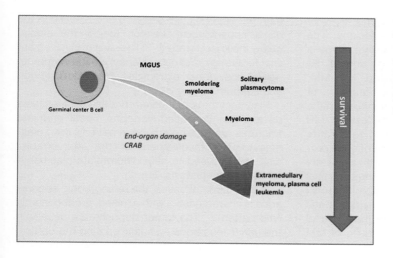

Fig. 1. Schematic representation of sequential progression of non-IgM MGUS and spectrum of plasma cell dyscrasias (IgM MGUS, on the other hand, progresses to WM). CRAB represents symptoms attributable to hypercalcemia, renal failure, anemia, and bone lesions.

(commonly called CRAB features—hypercalcemia, renal failure, anemia, and bone lesions). In patients with MGUS, serum M protein is less than 3g/dL, and a bone marrow biopsy shows clonal plasma cells less than 10%.

There are 3 distinct clinical types of MGUS: non-IgM (IgG or IgA) MGUS, IgM MGUS, and light chain MGUS. Serum immunofixation determines the type of M protein. Approximately 80% of MMs arise from non-IgM MGUS and 20% from light chain MGUS. Patients with IgM MGUS usually evolve into WM. Patients with IgM MGUS rarely progress to IgM MM.[9]

Imaging in patients with MGUS is not routinely used for patients who have low-risk disease (ie, IgG-type MGUS with serum M protein <1.5 g/dL) with no clinical concern for bone lesions or myeloma.[10,11] In patients with high-risk MGUS, skeletal survey is usually performed to exclude MM. MR imaging and/or PET-CT scan may be considered if there is concern for the presence of bone disease based on clinical features, because these techniques are more sensitive in detecting bone disease.

ASYMPTOMATIC SMOLDERING MYELOMA

SMM, also called asymptomatic MM, is an intermediate stage between MGUS and symptomatic MM. SMM is distinguished from MGUS based on the amount of circulating serum M protein and the percent plasma cells in the bone marrow. SMM is diagnosed in persons in whom serum monoclonal protein is greater than 3 g/dL and/or greater than 10% to less than 60% bone marrow clonal plasma cells and absence of myeloma defining events or amyloidosis (**Box 2**). Most patients with SMM progress to symptomatic

myeloma at a reported rate of 10% per year for the first 5 years, 3% per year for the next 5 years, and 1% to 2% per year for the following 10 years.[12]

Patients with SMM should be diagnosed from MM because these patients can remain stable over extended periods of time.[13–15] Hence, it is important to image these patients for presence of any bone lesions. Apart from laboratory tests, patients with SMM should receive imaging assessment, including a skeletal survey and/or any of PET-CT, whole-body MR imaging, or whole-body

---

Box 2
Myeloma-related organ or tissue impairment due to the plasma cell proliferative process

Calcium levels increased

Serum calcium >0.25 mmol/L above the upper limit of normal or >75 mmol/L

Renal insufficiency

Creatinine >173 mmol/L

Anemia

Hemoglobin 2 g/dL below the lower limit of normal or hemoglobin <10 g/dL

Bone lesions

Lytic lesions or osteoporosis with compression fractures (MR imaging or CT may clarify)

Other

Symptomatic hyperviscosity

Amyloidosis

Recurrent bacterial infections (>2 episodes in 12 months)

low-dose CT. PET-CT and MR imaging are very sensitive in detecting active bone lesions. The choice of test depends on availability.[9] Once a diagnosis is established, patients should be closely monitored for progression to MM, including annual metastatic radiographic or cross-sectional bone survey to monitor for the development of asymptomatic bone lesions. MR imaging may be performed 3 to 6 months after diagnosis in patients with a higher risk of bone progression. These include patients with a solitary focal lesion, those with equivocal findings on initial imaging, and those with 1 or more other high-risk factors. In patients with otherwise asymptomatic myeloma, the identification of more than 1 focal bone lesion on MR imaging is diagnostic of MM and an indication for therapy.

Patients with SMM are at increased risk of fracture and thromboembolic disease. Patients with SMM should be evaluated for osteoporosis with a dual-energy x-ray absorptiometry scan and have their vitamin D and calcium intake optimized. If osteoporosis is present, treatment with bisphosphonates may be considered. Persons with MGUS or SMM also have a higher incidence of developing second cancers.[16] No additional cancer screening has been recommended for this population apart from age-appropriate cancer screening.

SOLITARY PLASMACYTOMA

Solitary plasmacytoma (SP), defined as a proliferation of clonal plasma cells without evidence of significant bone marrow plasma cell infiltration, constitutes approximately 5% of cases of PCM.[17] Two separate entities have been described, based on presence in either bone or extramedullary soft tissue.[18] SP is most frequently seen in bones as a solitary lytic lesion due to clonal proliferation of plasma cells. it rarely present as extramedullary SP.[19] Adhesion molecule and chemokine receptor expression patterns determine the molecular basis of the differentiation between SP and MM.[20] The diagnostic criteria for SP are listed in **Boxes 1** and **2**.

Solitary Plasmacytoma of the Bone

In the United States, the incidence of solitary plasmacytoma of the bone (SPB) is approximately 0.15 cases/100,000 person-years or 450 cases per year. It is more common in men (2:1); incidence is highest in African Americans and lowest in Asians and Pacific Islanders. SPB commonly manifests as skeletal pain or a pathologic fracture of the affected bone. Bones are involved in active hematopoiesis; that is, the axial skeleton is more commonly involved

than the appendicular skeleton and disease in the distal appendicular skeleton (below the elbow/below the knee) is rare.[21,22] The sites of involvement (in decreasing order of frequency) are the vertebrae, pelvis, ribs, upper extremities, face, skull, femur, and sternum.[23]

Plasmacytoma of the vertebra usually manifests as a single collapsed vertebra. Focal endplate fractures are more common in patients with plasmacytoma.[24] Involvement of the intervertebral disk can be used to help differentiate plasmacytoma from metastasis (**Fig. 2**).

In two-thirds of cases, the radiographic appearance is characteristic, with a mixed, predominantly lytic pattern.[25] The tumor deposits are usually in the cancellous bone – usually sparing the cortical bone, which may occasionally be sclerotic[25] (**Fig. 3**).

In one-third of cases, the radiographic appearance is less characteristic, with a multicystic soap bubble, or a purely lytic appearance (see **Fig. 3A**). Solitary sclerotic plasmacytoma is extremely rare. On MR imaging, plasmacytoma has low signal intensity on T1–weighted imaging (WI), high signal intensity on T2-WI, and homogeneous intense enhancement on postcontrast T1-WI (see **Fig. 2**).[24,26,27] Because metastatic lesions are far more common than SPs, however, a biopsy is warranted to establish a definitive diagnosis. Another key role of radiology and nuclear medicine is to establish that the plasmacytoma is truly solitary once the pathologic diagnosis has been made, because this can have a considerable impact on the treatment. Skeletal survey alone is not adequate and national guidelines recommend sensitive studies, such as MR imaging survey or PET scan, to rule out other lesions (see **Fig. 2**).

Localized radiation therapy is the standard treatment of SPB. Surgery may be required for patients with structural instability of the bone or rapidly progressive symptoms from cord compression. The use of adjuvant of prophylactic chemotherapy in this population is controversial. The median survival of patients with SPB is 10 years. The overall survival rates at 5 years and 10 years are 75% and 45%, respectively. A little more than half of patients with SPB progress to MM.[21,22]

Solitary Extramedullary Plasmacytoma

By definition, solitary extramedullary plasmacytomas (SEPs) originate outside the bone marrow. Extramedullary plasmacytomas may arise in patients with MM at any time during the course of the disease and should not be confused with SEP. SEP constitutes approximately 3% of all

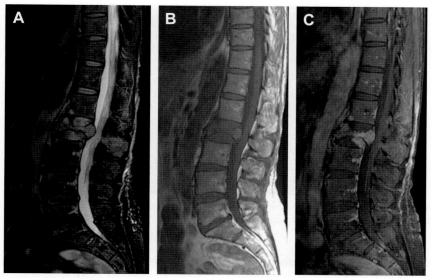

Fig. 2. SP of L2. (*A*) T2-weighted MR image shows increase in marrow signal intensity. (*B*) Precontrast and (*C*) post-contrast T1-WI showing decreased signal intensity (3b) with intense enhancement postcontrast and vertebral endplate fractures. Note the posterior extradural compression of the thecal sac.

plasma cell malignancies, with a median age of 55 to 60 years. Approximately two-thirds of patients are men. SEP usually presents with symptoms related to the location of mass. The most common location of SEP is in the upper respiratory tract (ie, oronasopharynx and paranasal sinuses) –

presenting with epistaxis, nasal discharge (rhinor-rhea), or nasal obstruction. Involvement of the gastrointestinal tract, liver, or lymph nodes is rare[28] (**Figs. 4** and **5**).

SP can be distinguished from most neoplasms based on the morphologic appearance of plasma

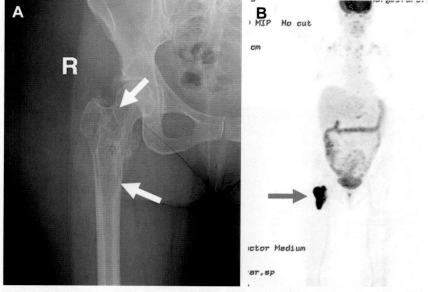

Fig. 3. A 54-year-old woman with an SP. (*A*) Frontal radiograph of the right hip with a well demarcated lytic lesion in the diaphysis (*white arrows*). Plasmacytomas (and MMs) are expansile lytic lesion with epicenter in the cancellous (medulla) bone. (*B*) Maximum intensity projection image of a PET-CT showing that the lesion is FDG avid (*red arrow*). No other metabolically avid lesions are seen in the axial or appendicular skeleton. A key role of imaging is to establish the disease burden.

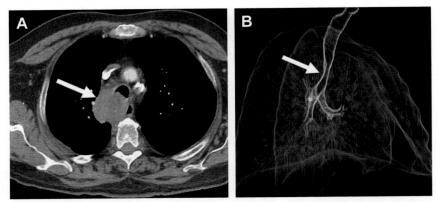

Fig. 4. SEP involving the trachea. (*A*) Axial contrast-enhanced CT scan showing a homogenous mass (*arrow*). (*B*) 3-D reconstruction from a virtual CT-bronchogram showing the degree of airway narrowing (*arrow*). The patient presented with dyspnea.

cells and on the clonal nature of the plasma cells, which can be established by immunostaining for kappa and lambda light chains or by flow cytometry. Typically, plasma cells in SEP are positive for CD138 and CD38 and show light chain restriction (ie, staining positive for either kappa or lambda but not both). Distinction between SEP and MM is made on basis of radiological and laboratory findings (see **Boxes 1** and **2**). Patients with SEP are less likely to progress to MM.[18]

MULTIPLE MYELOMA (SYMPTOMATIC MULTIPLE MYELOMA)

MM is a disseminated malignancy of postgerminal center plasma cells and is almost always preceded by MGUS and SMM, as discussed previously (see **Fig. 1**). MM accounts for 1.3% of all malignancies and 15% of hematologic cancers.[29] Men are affected more frequently than women; the incidence in Africans and African Americans is 2 to 3 times that in whites. The median age of diagnosis is 66 years.[30,31] Patients with plasma cell dyscrasia who present with symptoms attributable to CRAB features are suspected of having MM. MM is often discovered through routine blood screening or radiographic studies when patients are evaluated for unrelated problems. In one-third of patients, the condition is diagnosed after a pathologic fracture occurs, usually involving the axial skeleton. In a retrospective study of 1027 patients with MM in a single institution, 73% had anemia, 58% had symptoms of bone pain, and elevated creatinine was seen in 48%. Other systemic symptoms, such as fatigue and weight loss, were seen in 32% and 24%, respectively.[30]

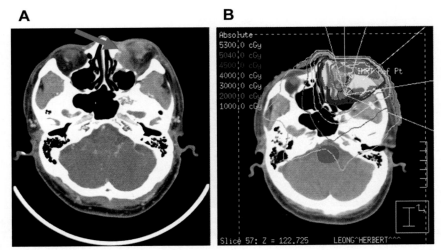

Fig. 5. Extramedullary plasmacytoma of the left orbit in a 52-year-old man with diplopia. (*A*) Note the diffuse soft tissue thickening/deposit (gadolinium). (*B*) The patient was treated with radiotherapy.

The International Myeloma Working Group diagnostic criteria for MM and SMM are shown in **Box 3**.

Myeloma bone disease: to meet the CRAB criteria, a bone lesion is defined as presence of an osteolytic lesion or presence of osteoporosis with compression fractures attributable to clonal plasma cell disorder.[32] Historically, skeletal surveys have been used in the diagnosis of MM. Whole-body skeletal surveys may not be suitable in identifying bone lesions because it is well established that to detect a lesion on a radiograph, at least 30% to 50% of the trabecular bone has to be resorbed.[33] This low sensitivity for identifying

---

Box 3
Revised International Myeloma Working Group diagnostic criteria for multiple myeloma and smoldering multiple myeloma

Definition of multiple myeloma: Clonal bone marrow plasma cells ≥10% or biopsy-proved bony or extramedullary plasmacytoma and any 1 or more of the following myeloma defining events:

Evidence of end-organ damage that can be attributed to the underlying plasma cell proliferative disorder, specifically:

- Hypercalcemia: serum calcium >2.75 mmol/L
- Renal insufficiency: creatinine clearance <40 mL/min
- Anemia: hemoglobin <100 g/L
- Bone lesions: 1 or more osteolytic lesions on skeletal radiography, CT, or PET-CT

Any 1 or more of the following biomarkers of malignancy:

- Clonal bone marrow plasma cell percentage* ≥60%
- Involved: uninvolved serum free light chain ratio ≥100
- >1 Focal bony lesions

Definition of smoldering multiple myeloma (both of these criteria should be met)

- Serum monoclonal protein (IgG or IgA) ≥30 g/L or urinary monoclonal protein ≥500 mg/24 h and/or clonal bone marrow plasma cells 10% to 60%
- Absence of myeloma defining events or amyloidosis

Adapted from Rajkumar SV, Dimopoulos MA, Palumbo A, et al. International myeloma working group updated criteria for the diagnosis of multiple myeloma. Lancet Oncol 2014;15(12):e538–48.

---

lesions can misclassify several patients without other CRAB symptoms as having SMM or asymptomatic myeloma.

MR imaging is more sensitive compared with whole-body skeletal survey for the detection of bone involvement in MM. In a series of 611 patients with MM, MR imaging and skeletal survey detected focal and osteolytic lesions in 74% and 56% of the imaged anatomic sites, respectively; 52% of 267 patients with normal skeletal survey had focal lesions on MR imaging.[34,35] Although MR imaging outperforms skeletal survey in the pelvis (**Fig. 6**), rib metastases and skull metastases (**Fig. 7**) are better seen on radiographs.[36]

Five MR imaging patterns of marrow involvement in myeloma have been recognized:

- Normal appearance of bone marrow
- Focal involvement (positive focal lesion is considered lesion of diameter ≥5 mm); see **Fig. 6**
- Homogeneous diffuse infiltration
- Combined diffuse and focal infiltration
- Variegated or salt-and-pepper pattern with inhomogeneous bone marrow with interposition of fat islands (**Fig. 8**)

Normal MR imaging pattern is associated with low tumor burden. A high tumor burden is usually suspected when there is diffuse hypointense change on T1-WI, diffuse hyperintensity on T2-WI, and enhancement after gadolinium injection. In several studies, the percentage of symptomatic patients with each of the abnormal MR imaging bone marrow patterns has ranged from 18% to 50% for focal pattern, 25% to 43% for diffuse pattern, and 1% to 5% for variegated pattern (**Fig. 6**).

The major advantage of MR imaging over other imaging modalities is assessment of spinal fractures and spinal cord compression, which is useful in treatment planning. MR imaging can help distinguish compression fractures due to myelomatous deposit from benign compression fractures. This may be especially valuable in patients without CRAB symptoms. Extramedullary lesions in myeloma may be diagnosed by whole-body MR imaging. Tumor burden can be assessed and monitored in patients with nonsecretory or oligosecretory MM (**Fig. 9**). MR imaging is found superior to whole-body CT in detecting skeletal lesions.[37] In a prospective study, Zamagni and colleagues[38] compared MR imaging of the spine and pelvis with skeletal survey versus PET-CT in 46 patients with MM at diagnosis. Although PET-CT was superior to skeletal survey in

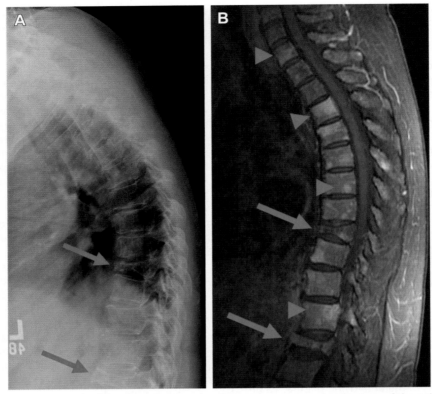

Fig. 6. (*A*) Lateral radiograph of the thoracic spine showing wedge compression fracture of thoracic and lumbar vertebrae (*red arrows*). (*B*) Contrast-enhanced T1-WI of the same area shows apart from the 2 wedge compression fractures, several enhancing bone lesions compatible with myelomatous deposits (*arrowheads*). MR imaging is more sensitive than radiographs in detecting bony lesions.

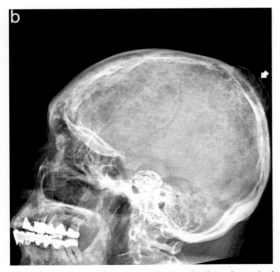

Fig. 7. Multiple lytic lesions in the skull and cervical spine in an 86-year-old woman. A lesion in the parietal skull (*arrow*) is associated with cortical expansion. Radiographs are more sensitive than MR imaging and PET-CT in detecting calvarial metastasis.

detecting lytic lesions in 46% of patients, it failed to reveal abnormal findings in 30% of patients who had abnormal MR imaging in the same areas, mainly of diffuse pattern. Most studies that find MR imaging nonsuperior to PET-CT or whole-body CT do not consider diffuse marrow involvement on MR imaging abnormal, which may explain such conclusions.[39] If whole-body MR imaging is not available, examination of the spine and pelvis may be performed.[40]

Changes in pattern of marrow involvement may provide information about response to therapy. It has been reported that complete response is characterized by complete resolution of the preceding marrow abnormality, whereas partial response is characterized by changeover of diffuse pattern to variegated or focal pattern. One of the disadvantages of MR imaging is that it often provides false-positive results because of persistent nonviable lesions.[41] PET-CT might be more suitable than MR imaging for determination of remission status. Improved access to PET–MR imaging may overcome some of the limitations of this modality.[42]

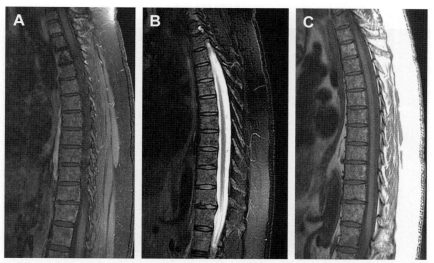

Fig. 8. (*A*) Sagittal T2-WI, (*B*) precontrast T1-WI, and (*C*) postcontrast T1-WI through the thoracic and upper lumbar spine showing a variegated (salt-and-pepper) pattern of diffuse myelomatous infiltration with interposition of fat islands. The areas of hypointensity on T1-WI show increased enhancement on the postcontrast images.

CT and PET-CT are also more sensitive than skeletal survey in detecting lesions in patients with MM, with up to 80% more lesions seen compared with skeletal survey.[36] According to the Durie/Salmon PLUS staging system, fludeoxyglucose F 18 [FDG] PET–CT imaging is necessary to confirm the staging of patients with MM. PET-CT is able to detect bone marrow involvement and hypermetabolic intramedullary and extramedullary lesions as well as to help differentiate between necrotic tissue and postradiation scar.[18] FDG-PET is superior to skeletal survey, with reported 85% sensitivity and 92% specificity in detecting myelomatous bone involvement.[43] PET-CT is useful in initial staging for baseline assessment to determine disease extent.[44,45] PET-CT might be more suitable than MR imaging for determination of remission status.[46] In a large study of 191 patients, PET-CT revealed faster change of imaging findings than MR imaging in patients who responded to therapy. Normalization of findings on PET-CT after treatment offers more information compared with MR imaging for better definition of complete response[47,48] (**Figs. 10** and **11**).

EXTRAOSSEOUS AND EXTRAMEDULLARY MANIFESTATIONS OF MYELOMA

As the name implies, extraosseous or extramedullary myeloma refers to the presence of myeloma deposits outside the skeletal system. Extramedullary manifestations often are seen in disseminated MM. Although considered rare, multiple autopsy series have noted the presence of extraosseous disease in approximately 63.5% of myeloma patients who died as a result of complications of the disease. The lymph nodes, the pleura, and the liver are commonly involved in extraosseous myeloma. Central nervous system involvement was also frequently found in patients with extraosseous disease, developing during the course of disease.[49] Clinical and radiological extraosseous disease is seen in almost 13% of myeloma patients[50] (**Figs. 12–14**).

Extraosseous disease is reported commonly after autologous or allogeneic stem cell transplantation. In a study following patterns of relapse after autologous peripheral stem cell transplantation, 14% of patients had extraosseous manifestations, with minimal or absent monoclonal protein, indicating the existence of sanctuary sites not reached by intensive chemoradiotherapy. In another study of 70 MM patients receiving reduced-intensity allogeneic stem cell transplantation, one-third had extraosseous relapse in the absence of marrow progression.[51,52] The presence of extraosseous involvement is also associated with poorer survival. The median survival after development of extraosseous disease in the course of MM in a single study was shown to be only 38 days.[53] The prognosis after an extraosseous relapse of myeloma is generally significantly worse than for medullary relapse.

A   B

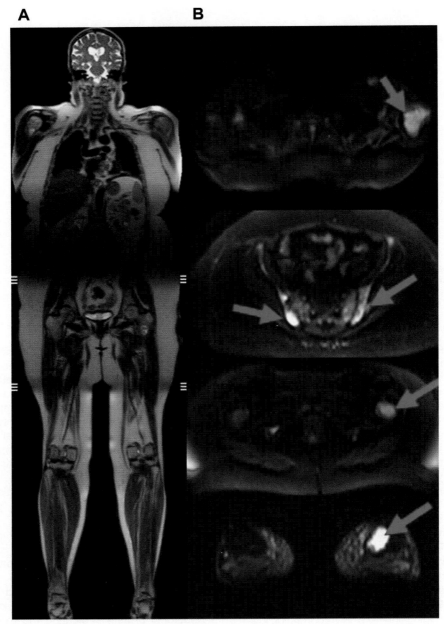

Fig. 9. 71 year-old man with MM. Whole-body MR imaging. (*A*) Coronal fast spin-echo T2. (*B*) Selected images of diffusion-weighted images show multiple lesions in the left humerus, bilateral iliac bone, left femur.

Nonsecretory Myeloma

As discussed previously, the clonal proliferation of plasma cells is typically associated with secretion of M protein. In 3% of patients, however, no monoclonal protein is detectable in either the serum or the urine with immunofixation.[1] In such cases, the monoclonal protein is usually identified in the plasma cells by immunoperoxidase or immunofluorescence. Two-thirds of patients with nonsecretory disease based on immunofixation, however, have an elevation of free monoclonal light chains in the serum by light chain assays. Patients with true nonsecretory myeloma need to be monitored mainly with imaging tests and bone marrow studies.[54] The survival of nonsecretory myeloma is superior to that of secretory myeloma.[55]

Oligosecretory Myeloma

Patients with myeloma and serum M protein less than 1 g/dL and urine M protein less than

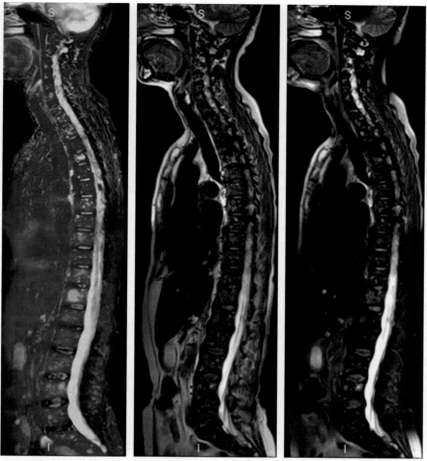

Fig. 10. Sagittal fused FDG PET-MRI and T1 and T2 fat-saturated images. There is diffusely heterogeneous marrow signal from variegated form of MM with a focal FDG-avid myeloma deposit in the T12 vertebral body.

200 mg/24 h are classified as having oligosecretory myeloma. Standard serum and urine electrophoretic tests in such patients are unreliable because it is difficult to determine if small variations are real or due to expected laboratory variability. These patients may also need to be monitored by imaging and bone marrow studies.[56]

POLYNEUROPATHY, ORGANOMEGALY, ENDOCRINOPATHY, MONOCLONAL PROTEIN, AND SKIN CHANGES SYNDROME

POEMS (polyneuropathy, organomegaly, endocrinopathy, monoclonal protein, and skin changes) syndrome is characterized by the presence of a

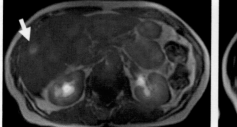
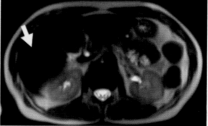

Fig. 11. Axial fused FDG-T1 and half-Fourier acquisition single-shot turbo spin-echo (HASTE) images through the liver demonstrate a focal hypermetabolic lesion in hepatic segment V (*arrow*) consistent with visceral involvement. Note is made of diffuse low signal intensity of the liver on T1 and T2 secondary to hemochromatosis (*arrow*).

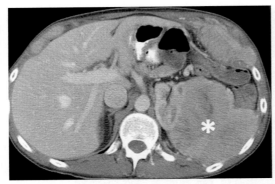

Fig. 12. Axial contrast-enhanced CT scan of the abdomen showing a large enhancing perinephric mass (*asterisk*) in a patient with MM. The mass was biopsy proved to be an extraosseous myelomatous deposit.

monoclonal plasma cell disorder, peripheral neuropathy, and one or more of the following features: osteosclerotic myeloma, Castleman disease, increased levels of serum vascular endothelial growth factor, organomegaly, endocrinopathy, typical skin changes, and papilledema.[57] All patients with POEMS syndrome by definition have peripheral neuropathy and a monoclonal plasma cell disorder. Physical examination reveals a symmetric sensorimotor neuropathy involving the extremities. Muscle weakness is more marked than sensory loss. Osteosclerotic lesions are seen in 97% of patients. Elevation of serum or plasma vascular endothelial growth factor levels is an important feature of the POEMS syndrome and can be followed to assess response to therapy[58] (**Fig. 15**).

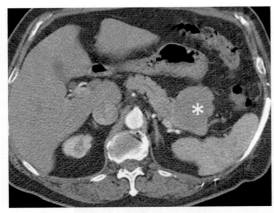

Fig. 13. Axial contrast-enhanced CT scan of the abdomen showing a large mass in the tail of the pancreas (*asterisk*) in a patient with MM. The mass was biopsy proved to be an extraosseous myelomatous deposit.

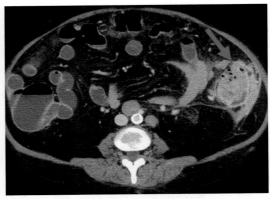

Fig. 14. Axial contrast-enhanced CT scan of the abdomen in a 72-year-old patient with MM shows a diffusely enhancing mass involving the descending colon with pericolonic deposit. This was biopsy proved to be an extraosseous myelomatous deposit.

OTHER
Waldenström Macroglobulinema

WM is a distinct subtype of plasma cell dyscrasia characterized by LPL in the bone marrow with an associated IgM monoclonal gammopathy. Patients with IgM MGUS usually develop into WM. Patients may present with symptoms related to the infiltration of the hematopoietic tissues or the effects of monoclonal IgM in the blood. WM is a rare disorder, with an incidence of approximately 3 per million people per year, with 1400 new cases diagnosed in the United States each year.[59] The median age at diagnosis is 64 years, with a slight male preponderance.[60] WM may show familial predisposition in up to 20% of cases.

Patients with WM commonly present with constitutional B symptoms, bleeding disorders, neuropathy, hyperviscosity syndrome, hepatosplenomegaly, and lymphadenopathy. Presence of dilated, segmented, and tortuous retinal veins on fundoscopic examination is a classic finding in WM related to hyperviscosity. The clinical presentation and radiological appearance of WM can have several features of lymphoma, such as bulky lymphadenopathy and hepatosplenomegaly. CT scans are also helpful in evaluating therapy response (**Fig. 16**).

Bing-Neel syndrome is a rare complication of WM characterized by CNS involvement by malignant cells. This can be a first manifestation of WM in up to a third of the patients. Subcortical and periventricular lesions with high signal on T2-WI and isointense to hypointense signal on T1-WI are usually seen[61] (**Fig. 17**).

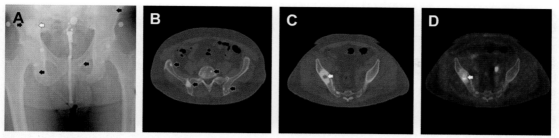

Fig. 15. Sclerotic lesions in MM. A 56-year-old man with tingling and numbness in the plantar aspects of both feet (POEMS syndrome). (*A*) Frontal radiograph of pelvis: multiple sclerotic lesions (*black arrows*). The largest located in the right iliac wing with a central lytic component (*white arrow*). (*B*) Axial CT: well-defined sclerotic lesions in the pelvis (*black arrows*). (*C*) Axial CT: central lytic component (*white arrow*) in the largest sclerotic lesion. (*D*) Axial fused FDG PET-CT: focal hypermetabolism (*white arrow*) associated with the lytic component but no metabolic activity associated with the sclerotic lesions.

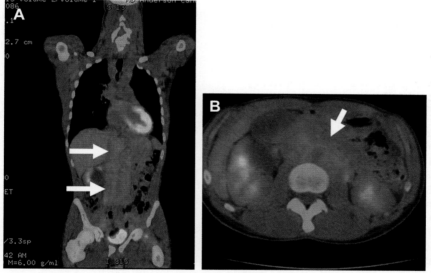

Fig. 16. Fused PET and CT images—coronal reconstruction; (*A*) axial images (*B*) in a patient with WM showing retroperitoneal lymphadenopathy with low-grade metabolic activity.

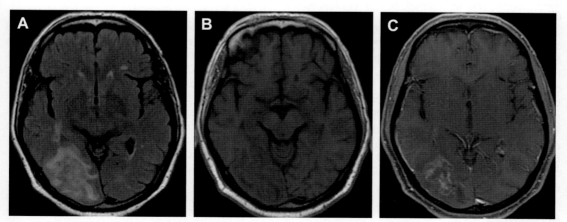

Fig. 17. (*A*) Axial T2, (*B*) precontrast, and (*C*) postcontrast axial T1-WI of the brain shows a hemorrhagic mass in the right occipital lobe with vasogenic edema. A craniotomy and resection showed small B-cell lymphoma with plasmacytic differentiation. The patient was later diagnosed with WM. Bing-Neel syndrome.

Amyloidosis and Monoclonal Immunoglobulin Deposition Diseases

Amyloidosis is a condition characterized by extracellular deposition of fibrils composed of a variety of normal serum proteins. These fibrils have an anti-parallel, β-pleated sheath configuration and typically bind to Congo red and thioflavin. The 2 most common types of amyloid are immunoglobulin light chain (AL) amyloidosis and AA amyloidosis, in which the fibrils are composed of fragments of acute phase reactant serum proteins. AA amyloidosis is generally secondary to chronic inflammation.

AL may occur de novo or in association with plasma cell dyscrasias, including MM and WM. All forms of systemic amyloidosis in which the fibrils are derived from monoclonal light chains are considered AL amyloidosis. AL amyloidosis is characterized by amyloid deposition in various organs, such as heart, kidneys, liver, lymph nodes, and periorbital tissues, leading to dysfunction.

Light Chain Deposition Disease and Heavy Chain Deposition Disease

Light chain deposition disease (LCDD) is similar pathogenetically to AL amyloidosis, but the light chain fragments do not have the necessary biochemical characteristics to form amyloid fibrils. It is, therefore, a nonamyloid monoclonal immunoglobulin LCDD (usually kappa) that is caused by a clonal plasma cell proliferative disorder. It is categorized as a monoclonal deposition disease in the World Health Organization classification of tumors of hematopoietic and lymphoid tissues. A single clone of plasma cells is responsible for overproduction of kappa chains and, rarely, lambda chains. Patients with LCDD usually present with renal, cardiac, or hepatic involvement and may have underlying MM or a lymphoproliferative disorder.

Heavy chain deposition disease (HCDD) is the least common of the monoclonal immunoglobulin deposition diseases. Renal involvement is the predominant feature in HCDD, with most patients presenting with renal failure (approximately 90% cases), recent-onset hypertension (approximately 70% cases), and nephrotic range proteinuria (80%).[62] Rarely, either light and heavy monoclonal immunoglobulin chains or only short (truncated) heavy chains cause nonamyloid tissue deposits [11–15]. HCDD and LCDD are collectively referred to as monoclonal immunoglobulin deposition disease.

REFERENCES

1. International Myeloma Working Group. Criteria for the classification of monoclonal gammopathies, multiple myeloma and related disorders: a report of the international myeloma working group. Br J Haematol 2003;121(5):749–57.

2. Campo E, Swerdlow SH, Harris NL, et al. The 2008 WHO classification of lymphoid neoplasms and beyond: evolving concepts and practical applications. Blood 2011;117(19):5019–32.

3. Plasma cell neoplasms. In: Swerdlow SH, Campo E, Harris NL, et al, editors. WHO classification of tumours of haematopoietic and lymphoid tissues. 4th edition. Lyon, IARC Press; 2008.

4. Greipp PR, San Miguel J, Durie BG, et al. International staging system for multiple myeloma. J Clin Oncol 2005;23(15):3412–20.

5. Palumbo A, Avet-Loiseau H, Oliva S, et al. Revised international staging system for multiple myeloma: a report from international myeloma working group. J Clin Oncol 2015;33(26):2863–9.

6. Mulligan ME. Skeletal abnormalities in multiple myeloma. Radiology 2005;234(1):313–4 [author reply: 314].

7. Durie BG, Kyle RA, Belch A, et al. Myeloma management guidelines: a consensus report from the scientific advisors of the international myeloma foundation. Hematol J 2003;4(6):379–98.

8. Kyle RA, Therneau TM, Rajkumar SV, et al. Prevalence of monoclonal gammopathy of undetermined significance. N Engl J Med 2006;354(13):1362–9.

9. Rajkumar SV, Dimopoulos MA, Palumbo A, et al. International myeloma working group updated criteria for the diagnosis of multiple myeloma. Lancet Oncol 2014;15(12):e538–48.

10. Mangiacavalli S, Cocito F, Pochintesta L, et al. Monoclonal gammopathy of undetermined significance: a new proposal of workup. Eur J Haematol 2013;91(4):356–60.

11. Rajan AM, Rajkumar SV. Diagnostic evaluation of monoclonal gammopathy of undetermined significance. Eur J Haematol 2013;91(6):561–2.

12. Kyle RA, Remstein ED, Therneau TM, et al. Clinical course and prognosis of smoldering (asymptomatic) multiple myeloma. N Engl J Med 2007;356(25): 2582–90.

13. Grignani G, Gobbi PG, Formisano R, et al. A prognostic index for multiple myeloma. Br J Cancer 1996;73(9):1101–7.

14. He Y, Wheatley K, Clark O, et al. Early versus deferred treatment for early stage multiple myeloma. Cochrane Database Syst Rev 2003;(1):CD004023.

15. Kyle RA, Greipp PR. Smoldering multiple myeloma. N Engl J Med 1980;302(24):1347–9.

16. Thomas A, Mailankody S, Korde N, et al. Second malignancies after multiple myeloma: from 1960s to 2010s. Blood 2012;119(12):2731–7.

17. Knowling MA, Harwood AR, Bergsagel DE. Comparison of extramedullary plasmacytomas with solitary

and multiple plasma cell tumors of bone. J Clin Oncol 1983;1(4):255–62.

18. Galieni P, Cavo M, Avvisati G, et al. Solitary plasmacytoma of bone and extramedullary plasmacytoma: two different entities? Ann Oncol 1995;6(7):687–91.

19. Soutar R, Lucraft H, Jackson G, et al. Guidelines on the diagnosis and management of solitary plasmacytoma of bone and solitary extramedullary plasmacytoma. Br J Haematol 2004;124(6):717–26.

20. Hughes M, Doig A, Soutar R. Solitary plasmacytoma and multiple myeloma: adhesion molecule and chemokine receptor expression patterns. Br J Haematol 2007;137(5):486–7.

21. Frassica DA, Frassica FJ, Schray MF, et al. Solitary plasmacytoma of bone: Mayo clinic experience. Int J Radiat Oncol Biol Phys 1989;16(1):43–8.

22. Bataille R, Sany J. Solitary myeloma: clinical and prognostic features of a review of 114 cases. Cancer 1981;48(3):845–51.

23. Ozsahin M, Tsang RW, Poortmans P, et al. Outcomes and patterns of failure in solitary plasmacytoma: a multicenter rare cancer network study of 258 patients. Int J Radiat Oncol Biol Phys 2006;64(1):210–7.

24. Shah BK, Saifuddin A, Price GJ. Magnetic resonance imaging of spinal plasmacytoma. Clin Radiol 2000;55(6):439–45.

25. Laredo JD, el Quessar A, Bossard P, et al. Vertebral tumors and pseudotumors. Radiol Clin North Am 2001;39(1):137–63, vi.

26. Major NM, Helms CA, Richardson WJ. The "mini brain": plasmacytoma in a vertebral body on MR imaging. AJR Am J Roentgenol 2000;175(1):261–3.

27. Rodallec MH, Feydy A, Larousserie F, et al. Diagnostic imaging of solitary tumors of the spine: what to do and say. Radiographics 2008;28(4):1019–41.

28. Gerry D, Lentsch EJ. Epidemiologic evidence of superior outcomes for extramedullary plasmacytoma of the head and neck. Otolaryngol Head Neck Surg 2013;148(6):974–81.

29. Siegel RL, Miller KD, Jemal A. Cancer statistics, 2015. CA Cancer J Clin 2015;65(1):5–29.

30. Kyle RA, Gertz MA, Witzig TE, et al. Review of 1027 patients with newly diagnosed multiple myeloma. Mayo Clin Proc 2003;78(1):21–33.

31. Waxman AJ, Mink PJ, Devesa SS, et al. Racial disparities in incidence and outcome in multiple myeloma: a population-based study. Blood 2010;116(25):5501–6.

32. Kyle RA, Rajkumar SV. Criteria for diagnosis, staging, risk stratification and response assessment of multiple myeloma. Leukemia 2009;23(1):3–9.

33. Durie BG, Salmon SE. A clinical staging system for multiple myeloma. Correlation of measured myeloma cell mass with presenting clinical features, response to treatment, and survival. Cancer 1975;36(3):842–54.

34. Ludwig H, Fruhwald F, Tscholakoff D, et al. Magnetic resonance imaging of the spine in multiple myeloma. Lancet 1987;2(8555):364–6.

35. Walker R, Barlogie B, Haessler J, et al. Magnetic resonance imaging in multiple myeloma: diagnostic and clinical implications. J Clin Oncol 2007;25(9):1121–8.

36. Regelink JC, Minnema MC, Terpos E, et al. Comparison of modern and conventional imaging techniques in establishing multiple myeloma-related bone disease: a systematic review. Br J Haematol 2013;162(1):50–61.

37. Baur-Melnyk A, Buhmann S, Becker C, et al. Whole-body MRI versus whole-body MDCT for staging of multiple myeloma. AJR Am J Roentgenol 2008;190(4):1097–104.

38. Zamagni E, Nanni C, Patriarca F, et al. A prospective comparison of 18F-fluorodeoxyglucose positron emission tomography-computed tomography, magnetic resonance imaging and whole-body planar radiographs in the assessment of bone disease in newly diagnosed multiple myeloma. Haematologica 2007;92(1):50–5.

39. Waheed S, Mitchell A, Usmani S, et al. Standard and novel imaging methods for multiple myeloma: correlates with prognostic laboratory variables including gene expression profiling data. Haematologica 2013;98(1):71–8.

40. Dimopoulos MA, Hillengass J, Usmani S, et al. Role of magnetic resonance imaging in the management of patients with multiple myeloma: a consensus statement. J Clin Oncol 2015;33(6):657–64.

41. Bannas P, Hentschel HB, Bley TA, et al. Diagnostic performance of whole-body MRI for the detection of persistent or relapsing disease in multiple myeloma after stem cell transplantation. Eur Radiol 2012;22(9):2007–12.

42. Lee IS, Jin YH, Hong SH, et al. Musculoskeletal applications of PET/MR. Semin Musculoskelet Radiol 2014;18(2):203–16.

43. Bredella MA, Steinbach L, Caputo G, et al. Value of FDG PET in the assessment of patients with multiple myeloma. AJR Am J Roentgenol 2005;184(4):1199–204.

44. Mihailovic J, Goldsmith SJ. Multiple myeloma: 18F-FDG-PET/CT and diagnostic imaging. Semin Nucl Med 2015;45(1):16–31.

45. van Lammeren-Venema D, Regelink JC, Riphagen II, et al. (1)(8)F-fluoro-deoxyglucose positron emission tomography in assessment of myeloma-related bone disease: a systematic review. Cancer 2012;118(8):1971–81.

46. Derlin T, Peldschus K, Munster S, et al. Comparative diagnostic performance of (1)(8)F-FDG PET/CT versus whole-body MRI for determination of remission status in multiple myeloma after stem cell transplantation. Eur Radiol 2013;23(2):570–8.

47. Bartel TB, Haessler J, Brown TL, et al. F18-fluoro-deoxyglucose positron emission tomography in the context of other imaging techniques and prognostic factors in multiple myeloma. Blood 2009;114(10): 2068–76.

48. Spinnato P, Bazzocchi A, Brioli A, et al. Contrast enhanced MRI and (1)(8)F-FDG PET-CT in the assessment of multiple myeloma: a comparison of results in different phases of the disease. Eur J Radiol 2012;81(12):4013–8.

49. Damaj G, Mohty M, Vey N, et al. Features of extra-medullary and extraosseous multiple myeloma: a report of 19 patients from a single center. Eur J Haematol 2004;73(6):402–6.

50. Varettoni M, Corso A, Pica G, et al. Incidence, presenting features and outcome of extramedullary disease in multiple myeloma: a longitudinal study on 1003 consecutive patients. Ann Oncol 2010;21(2): 325–30.

51. Alegre A, Granda A, Martinez-Chamorro C, et al. Different patterns of relapse after autologous peripheral blood stem cell transplantation in multiple myeloma: clinical results of 280 cases from the Spanish Registry. Haematologica 2002;87(6): 609–14.

52. Perez-Simon JA, Sureda A, Fernandez-Aviles F, et al. Reduced-intensity conditioning allogeneic transplantation is associated with a high incidence of extramedullary relapses in multiple myeloma patients. Leukemia 2006;20(3):542–5.

53. Cerny J, Fadare O, Hutchinson L, et al. Clinicopathological features of extramedullary recurrence/relapse of multiple myeloma. Eur J Haematol 2008; 81(1):65–9.

54. Tan CH, Wang M, Fu WJ, et al. Nodular extramedullary multiple myeloma: hepatic involvement presenting as hypervascular lesions on CT. Ann Acad Med Singapore 2011;40(7):329–31.

55. Chawla SS, Kumar SK, Dispenzieri A, et al. Clinical course and prognosis of non-secretory multiple myeloma. Eur J Haematol 2015;95(1):57–64.

56. Larson D, Kyle RA, Rajkumar SV. Prevalence and monitoring of oligosecretory myeloma. N Engl J Med 2012;367(6):580–1.

57. Dispenzieri A, Kyle RA, Lacy MQ, et al. POEMS syndrome: definitions and long-term outcome. Blood 2003;101(7):2496–506.

58. Kuwabara S, Dispenzieri A, Arimura K, et al. Treatment for POEMS (polyneuropathy, organomegaly, endocrinopathy, M-protein, and skin changes) syndrome. Cochrane Database Syst Rev 2012;(6):CD006828.

59. Groves FD, Travis LB, Devesa SS, et al. Waldenstrom's macroglobulinemia: incidence patterns in the United States, 1988-1994. Cancer 1998;82(6): 1078–81.

60. Garcia-Sanz R, Montoto S, Torrequebrada A, et al. Waldenstrom macroglobulinaemia: presenting features and outcome in a series with 217 cases. Br J Haematol 2001;115(3):575–82.

61. Simon L, Fitsiori A, Lemal R, et al. Bing-Neel syndrome, a rare complication of Waldenstrom's macroglobulinemia: analysis of 44 cases and review of the literature. A study on behalf of the French Innovative Leukemia Organization (FILO). Haematologica 2015;100(12):1587–94.

62. Rane S, Rana S, Mudrabettu C, et al. Heavy-chain deposition disease: a morphological, immunofluorescence and ultrastructural assessment. Clin Kidney J 2012;5(5):383–9.

Taxonomy and Imaging Manifestations of Systemic Amyloidosis

Naoki Takahashi, MD[a],*, James Glockner, MD, PhD[a],
Benjamin M. Howe, MD[a], Robert P. Hartman, MD[a],
Akira Kawashima, MD, PhD[b]

KEYWORDS

- Amyloidosis • Heart • Lung • Urinary tract • Joint • Computed tomography • MR imaging

KEY POINTS

- Amyloid light-chain amyloidosis is the most common type of amyloidosis, and cardiac involvement is often a major determinant of prognosis.
- Global subendocardial to transmural cardiac wall enhancement is the most common pattern of cardiac amyloidosis on late gadolinium enhancement on MR images.
- The localized form of amyloidosis most commonly involves urinary tract or respiratory tract, and usually has a benign clinical course.
- Amyloid arthropathy is most commonly owing to Aβ2M (dialysis-related) amyloid deposition.
- Amyloid deposits commonly exhibit decreased T1- and T2-weighted signal on MR images.

INTRODUCTION

Amyloidosis is a heterogeneous group of multisystem disorders that are characterized by extracellular deposition of amyloid fibrils in β-pleated sheets resulting in organ dysfunction. Although approximately 25 different amyloid proteins have been identified, 5 types of amyloidosis account for 99% of all amyloidosis. Amyloid of all types shares the same physical properties: apple-green birefringence after Congo red staining. Amyloid deposits produce diverse clinical syndromes depending on their type, location, and the amount of deposition.

AMYLOID TYPES AND MANAGEMENT

There are several forms of amyloidosis. The 2 most common types of amyloidosis are amyloid light-chain (AL) amyloidosis (previously referred to as primary amyloidosis) and amyloid A (AA) amyloidosis (previously referred to as secondary amyloidosis).[1] AL amyloidosis is owing to deposition of protein derived from immunoglobulin light chain fragments. Patients with AL amyloidosis have monoclonal B-cell dyscrasia, which generally has low-level activity. However, 10% to 50% of patients are associated with multiple myeloma or other plasma cell neoplasia, such as B-cell lymphoma and Waldenström macroglobulinemia.[2] Similar to other plasma cell dyscrasias, AL amyloidosis is a disease of older adults with a median age at diagnosis of 65 years old. AL amyloidosis is mostly a systemic disorder that can present with a variety of symptoms or signs depending on the predominant sites of involvement. Nonspecific systemic symptoms include fatigue and weight loss. Other common clinical presentations of AL amyloidosis include proteinuria or nephrotic syndrome, heart failure, hepatosplenomegaly, and neuropathy. Without treatment, systemic AL amyloidosis is a fatal disease owing to uncontrolled organ damage. Treatment is aimed at control of plasma cell

[a] Department of Radiology, Mayo Clinic, 200 First Street Southwest, Rochester, MN 55905, USA; [b] Department of Radiology, Mayo Clinic, Scottsdale, Az, USA
* Corresponding author.
E-mail address: takahashi.naoki@mayo.edu

Radiol Clin N Am 54 (2016) 597–612
http://dx.doi.org/10.1016/j.rcl.2015.12.012
0033-8389/16/$ – see front matter © 2016 Elsevier Inc. All rights reserved.

dyscrasia in the form of chemotherapy and/or hematopoietic stem cell transplantation.

In AL amyloidosis, amyloid deposition can be isolated to a single organ resulting in specific syndromes. Localized amyloidosis is attributed to a local immunocyte dyscrasia and resulting in deposition of immunoglobulin light chain. The location of the amyloid deposits can be a clue to its localized nature. Respiratory tract, skin, and urinary tract are common sites of localized amyloidosis. Patients with localized amyloidosis do not have monoclonal protein in the serum or urine or bone marrow plasmacytosis. Patients with localized amyloidosis do not require systemic therapy, and surgical excision may be the only treatment needed.

AA amyloidosis is a result of chronic inflammatory conditions such as rheumatoid arthritis, Crohn's disease, tuberculosis, bronchiectasis, and chronic osteomyelitis. It may occur in association with other causes, including neoplasms (renal cell carcinoma and Hodgkin's disease). Amyloid is composed of fragments of the acute phase protein, serum AA. The most common organ involved is the kidney, leading to nephrotic syndrome. If untreated, secondary amyloidosis may be fatal owing to end-stage renal disease, infection, or heart failure. Treatment is aimed at control of the underlying inflammatory or infectious process. AA amyloidosis is more common in underdeveloped countries, whereas AL amyloidosis is the most common type of amyloidosis in the developed countries.

Two other major forms of amyloidosis are transthyretin-related amyloidosis (ATTR) and Aβ2M amyloidosis. ATTR amyloidosis is owing to deposition of wild-type transthyretin (TTR) or mutant TTR. Wild-type ATTR amyloidosis is commonly referred to as age-related or senile amyloidosis. The predominant site of involvement is heart and it almost exclusively affects older men; most patients are older than 70 years at diagnosis, with a 10-fold greater incidence in men. Autopsy series suggests asymptomatic amyloid deposition is common in heart and gastrointestinal tract.[3,4] Mutant ATTR amyloidosis is a hereditary disease, and commonly referred to as familial amyloid polyneuropathy. It has predilection for involvement of the peripheral and autonomic nerves. Inheritance is autosomal dominant with variable penetrance, and at least 120 point mutations of the TTR gene have been described. Aβ2M amyloidosis (dialysis related) occurs in patients undergoing long-term hemodialysis owing to deposition of β2 microalbumin. It has a predilection for deposition in the bones and joints.

Although amyloidosis may be suggested by the history and clinical manifestations (eg, nephrotic syndrome in patients with myeloma), tissue biopsy is often necessary to confirm the diagnosis. Biopsies can be obtained from either clinically uninvolved site, such as subcutaneous fat, or from dysfunctional organs. Abdominal fat pad biopsy is preferred in patients with suspected systemic amyloidosis because it is less invasive. Biopsy of an involved organ is often necessary when a limited number of organs is affected, such as in localized amyloidosis.

GENERAL IMAGING FEATURES OF AMYLOID DEPOSITION

On computed tomography (CT), amyloid deposition is commonly associated with calcification, and it is attributed to an affinity of amyloid fibrils for calcium.[5] On CT and MR imaging, the enhancement of the affected organs is often decreased in the parenchymal phase and increased in the delayed phase. This enhancement pattern is considered owing to expansion of the extracellular space by amyloid deposition causing delayed inflow and washout of contrast material.[6,7] Amyloid deposits often shows decreased T1 signal (T1 prolongation) and decreased T2 signal (T2 shortening) on MR imaging likely related to physical properties of amyloid fibrils, but the exact cause of these signal changes are unknown.[8]

HEART
Amyloid Variants Affecting the Heart

The heart can be affected by several amyloid types, and cardiac involvement is often a major determinant of prognosis. The 2 most common forms of cardiac amyloidosis are the AL and ATTR types. AL amyloid is the most commonly diagnosed form of cardiac amyloidosis. It may involve almost any organ in the body, with cardiac disease seen in 50% to 70% of patients.[9] The prevalence of wild-type ATTR amyloidosis is uncertain; although fewer cases are diagnosed annually in comparison with AL amyloidosis, autopsy series have noted ATTR deposits in up to 25% of individuals greater than 80 years of age in the heart,[3] suggesting that the disease is underdiagnosed, or that perhaps there is a spectrum of disease including asymptomatic or minimally symptomatic disease. Cardiac involvement is the predominant clinical feature of wild-type ATTR amyloidosis, although carpal tunnel syndrome is common and may precede development of cardiac symptoms by 10 to 15 years. Isolated atrial amyloidosis occurs when atrial natriuretic peptide serves as the precursor protein for amyloid formation and deposition into the atrial walls. Isolated atrial amyloidosis typically occurs in elderly women, with prevalence increasing with advancing age; 1 autopsy study found 95% of subjects aged 81 to 90 years had atrial amyloid deposits.[10] Isolated atrial amyloidosis is almost always asymptomatic and an incidental diagnosis, although some authors have suggested a role in the development of atrial conduction defects.

Clinical Features and Pathophysiology

Cardiac amyloidosis represents the classic prototype of restrictive cardiomyopathy, and is characterized initially by diastolic dysfunction with symptoms of exercise intolerance, fatigue, and shortness of breath. Myocardial deposition of amyloid results in progressive thickening of ventricular walls, thereby increasing myocardial stiffness and ventricular filling pressures. Chronic elevation of ventricular filling pressures leads to atrial enlargement and subsequent paroxysmal or persistent atrial fibrillation—atrial thrombi are relatively common in cardiac amyloidosis[11] and can cause systemic embolic events. Pericardial effusions are found in 40% to 60% of patients and are thought to occur because of increased right atrial pressures as well as pericardial amyloid infiltration. Valve thickening and subsequent regurgitation is a common finding, although the level of dysfunction is typically mild. The most common causes of death in cardiac amyloidosis are progressive heart failure and sudden cardiac death.[12]

Laboratory and Electrocardiographic Findings

The presence of low-voltage QRS complexes in a patient with increased left ventricular wall thickness is a classic finding in cardiac amyloidosis; however, the sensitivity of this finding is probably not high, and low-voltage QRS complexes are less frequent in patients with ATTR amyloid. On the other hand, conduction system abnormalities are relatively common in ATTR amyloid and are infrequent in patients with AL amyloidosis. The combination of elevated serum N-terminal pro-brain natriuretic peptide (NT-proBNP) and cardiac troponin T is associated with a poor prognosis, and is the basis of the Mayo Clinic staging system widely used in clinical practice.

Prognosis

The prognosis for patients with cardiac amyloidosis is generally poor; however, innovative treatment strategies have led to improved survival in patients with cardiac amyloidosis. AL cardiac amyloidosis has the worst prognosis, with greater than 50% mortality within 6 months of the initial diagnosis and an overall survival of 33% at 4 years from diagnosis.[13] ATTR cardiac amyloid has a more favorable prognosis of 3 to 5 years, with nearly 100% survival at 2 years.[14]

Echocardiography

Echocardiography is usually the first imaging study performed in patients with cardiac amyloidosis, and can often suggest the diagnosis, particularly in patients with advanced disease. The classic appearance of amyloid includes concentric thickening of the left ventricular walls (>12 mm at end diastole) with a normal or small left ventricular cavity and preserved left ventricular ejection fraction (>50%; **Fig. 1**). The right ventricle may also be thickened. The myocardium in cardiac amyloidosis has been described as having a brilliant speckled appearance, although the sensitivity and specificity of this sign are probably low. Diastolic dysfunction is indicated by an abnormal mitral filling pattern and associated atrial enlargement. Thickening of valve leaflets, thickening of the interatrial septum, and small pericardial and pleural effusions are also common findings.

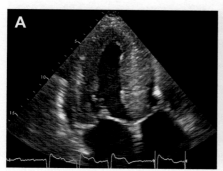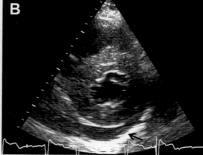

Fig. 1. Horizontal long axis (A) and midventricular short axis (B) images in a patient with cardiac amyloidosis demonstrate diffuse thickening of the left ventricle, biatrial enlargement, and a small pericardial effusion (*arrow* in B).

Myocardial strain imaging has recently emerged as an important technique in assessing patients with known or suspected cardiac amyloid. Speckle tracking echocardiography uses automatic frame by frame tracking of natural acoustic markers to track myocardial deformation over the cardiac cycle. A recent study of 200 patients with AL cardiac amyloid showed that longitudinal strain was strongly correlated with NT-proBNP levels, and that longitudinal strain was independently correlated with survival.[15] An apical sparing pattern of longitudinal strain has been noted in cardiac amyloid,[16] which can be very helpful in distinguishing amyloidosis from other causes of myocardial thickening, such as hypertrophic cardiomyopathy and hypertensive cardiomyopathy (**Fig. 2**).

MR Imaging

Cardiac MR imaging is one of the most useful and comprehensive techniques available for assessing cardiac amyloidosis. Demonstration of left and right ventricular myocardial thickening, increased myocardial mass, atrial enlargement, and pleural and pericardial effusions can all be accomplished with standard electrocardiograph-gated cine steady-state free precession images (**Fig. 3**). These series can also be used to quantify chamber size and ventricular function, with greater accuracy and reproducibility in comparison to echocardiography.

Postgadolinium images are often strikingly abnormal in cardiac amyloid patients. Late gadolinium enhancement (LGE) images are typically obtained 10 to 20 minutes after gadolinium injection using electrocardiograph-gated inversion recovery spoiled gradient echo T1-weighted pulse sequences. The marked expansion of the extracellular myocardial space caused by amyloid deposition leads to slower washout of gadolinium, with corresponding extensive myocardial enhancement (in contrast with the usual dark signal of normal myocardium; **Fig. 4**). Global subendocardial to transmural enhancement is the most commonly described pattern; however, enhancement can be patchy, usually predominant in the basal left ventricle.[7,17,18] A recent study showed that LGE had a sensitivity and specificity of 88% and 95% for detecting cardiac amyloidosis, respectively.[19] Right ventricular enhancement is often seen, and its presence can help to distinguish amyloid from other nonischemic cardiomyopathies. Diffuse atrial wall enhancement and thickening may also be noted.

Gadolinium contrast agents often are cleared from the blood pool more quickly in amyloidosis patients, with the blood pool often appearing dark on LGE images, and the altered kinetics of both myocardium and blood pool cause difficulties in determining the correct inversion time (TI) for LGE acquisitions. This general observation has been termed abnormal myocardial nulling. A more specific finding is myocardium reaching its null point before the blood pool on a cine inversion recovery spoiled gradient recalled echo acquisition used to select the optimal TI for LGE imaging, where each successive cardiac phase has an incrementally longer TI (**Fig. 5**).[18,20]

The abnormal nulling phenomenon is a reflection of the reduced myocardial T1 owing to retention of gadolinium, which in turn results from expansion of the extracellular space by amyloid deposition. T1 mapping offers an attractive means of quantifying the extent of myocardial disease in comparison to LGE imaging, in which the amount of apparent enhancement depends on the choice of TI. T1 mapping is typically performed with a shortened modified Look Locker inversion recovery sequence. Measurement of myocardial and

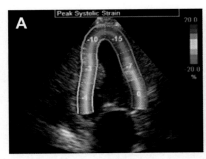
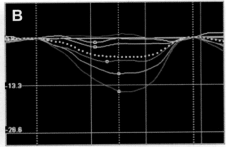

Fig. 2. Echocardiographic longitudinal strain measurements in a patient with cardiac amyloidosis. Parametric image of longitudinal strain superimposed over a long axis echocardiography view (*A*) reveals reduced longitudinal strain values (normal, less than -16), with relative sparing of apical segments. Two-dimensional plot of strain in color-coded cardiac segments (*B*) again demonstrates markedly reduced strain in basal segments with preserved strain in apical segments.

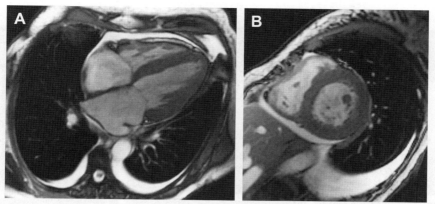

Fig. 3. Horizontal long axis (*A*) and midventricular short axis (*B*) electrocardiographic-gated cine steady state free precession MR images in a patient with cardiac amyloidosis demonstrate mild diffuse left ventricular thickening, biatrial enlargement, and small pericardial and pleural effusions.

blood pool T1 before and after gadolinium administration along with knowledge of the hematocrit allows calculation of the myocardial extracellular volume. A recent investigation found that an increased extracellular volume was associated with an increased hazard ratio for death.[21] An additional important result of this research is that T1 mapping of native myocardium (ie, without gadolinium contrast) is also strongly predictive of the presence of amyloid, with increasing T1 values associated with a larger amyloid burden and predictive of increased mortality.[21,22] Because many patients with AL amyloid also have renal involvement and reduced renal function, the ability to perform a quantitative assessment of disease burden without using gadolinium contrast agents is very attractive.

Nuclear Medicine

Radiolabeled serum amyloid P component scintigraphy is useful for evaluating the whole-body amyloid burden; however, it cannot assess cardiac involvement owing to blood pool uptake.[23] There has been much recent interest in off-label use of the bone scintigraphy tracers technetium-3,3-diphosphono-1,2-propanodicarboxylic acid (^{99m}Tc-DPD) and technetium pyrophosphate (^{99m}Tc-PYP) for diagnosis of cardiac ATTR amyloidosis.[24–26] The ^{99m}Tc phosphate derivatives can bind to TTR in the myocardium, but not to immunoglobulin light chains, and therefore a positive scan provides strong evidence for ATTR cardiac amyloidosis (**Fig. 6**). Both ^{99m}Tc-DPD and ^{99m}Tc-PYP seem to be very sensitive for the detection of ATTR amyloid deposits, and have identified presymptomatic disease.

Computed Tomography

CT has played a limited role in diagnosis of cardiac amyloidosis, and has generally been used in our practice as an alternative technique in patients who are not candidates for MR imaging. CT can

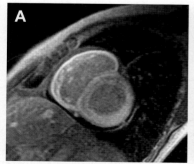
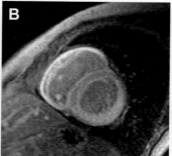
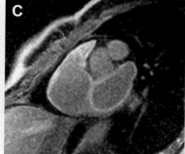

Fig. 4. Short axis late gadolinium enhancement MR images in a patient with cardiac amyloidosis. Midventricular short axis images (*A*, *B*) reveal marked diffuse enhancement of the right ventricular free wall as well as patchy near transmural enhancement of the lateral and inferior left ventricular walls. Short axis image through the atria (*C*) demonstrates diffuse enhancement and mild thickening of right and left atrial walls.

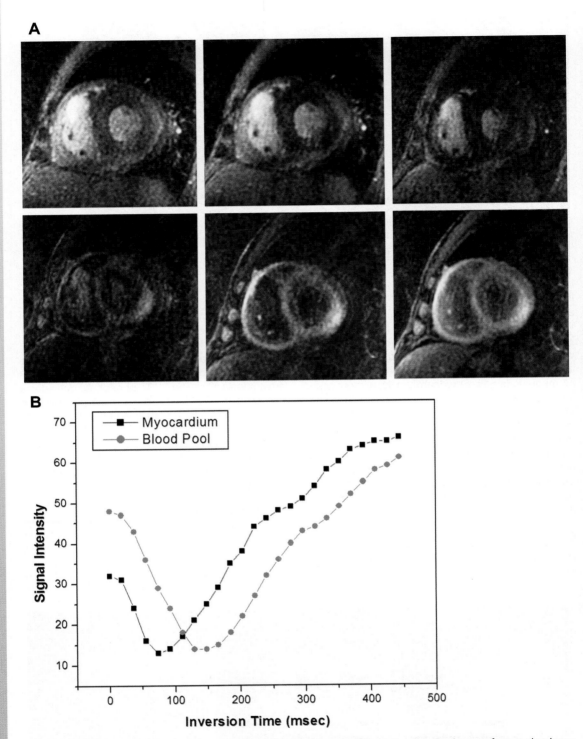

Fig. 5. Abnormal myocardial nulling in a patient with cardiac amyloidosis. Consecutive images from a cine inversion recovery spoiled gradient recalled echo acquisition (*A*) with increasing inversion times show the myocardium reaching its null point and then becoming hyperintense before the blood pool. This is graphically illustrated in (*B*) where signal intensity of regions of interest placed in the myocardium and blood pool are plotted versus inversion time.

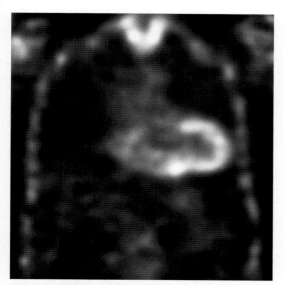

Fig. 6. Nuclear medicine ⁹⁹ᵐTc-PYP coronal image from a patient with transthyretin-related cardiac amyloidosis demonstrates diffuse activity in the left ventricle and mild right ventricular activity.

demonstrate many of the signs of cardiac involvement, including myocardial thickening, pericardial and pleural effusions, and atrial enlargement. Soft tissue characterization is limited in comparison with MR imaging, however, and a definitive diagnosis of myocardial amyloid may not be possible in some cases. Quantification of extracellular volume expansion can be performed with contrast-enhanced CT using methods very similar to the MR imaging techniques, and 1 recent investigation has shown promising results in this regard.[27]

THORAX

Amyloid can deposit in many structures in the chest, including the walls of the blood vessels, lymph nodes, alveolar septa, airways, and pleura.[28] The resulting changes can be identified on chest radiographs and/or chest CT. The findings are often nonspecific and in many cases can mimic infectious or neoplastic etiologies.

Changes within the chest are often associated with systemic amyloidosis, but may uncommonly be related to localized disease.[29] Localized amyloid deposition may involve the tracheobronchial tree or pulmonary parenchyma. The most common types of amyloid encountered in the thorax are composed of AL amyloidosis and AA amyloidosis.[29] ATTR amyloidosis (senile amyloidosis) often involves the heart, but sometimes is evident in the lungs.

Tracheobronchial Amyloidosis

Localized amyloidosis of the tracheobronchial system is relatively uncommon. When the airway is involved, the site of deposition is often categorized as either proximal, mid, or distal.[30,31] The amyloid deposits may present as multifocal submucosal plaques or tumorlike amyloid masses. These may contain identifiable higher attenuation on CT from either calcification or ossification (Fig. 7). The change may be localized or multifocal and a long segment tracheal narrowing may be evident.[32–36] Although localized tracheobronchial amyloidosis is not associated with systemic disease, it may have a poor prognosis. Proximal airway involvement tends to be worse than mid or distal affection. Ultimately, patients may die of respiratory failure or recurrent pneumonia secondary to bronchial obstruction.[32]

Parenchymal Amyloidosis

Localized parenchymal amyloidosis exists in 2 distinct patterns: nodular parenchymal and alveolar septal. Nodular parenchymal amyloid lesions are often termed amyloidomas. These may be solitary or multiple and occur more frequently in the lower lobes[32] (Fig. 8). These can be obvious on chest radiographs and may be present in to 60%

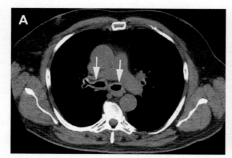
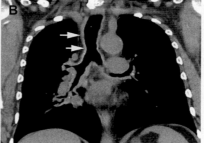

Fig. 7. (A, B) Axial and coronal computed tomography images demonstrating diffuse circumferential thickening of the wall of the trachea and central bronchi in a patient with localized amyloidosis (arrows).

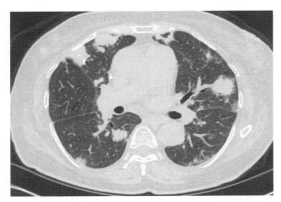

Fig. 8. Axial computed tomography scan demonstrates multiple, bilateral pulmonary nodules of varying configurations ranging from well-defined to spiculated. Tiny foci of calcification/ossification are present in the nodules in the anterior right lung. Transbronchial biopsy confirmed amyloid light-chain amyloidosis.

of patients.[36] Solitary or multiple nodules may mimic other diseases including granulomatous disease or malignancy. The nodules can be smooth, lobulated, or spiculated. Calcification or ossification may be identifiable within the nodules. This may help to suggest the diagnosis.[37,38] However, given the nonspecific appearance, the diagnosis is often difficult based on imaging alone. Confirmatory biopsy is often required. The prognosis for localized nodular parenchymal amyloidosis is benign. Although the nodules may progress, treatment is usually not necessary.

Alveolar septal amyloidosis is rare as a localized disease and is more often associated with systemic AL or AA amyloidosis.[30] Although it is less common than nodular parenchymal amyloidosis,

it is more significant clinically. It is often symptomatic, resulting in pulmonary hypertension and respiratory failure. The median survival is 16 months with gradual worsening of pulmonary function over time.[29] Alveolar septal amyloidosis presents as a diffuse interstitial pattern with interlobular septal thickening, reticulation and associated 2 to 4 mm micronodules (**Fig. 9**). This is often in a peripheral basal distribution.[39,40] Associated lung cysts have been described rarely. When present, these often occur in patients with systemic amyloidosis owing to Sjögren syndrome.[39] Alveolar septal walls are the common sites of ATTR deposition (senile amyloidosis). Despite the presence of amyloid, there are seldom clinical manifestations and chest radiographs are commonly normal or nonspecific (**Fig. 10**).[30,41,42]

Mediastinal or Hilar Adenopathy

Rarely, amyloidosis may present with asymptomatic lymphadenopathy or a solitary mediastinal mass in any of the compartments[43] (**Fig. 11**). The appearance is nonspecific and can mimic other causes of adenopathy, such as lymphoma, sarcoidosis, or a mediastinal neoplasm.

GASTROINTESTINAL AND GENITOURINARY TRACTS

Amyloid deposits may occur in many organs in the gastrointestinal and genitourinary tracts. In systemic amyloidosis, the liver, spleen, intestinal tract, and kidneys are commonly involved, but renal involvement is the major source of morbidity, often manifesting as nephrotic-range proteinuria.

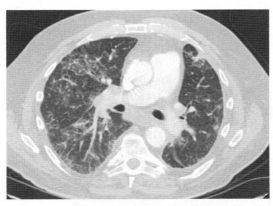

Fig. 9. Axial computed tomography demonstrates the pattern of micronodularity and septal thickening found in alveolar septal amyloidosis. Transbronchial biopsy confirmed amyloid light-chain amyloidosis.

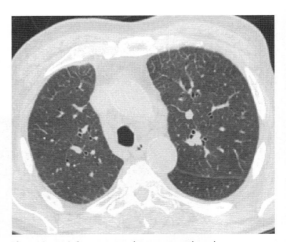

Fig. 10. Axial computed tomography demonstrates diffuse ground glass opacity and peripheral reticular changes in a patient with transthyretin-related amyloidosis.

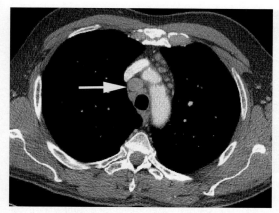

Fig. 11. Axial computed tomography image demonstrates mediastinal adenopathy (*arrow*) in a patient with amyloid light-chain amyloidosis.

Luminal gastrointestinal tract involvement may result in a variety of nonspecific gastrointestinal symptoms. Involvement of the urinary tract, including the bladder, ureter, renal pelvis, and urethra, are often owing to localized amyloidosis, which may cause hematuria or urinary tract obstruction.

Liver

Hepatic involvement is very common in patients with systemic amyloidosis, but the clinical manifestations of hepatic involvement are usually mild. Symptomatic involvement, such as rupture, portal hypertension, or hepatic failure, is rare. Hepatomegaly and a mild abnormal liver function test are the most frequent findings in patients with hepatic amyloidosis.[44] Amyloid deposition occurs along the sinusoids within the space of Disse or in blood vessel walls. Hepatocytes are compressed by accumulation of amyloid and they may atrophy. Frequent imaging findings of hepatic amyloidosis are hepatomegaly. On unenhanced CT, the liver may show decreased attenuation. Calcification may be present. On contrast-enhanced CT, the liver shows delayed enhancement, probably as a result of impairment of blood flow secondary to diffuse parenchymal infiltration of amyloid.[6,45,46]

Spleen

Splenic involvement is common in systemic amyloidosis, but symptomatic involvement is uncommon. Pathologically, the amyloid deposition occurs in red/white pulp or blood vessels, which can cause splenic swelling and hardening when it is massive. Splenomegaly, calcification, and poor contrast enhancement of the parenchyma are

common findings on contrast-enhanced CT (**Fig. 12**).[6,47]

Gastrointestinal Tract

Although amyloid deposition in the luminal gastrointestinal tract is very common in patients with systemic amyloidosis, only 30% to 60% of patients develop gastrointestinal symptoms.[48–50] Common manifestations include gastrointestinal bleeding, gut dysmotility, malabsorptive diarrhea, spontaneous perforation, and obstructive symptoms.[48,49] In most cases, these presentations result from ischemic and infiltrative damage caused by accumulation of amyloid in the confined tissue spaces. Hereditary ATTR amyloidosis may manifest with gastrointestinal symptoms such as diarrhea and weight loss owing to autonomic neuropathy. Wild-type ATTR deposition is common in autopsy series, but usually asymptomatic.[4] Similar to gastrointestinal complaints, many of the endoscopic features of amyloidosis are not specific to the disease. Findings described include thickened folds, erosions, ulcerations, friability, and edema.[49]

On barium study, the esophagus may initially seem to be dilated with decreased peristalsis and eventually reveals evidence of reflux.[50] The stomach can show barium retention, pyloric obstruction, diminished or rigid rugae, and a mass or diffuse thickening.[50] The small intestine may exhibit thickened valvulae conniventes, dilated loops, nodules, hypotonia, or delayed transit time. Findings on CT scans include marked thickening of the walls of the stomach or small intestine, observed in 17% of patients (**Fig. 13**).[6,51]

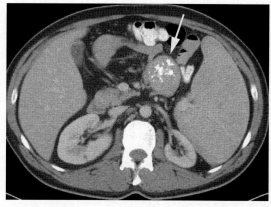

Fig. 12. Axial computed tomography image demonstrates splenomegaly and 5-cm partially calcified mass in the small bowel mesentery (*arrow*). Splenic involvement by amyloid A amyloidosis secondary to Castleman's disease (mesenteric mass) was confirmed at surgery.

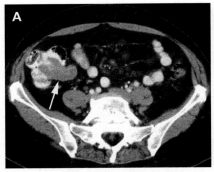
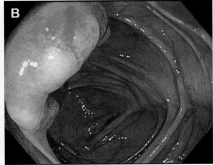

Fig. 13. Axial computed tomography image demonstrates 6-cm-long circumferential mass involving the terminal ileum (*arrow, A*). Endoscopy showed multiple submucosal masses in the terminal ileum and ileocecal valve (*B*). Ileocecal resection confirmed amyloid light-chain amyloidosis. The patient later developed follicular B-cell lymphoma.

Clusters of calcifications and ulcerated mucosa reveal high attenuation. MR imaging may demonstrate normal T2-weighted images with an increased signal on T1-weighted images.

Kidney

Renal involvement is very common in patients with systemic amyloidosis and often is a major source of morbidity. Common clinical manifestation of renal involvement is nephrotic-range proteinuria. Varying degrees of renal insufficiency is often present.[52] Pathologically, amyloid can be found anywhere in the kidney, but glomerular deposition typically predominates. The most common imaging finding of renal amyloidosis is atrophy of renal parenchyma and cortical thinning.[53] Renal enlargement also may be seen in the acute stage of disease.[53] On ultrasound imaging, the renal parenchyma often shows diffusely increased echogenicity with preservation of corticomedullary differentiation.[6] Other rare manifestations of renal involvement include amorphous renal parenchymal calcifications and focal renal mass lesions.[54]

Urinary Bladder

Amyloidosis of the urinary tract is most commonly a localized form, and the urinary bladder is the most common target site of involvement. Amyloidosis deposition primarily affects posterior and lateral walls of the bladder.[55] Pathologically, deposits of amyloid are found in the vessels and sub-urothelial connective tissue. Patients often present with gross painless hematuria or irritative symptoms. Amyloidosis of the bladder presents a great challenge to the urologist because of its close resemblance to an infiltrating neoplasm of bladder on cystoscopy. On CT and MR imaging, bladder amyloidosis often demonstrates focal thickening

of bladder wall or less commonly filling defect in the bladder lumen. Linear intramural calcification of the bladder wall is characteristic of amyloidosis, whereas superficial calcification along the urothelial lining may be seen in encrustation cystitis or urothelial carcinoma.[56] Other uncommon causes of intramural calcifications include schistosomiasis and tuberculosis. The bladder lesion may show decreased signal on T2-weighted images, which is useful in differentiating amyloidosis from urothelial carcinoma. However, desmoplastic metastases or lymphomatous involvement of the bladder may demonstrate similar decreased T2 signal. The bladder lesion often demonstrates decreased contrast enhancement in contrast with avidly enhancing urothelial carcinoma. However, the degree of enhancement may vary.[57–60]

Ureter and Renal Pelvis

Patients with amyloidosis of the renal pelvis and ureter often present with hematuria or symptoms related to ureteral obstruction. Amyloid deposition in the upper urinary tract is usually unifocal and often involves the lower ureter.[61] Typical imaging findings include focal or diffuse wall thickening and irregular ureteral narrowing, which often results in obstruction.[61] Linear intramural calcification is typical of amyloidosis, but often is indistinguishable from calcification associated with urothelial carcinoma (**Fig. 14**).

Urethra

Amyloidosis of the urethra is most commonly a localized form and amyloid deposition occurs in the urethral stroma. Patients with urethral amyloidosis may present with hematuria, dysuria, or urethral obstruction, and may mimic urethral malignancy. Penile ultrasound imaging may depict urethral and periurethral foci intramural

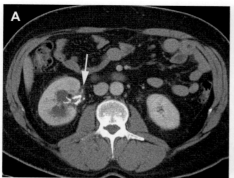
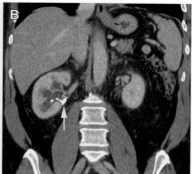

Fig. 14. (*A, B*) Axial and coronal computed tomography images demonstrate thick curvilinear calcifications along the right renal pelvis wall (*arrows*) resulting in moderate pyelocaliectasis. Ureteroscopic biopsy confirmed amyloid light-chain amyloidosis related to Waldenström macroglobulinemia.

calcifications as echogenic foci with posterior shadowing. On MR imaging, amyloid deposit often appears as an area of decreased signal on T2-weighted images. The finding may be useful in differentiating from malignant lesions[62] (**Fig. 15**).

Seminal Vesicle

Amyloid deposition in the seminal vesicles is mostly owing to localized amyloidosis. The prevalence of amyloid deposition in the seminal vesicles is high in older malea, occurring in 20% of patients over 75 years old at autopsy.[63,64] On T2-wegihted MR imaging, the seminal vesicle wall becomes thick and appears as low signal intensity with reduced volume of intravesicular fluid. The appearance may mimic tumor invasion from prostate carcinoma.[65]

Retroperitoneum and Mesentery

Amyloid may diffusely infiltrate the retroperitoneal and mesenteric fat. On CT and MR imaging,

amyloid deposition manifests as diffuse replacement of normal retroperitoneal fat with soft tissues.[66] Diffuse amyloid deposition may undergo calcification that gradually progresses over time[5] (**Fig. 16**). A focal mass (amyloidoma) may be formed mimicking plasmacytoma or lymphoma.

MUSCULOSKELETAL SYSTEM

Systemic amyloidosis results in amyloid deposition within the musculoskeletal system. Most commonly, the accumulation in the musculoskeletal system becomes clinically apparent with deposition in the joints, where it may mimic inflammatory arthritis.[67,68] Amyloid deposition may be seen within bones, muscles, ligaments, tendons, and fat, but is less likely to come to clinical attention than joint-related disease. The less common musculoskeletal manifestations of systemic amyloidosis are bone and soft tissue amyloidomas, amyloid myopathy, and peripheral neuropathy.

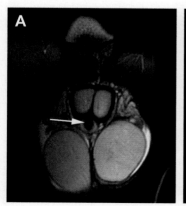
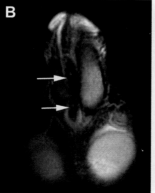
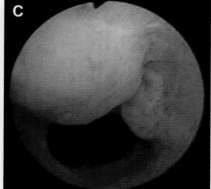

Fig. 15. Axial and coronal T2-weighted MR images show areas of decreased signal intensity in the corpus spongiosum centered in the urethra (*arrows; A, B*). Urethroscopic image demonstrates multiple submucosal masses causing urethral stricture (*C*). Biopsy confirmed amyloid deposition.

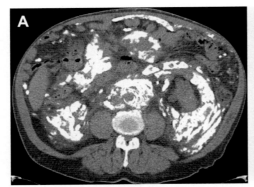
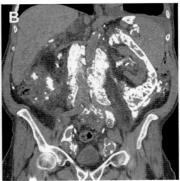

Fig. 16. (*A, B*) Axial and coronal computed tomography images demonstrate extensive calcifications in the retroperitoneal, mesenteric and omental fat. Biopsy confirmed amyloid light-chain amyloidosis associated with marginal zone lymphoma.

Amyloid Arthropathy

Amyloid arthropathy is a well-known musculoskeletal complication of amyloidosis.[67–69] Arthropathy is most common with Aβ2M (dialysis-related) amyloidosis.[70,71] Amyloid arthropathy also occurs with AL amyloidosis and is most commonly reported in the knee, followed by the joints of the hands, wrist, elbow, hip, and ankle.[68]

Massive amounts of amyloid may deposit in the joints resulting in amyloid arthropathy. Radiographs often demonstrate well-marginated erosions with the radiographic differential diagnosis, including rheumatoid arthritis, gout, and chronic infection (**Fig. 17**A). Amyloid deposition in the joints has a relative specific MR appearance with the amyloid tissue demonstrating decreased T1 and T2-weighted signal (**Fig. 17**B, C). Pigmented villonodular synovitis is an intraarticular synovial proliferative process that also demonstrates decreased T1- and T2-weighted signal and might have a similar appearance; however, pigmented villonodular synovitis is almost exclusively monoarticular[72] as opposed to amyloid arthropathy, which is typically polyarticular. Pigmented villonodular synovitis contains hemosiderin and often demonstrates blooming artifact on gradient echo MR sequences, a feature that is absent in amyloid arthropathy. Spinal amyloid depositions can also occur and radiographically may mimic an inflammatory spondyloarthropathy.[73]

Amyloidoma

An amyloidoma is a focal, masslike collection of amyloid that may occur in soft tissue or bone.[74] Amyloidomas are most associated with AL amyloidosis.[74,75] Extremity amyloidomas are

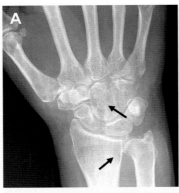
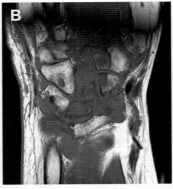
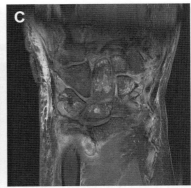

Fig. 17. Frontal radiograph of the wrist (*A*) demonstrates osseous erosions throughout the wrist with arrows indicating the largest erosions. Coronal T1 (*B*) and T2 fat-saturated (*C*) MR images of the wrist confirm the extensive osseous erosions. The MR images demonstrated extensive soft tissue throughout all compartments of the wrist with decreased T1- and T2-weighted signal. MR images and radiographs of the contralateral wrist demonstrated similar findings consistent with amyloid arthropathy. The patient underwent carpal tunnel release and flexor tenosynovectomy for median nerve symptoms with pathologic confirmation of amyloid deposition secondary to chronic hemodialysis.

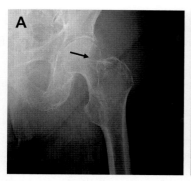
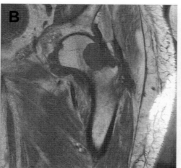
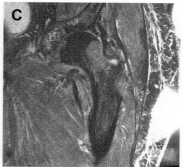

Fig. 18. Frontal radiograph of the left hip (*A*) demonstrates an indeterminate lytic lesion in the left femoral neck (*A, arrow*). Coronal T1 (*B*) and T2 (*C*) fat saturated MR images of the left hip demonstrate features of amyloid arthropathy with decreased T1 and T2-weighted soft tissue in the hip joint. The large lytic lesion in the femoral neck demonstrates similar MR signal characteristics. A bipolar femoral endoprosthesis was placed for a pathologic fracture and pathology and laboratory studies confirmed amyloid light-chain amyloidosis. Subsequent bone marrow biopsy and laboratory studies confirmed multiple myeloma.

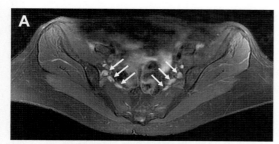

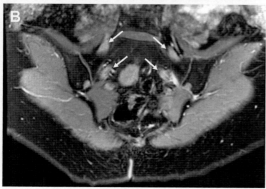

Fig. 19. Axial T2-weighted fat saturated image of the pelvis in a patient with immunoglobulin G lymphoplasmacytic lymphoma (*A*) demonstrates diffuse enlargement and T2-weighted hyperintensity of the lumbosacral plexus (*A, arrows*). This is a nonspecific appearance that can be seen with infectious or inflammatory neuropathies. A coronal oblique fat saturated postgadolinium MR image (*B*) demonstrates fusiform nerve enhancement (*B, arrows*) raising concern for an infiltrative process, including lymphoma. An open sciatic nerve biopsy demonstrated amyloid deposition in the nerve.

exceedingly rare and have indeterminate imaging features that may raise concern for soft tissue sarcoma. Osseous amyloidomas present on radiographs as indeterminate lytic lesions (**Fig. 18**A). MR imaging may demonstrate similar features to amyloid deposition in the joints with decreased T1-weighted and intermediate to decreased T2-weighted signal (**Fig. 18**B, C).

Amyloid Myopathy

Intramuscular amyloid deposition may occur, leading to the clinical signs of macroglossia and muscle pseudohypertrophy. Amyloid myopathy is rare, with significant clinical overlap with inflammatory myopathies.[76,77] It is most often reported in association with AL amyloidosis.[78] Similar to inflammatory myopathies, symptoms include proximal muscle weakness and increased serum creatine kinase.[76,78] Case reports suggest decreased T1- and T2-weighted signal of the muscles secondary to amyloid deposition, but the utility of this MR imaging feature in the prospective evaluation of amyloid myopathy is unknown.[79]

Peripheral Nerve Amyloid

Peripheral neuropathy is a well-known manifestation of systemic amyloidosis, particularly AL amyloidosis and mutant ATTR amyloidosis (familial).[77,80] Symptoms are typically sensory predominant with a peripheral distribution, often associated with pain.[81] Peripheral nerve amyloid involvement is traditionally a clinical diagnosis; however, advancement in MR imaging techniques now allow for direct evaluation of the peripheral nerves. Amyloid involvement of the peripheral nerves is most often diffuse with nerve enlargement, T2-weighted hyperintensity, and variable postgadolinium enhancement[82] (Fig. 19). Kollmer and colleagues[83] evaluated sciatic nerves with MR imaging quantitative volumetric and T2-weighted signal analysis and found significant differences between symptomatic individuals with familial amyloid and asymptomatic gene carriers and controls.[83] A significant difference was also present between asymptomatic gene carriers and controls. MR may prove helpful for prognosis and monitoring treatment response of peripheral nerve involvement in familial amyloidosis.[83] Peripheral nerve amyloidomas are exceedingly rare.[84]

Patients with systemic amyloidosis commonly develop carpal tunnel syndrome, particularly in amyloidosis secondary to chronic dialysis (Aβ2M amyloidosis). The incidence increases with increased duration of dialysis.[85] Carpal tunnel syndrome associated with amyloidosis results from median nerve compression and entrapment in the carpal tunnel rather than direct amyloid peripheral nerve deposition. Treatment of carpal tunnel syndrome secondary to dialysis associated amyloidosis is carpal tunnel release; however, recurrence of carpal tunnel symptoms are more common in chronic hemodialysis patients.[85]

REFERENCES

1. Sipe JD, Benson MD, Buxbaum JN, et al. Nomenclature 2014: Amyloid fibril proteins and clinical classification of the amyloidosis. Amyloid 2014;21(4):221–4.
2. Gertz MA, Kyle RA, Noel P. Primary systemic amyloidosis: a rare complication of immunoglobulin M monoclonal gammopathies and Waldenstrom's macroglobulinemia. J Clin Oncol 1993; 11(5):914–20.
3. Cornwell GG 3rd, Murdoch WL, Kyle RA, et al. Frequency and distribution of senile cardiovascular amyloid. A clinicopathologic correlation. Am J Med 1983;75(4):618–23.
4. Ueda M, Horibata Y, Shono M, et al. Clinicopathological features of senile systemic amyloidosis: an ante- and post-mortem study. Mod Pathol 2011;24(12):1533–44.
5. Georgiades CS, Neyman EG, Barish MA, et al. Amyloidosis: review and CT manifestations. Radiographics 2004;24(2):405–16.
6. Kim SH, Han JK, Lee KH, et al. Abdominal amyloidosis: spectrum of radiological findings. Clin Radiol 2003;58(8):610–20.
7. Maceira AM, Prasad SK, Hawkins PN, et al. Cardiovascular magnetic resonance and prognosis in cardiac amyloidosis. J Cardiovasc Magn Reson 2008;10:54.
8. Gean-Marton AD, Kirsch CF, Vezina LG, et al. Focal amyloidosis of the head and neck: evaluation with CT and MR imaging. Radiology 1991;181(2):521–5.
9. Patel KS, Hawkins PN. Cardiac amyloidosis: where are we today? J Intern Med 2015;278(2):126–44.
10. Steiner I. The prevalence of isolated atrial amyloid. J Pathol 1987;153(4):395–8.
11. Feng D, Edwards WD, Oh JK, et al. Intracardiac thrombosis and embolism in patients with cardiac amyloidosis. Circulation 2007;116(21):2420–6.
12. Selvanayagam JB, Hawkins PN, Paul B, et al. Evaluation and management of the cardiac amyloidosis. J Am Coll Cardiol 2007;50(22):2101–10.
13. Kumar SK, Gertz MA, Lacy MQ, et al. Recent improvements in survival in primary systemic amyloidosis and the importance of an early mortality risk score. Mayo Clin Proc 2011;86(1):12–8.
14. Ruberg FL, Maurer MS, Judge DP, et al. Prospective evaluation of the morbidity and mortality of wild-type and V122I mutant transthyretin amyloid cardiomyopathy: the Transthyretin Amyloidosis Cardiac Study (TRACS). Am Heart J 2012;164(2):222–8.e1.
15. Buss SJ, Emami M, Mereles D, et al. Longitudinal left ventricular function for prediction of survival in systemic light-chain amyloidosis: incremental value compared with clinical and biochemical markers. J Am Coll Cardiol 2012;60(12):1067–76.
16. Phelan D, Collier P, Thavendiranathan P, et al. Relative apical sparing of longitudinal strain using two-dimensional speckle-tracking echocardiography is both sensitive and specific for the diagnosis of cardiac amyloidosis. Heart 2012;98(19):1442–8.
17. Ruberg FL, Appelbaum E, Davidoff R, et al. Diagnostic and prognostic utility of cardiovascular magnetic resonance imaging in light-chain cardiac amyloidosis. Am J Cardiol 2009;103(4):544–9.
18. Syed IS, Glockner JF, Feng D, et al. Role of cardiac magnetic resonance imaging in the detection of cardiac amyloidosis. JACC Cardiovasc Imaging 2010; 3(2):155–64.
19. Austin BA, Tang WH, Rodriguez ER, et al. Delayed hyper-enhancement magnetic resonance imaging provides incremental diagnostic and prognostic utility in suspected cardiac amyloidosis. JACC Cardiovasc Imaging 2009;2(12):1369–77.
20. White JA, Kim HW, Shah D, et al. CMR imaging with rapid visual T1 assessment predicts mortality in patients suspected of cardiac amyloidosis. JACC Cardiovasc Imaging 2014;7(2):143–56.
21. Banypersad SM, Fontana M, Maestrini V, et al. T1 mapping and survival in systemic light-chain amyloidosis. Eur Heart J 2015;36(4):244–51.
22. Karamitsos TD, Piechnik SK, Banypersad SM, et al. Noncontrast T1 mapping for the diagnosis of

cardiac amyloidosis. JACC Cardiovasc Imaging 2013;6(4):488–97.

23. Hazenberg BP, van Rijswijk MH, Piers DA, et al. Diagnostic performance of 123I-labeled serum amyloid P component scintigraphy in patients with amyloidosis. Am J Med 2006;119(4):355.e15–24.

24. Perugini E, Guidalotti PL, Salvi F, et al. Noninvasive etiologic diagnosis of cardiac amyloidosis using 99mTc-3,3-diphosphono-1,2-propanodicarboxylic acid scintigraphy. J Am Coll Cardiol 2005;46(6): 1076–84.

25. Rossi P, Tessonnier L, Frances Y, et al. 99mTc DPD is the preferential bone tracer for diagnosis of cardiac transthyretin amyloidosis. Clin Nucl Med 2012;37(8): e209–10.

26. de Haro-del Moral FJ, Sanchez-Lajusticia A, Gomez-Bueno M, et al. Role of cardiac scintigraphy with 99mTc-DPD in the differentiation of cardiac amyloidosis subtype. Rev Esp Cardiol (Engl Ed) 2012;65(5): 440–6.

27. Treibel TA, Bandula S, Fontana M, et al. Extracellular volume quantification by dynamic equilibrium cardiac computed tomography in cardiac amyloidosis. J Cardiovasc Comput Tomogr 2015; 9(6):585–92.

28. Berk JL, O'Regan A, Skinner M. Pulmonary and tracheobronchial amyloidosis. Semin Respir Crit Care Med 2002;23(2):155–65.

29. Czeyda-Pommersheim F, Hwang M, Chen SS, et al. Amyloidosis: modern cross-sectional imaging. Radiographics 2015;35(5):1381–92.

30. Utz JP, Swensen SJ, Gertz MA. Pulmonary amyloidosis. The Mayo Clinic experience from 1980 to 1993. Ann Intern Med 1996;124(4):407–13.

31. O'Regan A, Fenlon HM, Beamis JF Jr, et al. Tracheobronchial amyloidosis. The Boston University experience from 1984 to 1999. Medicine (Baltimore) 2000; 79(2):69–79.

32. Hui AN, Koss MN, Hochholzer L, et al. Amyloidosis presenting in the lower respiratory tract. Clinicopathologic, radiologic, immunohistochemical, and histochemical studies on 48 cases. Arch Pathol Lab Med 1986;110(3):212–8.

33. Rubinow A, Celli BR, Cohen AS, et al. Localized amyloidosis of the lower respiratory tract. Am Rev Respir Dis 1978;118(3):603–11.

34. Thompson PJ, Citron KM. Amyloid and the lower respiratory tract. Thorax 1983;38(2):84–7.

35. Cordier JF, Loire R, Brune J. Amyloidosis of the lower respiratory tract. Clinical and pathologic features in a series of 21 patients. Chest 1986;90(6):827–31.

36. Pickford HA, Swensen SJ, Utz JP. Thoracic cross-sectional imaging of amyloidosis. AJR Am J Roentgenol 1997;168(2):351–5.

37. Urban BA, Fishman EK, Goldman SM, et al. CT evaluation of amyloidosis: spectrum of disease. Radiographics 1993;13(6):1295–308.

38. Ohdama S, Akagawa S, Matsubara O, et al. Primary diffuse alveolar septal amyloidosis with multiple cysts and calcification. Eur Respir J 1996;9(7): 1569–71.

39. Lee AY, Godwin JD, Pipavath SN. Case 182: pulmonary amyloidosis. Radiology 2012;263(3):929–32.

40. Graham CM, Stern EJ, Finkbeiner WE, et al. High-resolution CT appearance of diffuse alveolar septal amyloidosis. AJR Am J Roentgenol 1992;158(2): 265–7.

41. Westermark P, Bergstrom J, Solomon A, et al. Transthyretin-derived senile systemic amyloidosis: clinicopathologic and structural considerations. Amyloid 2003;10(Suppl 1):48–54.

42. Roden AC, Aubry MC, Zhang K, et al. Nodular senile pulmonary amyloidosis: a unique case confirmed by immunohistochemistry, mass spectrometry, and genetic study. Hum Pathol 2010;41(7):1040–5.

43. Fiorelli A, Accardo M, Ciancia G, et al. Isolated mediastinal amyloidosis mimicking a neoplastic lesion. Gen Thorac Cardiovasc Surg 2014;62(5): 324–6.

44. Park MA, Mueller PS, Kyle RA, et al. Primary (AL) hepatic amyloidosis: clinical features and natural history in 98 patients. Medicine (Baltimore) 2003; 82(5):291–8.

45. Monzawa S, Tsukamoto T, Omata K, et al. A case with primary amyloidosis of the liver and spleen: radiologic findings. Eur J Radiol 2002;41(3):237–41.

46. Shin YM. Hepatic amyloidosis. Korean J Hepatol 2011;17(1):80–3.

47. Mainenti PP, Cantalupo T, Nicotra S, et al. Systemic amyloidosis: the CT sign of splenic hypoperfusion. Amyloid 2004;11(4):281–2.

48. Friedman S, Janowitz HD. Systemic amyloidosis and the gastrointestinal tract. Gastroenterol Clin North Am 1998;27(3):595–614, vi.

49. James DG, Zuckerman GR, Sayuk GS, et al. Clinical recognition of Al type amyloidosis of the luminal gastrointestinal tract. Clin Gastroenterol Hepatol 2007;5(5):582–8.

50. Petre S, Shah IA, Gilani N. Review article: gastrointestinal amyloidosis - clinical features, diagnosis and therapy. Aliment Pharmacol Ther 2008;27(11): 1006–16.

51. Araoz PA, Batts KP, MacCarty RL. Amyloidosis of the alimentary canal: radiologic-pathologic correlation of CT findings. Abdom Imaging 2000;25(1):38–44.

52. Dember LM. Amyloidosis-associated kidney disease. J Am Soc Nephrol 2006;17(12):3458–71.

53. Ekelund L. Radiologic findings in renal amyloidosis. AJR Am J Roentgenol 1977;129(5):851–3.

54. Levine E. Abdominal visceral calcification in secondary amyloidosis: CT findings. Abdom Imaging 1994;19(6):554–5.

55. Tirzaman O, Wahner-Roedler DL, Malek RS, et al. Primary localized amyloidosis of the urinary bladder:

a case series of 31 patients. Mayo Clin Proc 2000; 75(12):1264–8.

56. Thomas SD, Sanders PW 3rd, Pollack H. Primary amyloidosis of urinary bladder and ureter: cause of mural calcification. Urology 1977;9(5):586–9.

57. Zhou F, Lee P, Zhou M, et al. Primary localized amyloidosis of the urinary tract frequently mimics neoplasia: a clinicopathologic analysis of 11 cases. Am J Clin Exp Urol 2014;2(1):71–5.

58. Merrimen JL, Alkhudair WK, Gupta R. Localized amyloidosis of the urinary tract: case series of nine patients. Urology 2006;67(5):904–9.

59. Kato H, Toei H, Furuse M, et al. Primary localized amyloidosis of the urinary bladder. Eur Radiol 2003;13(Suppl 4):L109–12.

60. Amano Y, Kumazaki T. MR appearances of urinary bladder in amyloidosis associated with multiple myeloma. Abdom Imaging 1996;21(5):468–9.

61. Mark IR, Goodlad J, Lloyd-Davies RW. Localized amyloidosis of the genito-urinary tract. J R Soc Med 1995;88(6):320–4.

62. Ichioka K, Utsunomiya N, Ueda N, et al. Primary localized amyloidosis of urethra: magnetic resonance imaging findings. Urology 2004;64(2):376–8.

63. Pitkanen P, Westermark P, Cornwell GG 3rd, et al. Amyloid of the seminal vesicles. A distinctive and common localized form of senile amyloidosis. Am J Pathol 1983;110(1):64–9.

64. Kee KH, Lee MJ, Shen SS, et al. Amyloidosis of seminal vesicles and ejaculatory ducts: a histologic analysis of 21 cases among 447 prostatectomy specimens. Ann Diagn Pathol 2008;12(4):235–8.

65. Ramchandani P, Schnall MD, LiVolsi VA, et al. Senile amyloidosis of the seminal vesicles mimicking metastatic spread of prostatic carcinoma on MR images. AJR Am J Roentgenol 1993;161(1):99–100.

66. Glynn TP Jr, Kreipke DL, Irons JM. Amyloidosis: diffuse involvement of the retroperitoneum. Radiology 1989;170(3 Pt 1):726.

67. Wiernik PH. Amyloid joint disease. Medicine (Baltimore) 1972;51(6):465–79.

68. Elsaman AM, Radwan AR, Akmatov MK, et al. Amyloid arthropathy associated with multiple myeloma: a systematic analysis of 101 reported cases. Semin Arthritis Rheum 2013;43(3):405–12.

69. Kurer MH, Baillod RA, Madgwick JC. Musculoskeletal manifestations of amyloidosis. A review of 83 patients on haemodialysis for at least 10 years. J Bone Joint Surg Br 1991;73(2):271–6.

70. Gisserot O, Landais C, Cremades S, et al. Amyloid arthropathy and Waldenstrom macroglobulinemia. Joint Bone Spine 2006;73(4):456–8.

71. Buxbaum JN. The systemic amyloidoses. Curr Opin Rheumatol 2004;16(1):67–75.

72. Wagner ML, Spjut HJ, Dutton RV, et al. Polyarticular pigmented villonodular synovitis. AJR Am J Roentgenol 1981;136(4):821–3.

73. Lim CY, Ong KO. Various musculoskeletal manifestations of chronic renal insufficiency. Clin Radiol 2013;68(7):e397–411.

74. Krishnan J, Chu WS, Elrod JP, et al. Tumoral presentation of amyloidosis (amyloidomas) in soft tissues. A report of 14 cases. Am J Clin Pathol 1993; 100(2):135–44.

75. Verhoeven F, Prati C, Wendling D. Amyloidoma, an unusual cause of fracture. Case Rep Rheumatol 2014;2014:424056.

76. Tuomaala H, Karppa M, Tuominen H, et al. Amyloid myopathy: a diagnostic challenge. Neurol Int 2009; 1(1):e7.

77. Gertz MA, Kyle RA. Myopathy in primary systemic amyloidosis. J Neurol Neurosurg Psychiatry 1996; 60(6):655–60.

78. Chapin JE, Kornfeld M, Harris A. Amyloid myopathy: characteristic features of a still underdiagnosed disease. Muscle Nerve 2005;31(2):266–72.

79. Metzler JP, Fleckenstein JL, White CL 3rd, et al. MRI evaluation of amyloid myopathy. Skeletal Radiol 1992;21(7):463–5.

80. Falk RH, Skinner M. The systemic amyloidoses: an overview. Adv Intern Med 2000;45:107–37.

81. Matsuda M, Gono T, Morita H, et al. Peripheral nerve involvement in primary systemic AL amyloidosis: a clinical and electrophysiological study. Eur J Neurol 2011;18(4):604–10.

82. Thawait SK, Chaudhry V, Thawait GK, et al. High-resolution MR neurography of diffuse peripheral nerve lesions. AJNR Am J Neuroradiol 2011;32(8): 1365–72.

83. Kollmer J, Hund E, Hornung B, et al. In vivo detection of nerve injury in familial amyloid polyneuropathy by magnetic resonance neurography. Brain 2015;138(Pt 3):549–62.

84. Consales A, Roncaroli F, Salvi F, et al. Amyloidoma of the brachial plexus. Surg Neurol 2003;59(5):418–23 [discussion: 23].

85. Kopec J, Gadek A, Drozdz M, et al. Carpal tunnel syndrome in hemodialysis patients as a dialysis-related amyloidosis manifestation–incidence, risk factors and results of surgical treatment. Med Sci Monit 2011;17(9):CR505–9.

Systemic Vasculopathies
Imaging and Management

Ankaj Khosla, MD[a], Brice Andring, MD[a], Benjamin Atchie, MD[a], Joseph Zerr, MD[a], Benjamin White, MD[a], Jarrod MacFarlane, MD[a], Sanjeeva P. Kalva, MD[a,b,*]

KEYWORDS

- Vasculitis • Vasculopathy • Arteritis • Connective tissue disease

KEY POINTS

- Systemic vasculopathies represent a wide variety of vascular disorders characterized by vessel wall thickening, luminal irregularities, stenosis, occlusion, dissection, and aneurysm formation.
- Imaging plays an important role in the management of systemic vasculopathies by identifying the involved vessels and vascular abnormalities, assessing disease progression and the risk of complications, localizing active areas of vascular inflammation, and recognizing end organ damage.
- This article discusses various common systemic vasculopathies emphasizing the salient vascular imaging findings and the role of endovascular therapy for management of these conditions.

INTRODUCTION

Systemic vasculopathies represent multifocal vascular disorders that occur either in isolation (of unknown etiology) or are associated with systemic inflammatory/infective/neoplastic conditions, connective tissue disorders, or chemical toxicity (**Box 1**).[1] These vasculopathies are often classified according to the size of the vessels involved (**Box 2**) to facilitate practical approach for diagnosis and management.[2] Despite varied etiologies and vessels involved, the pathologic manifestations of various systemic vasculopathies remain similar, making it difficult to diagnose these conditions solely on imaging morphology. Associated clinical manifestations, involvement of other organs, laboratory findings, and other radiologic tests help distinguish these entities. Some conditions require histopathologic confirmation for definitive diagnosis. Imaging plays an important role in the management of systemic vasculopathies by identifying the involved vessels and vascular abnormalities, assessing disease progression and the risk of complications, localizing active areas of vascular inflammation, and recognizing end organ damage. This review briefly discusses various common systemic vasculopathies emphasizing the salient vascular imaging findings and the role of endovascular therapy for management of these conditions.

LARGE-VESSEL VASCULITIS
Takayasu Arteritis

Also known as *pulseless disease* and *aortic arch syndrome*, Takayasu arteritis is an idiopathic large-vessel arteritis that involves the aorta and its major branches, pulmonary arteries, and coronary arteries. The disease often manifests before the age of 40 years with a distinct female preponderance. Patients typically present with nonspecific constitutional symptoms during initial phase of the disease. Active inflammatory phase is associated with elevated erythrocyte sedimentation rate (ESR) and C-reactive protein (CRP) levels. Chronic granulomatous and lymphocytic

Disclosure: No relevant financial disclosures by any authors.
[a] Department of Radiology, University of Texas Southwestern Medical Center, 5393 Harry Hines Boulevard, Dallas, TX 75390, USA; [b] Interventional Radiology, UT Southwestern Medical Center, 5393 Harry Hines Boulevard, Dallas, TX 75390-8834, USA
* Corresponding author. Interventional Radiology, UT Southwestern Medical Center, 5393 Harry Hines Boulevard, Dallas, TX 75390-8834.
E-mail address: Sanjeeva.Kalva@UTSouthwestern.edu

Radiol Clin N Am 54 (2016) 613–628
http://dx.doi.org/10.1016/j.rcl.2015.12.011
0033-8389/16/$ – see front matter © 2016 Elsevier Inc. All rights reserved.

Box 1
Systemic vasculopathies

Inflammatory/immune complex conditions
Takayasu arteritis
GCA
Systemic lupus erythematosus
Sjögren's syndrome and scleroderma
Rheumatoid arthritis
Seronegative arthritis
Behçet disease–associated vasculitis
PAN
Kawasaki disease
Thromboangiitis obliterans
Churg Strauss syndrome
Leukocytoclastic vasculitis
Henoch-Schonlein purpura
Wegener granulomatosis (granulomatosis with polyangiitis)

Connective tissue disorders
Marfan syndrome
LDS
EDS

Infective
Septic emboli
Viral infections (eg, herpes, hepatitis B and C, human immunodeficiency virus)
Bacterial infections

Neoplastic
Hematologic malignancies
Solid organ malignancies

Unknown etiology
Fibromuscular dysplasia
Segmental arterial mediolysis

Chemical toxicity
Antimicrobials (penicillins, cephalosporins, tetracyclines, gentamicin, sulfasalazine, quinolones)
Antithyroid medications (Propylthiouracil, methimazole)
Drugs of abuse (cocaine, heroin, methamphetamine, ecstasy)
Psychotropic medications (olanzapine, trazodone, clozapine)
Analgesics (naproxen, ketorolac, sulindac, indomethacin)
Cardiovascular drugs (Digitalis, Hydralazine, Methyldopa, Thiazides)
Anticonvulsants (Phenytoin, Carbamazepine)
Anti–tumor necrosis factor–α agents (infliximab, etanercept, adalimumab)
Others (phenylpropanolamine, sulfonamides, leukotriene inhibitors)

**Box 2
Classification of vasculopathies**

Large-vessel vasculitis
Takayasu arteritis
GCA

Medium-sized vessel vasculitis
PAN
Kawasaki disease

Small-vessel vasculitis
ANCA-associated vasculitis (microscopic polyangiitis, granulomatosis with polyangiitis, eosinophilic granulomatosis with polyangiitis)
Immune complex vasculitis (antiglomerular basement membrane disease, cryoglobulinemic vasculitis, IgA vasculitis, hypocomplementemic urticarial vasculitis)

Variable-vessel vasculitis
Behçet disease
Cogan syndrome

Single-organ vasculitis
Cutaneous leukocytoclastic vasculitis
Cutaneous arteritis
Primary central nervous system vasculitis
Isolated aortitis

Vasculitis associated with systemic disease
Lupus vasculitis
Rheumatoid vasculitis
Sarcoid vasculitis
Others

Vasculitis associated with probable etiology
Hepatitis C–associated cryoglobulinaemic vasculitis
Hepatitis B–associated vasculitis
Syphilitic aortitis
Drug-associated immune complex vasculitis
Drug-associated ANCA-associated vasculitis
Cancer-associated vasculitis
Others

---

inflammation affects the intima and media leading to arterial wall thickening, focal stenosis, occlusion, or aneurysm formation. Severe stenosis and occlusion of the proximal carotid and subclavian arteries commonly leads to absence of the pulses, hence, the disease moniker. Other characteristic clinical presentations of Takayasu arteritis include claudication, vascular bruits, renal hypertension, and limb blood pressure discrepancies.

Diagnosis and classification of Takayasu arteritis is based largely on imaging findings (**Table 1**).[3,4] Stenosis, occlusion, vessel wall thickening, dilation, and aneurysms of the characteristic arteries are identified on catheter angiography, computed tomography (CT) angiography, and magnetic resonance (MR) imaging/MR angiography (**Fig. 1**). Enhancement of the arterial wall on contrast-enhanced CT and MR images suggests active inflammation, although chronic fibrosis may also enhance.[5,6] Ultrasound scan can diagnose regions of stenosis and dilation. Ultrasound scan is also shows wall thickening

Table 1 Angiographic classification of Takayasu arteritis	
Type	**Vessels Involved**
Type 1	Branches of the aortic arch
Type 2a	Ascending aorta, aortic arch and its branches
Type 2b	Ascending aorta, aortic arch and its branches, descending thoracic aorta
Type 3	Descending thoracic aorta, abdominal aorta, or renal arteries
Type 4	Abdominal aorta or renal arteries
Type 5	Combined features of types 2b and 4

and edema with acute flares.[7,8] PET/CT can show increased ^{18}F-flourodeoxyglucose uptake in the affected arteries, although the clinical utility of this finding has not been well established.[9]

Management of Takayasu arteritis involves controlling the disease activity through medical therapy and decreasing the effects of vascular compromise through surgical or endovascular interventions. Corticosteroid therapy is the mainstay of medical therapy. Other immune-modulating drugs (eg, methotrexate, azathioprine) are used in patients who do not respond to steroid therapy. Endovascular therapy through angioplasty and stenting are used in patients with symptomatic claudication and severe renovascular hypertension recalcitrant to medical therapy. Stenting is used for ostial lesions, long-segment stenosis/occlusion, failed angioplasty, and angioplasty complicated by recurrent stenosis or dissection.

Surgical bypass and reconstructive surgery are reserved for patients with severe aortic stenosis, thoraco-abdominal aortic aneurysms and arch vessel stenosis.[10]

Giant Cell Arteritis

Giant cell arteritis (GCA) is a chronic, immune-mediated, inflammatory vasculopathy that commonly affects medium and large arteries with resultant ischemic complications. The common target vascular beds of involvement include branches of the external carotid artery and the thoracic aorta and its branches. GCA typically affects older women (accounting for 65%–75% of cases), with a peak incidence in the seventh decade. Temporal arteritis is the classic presentation of the disease with palpable, tender, temporal arteries associated with constitutional symptoms and elevated ESR (usually >100) and CRP level. Ischemic optic neuropathy from ophthalmic artery involvement is a complication that may lead to blindness in 10% to 15% of patients. Large-vessel vasculitis (aortitis) occurs in 25% of patients and may be complicated by dissection or aneurysm formation. Approximately 50% of patients with GCA may manifest polymyalgia rheumatica, a symptomatic, symmetric, myalgia syndrome that commonly involves select muscle groups in the neck, proximal upper extremities, and pelvic girdle. For patients with suspected GCA, temporal artery biopsy is performed and high-dose glucocorticoids administered on an emergent basis to avoid acute blindness. Long-term glucocorticoid therapy is continued if the biopsy result shows giant, mononuclear, and lymphocytic cell infiltrate

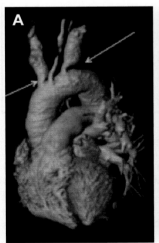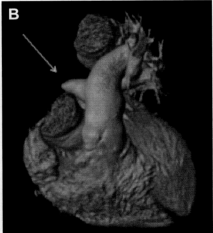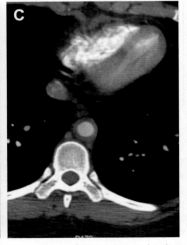

Fig. 1. A 26-year-old man with Takayasu arteritis. (*A*) Three-dimensional reconstructions of CT angiography data set show stenosis and aneurysmal dilation of the brachiocephalic artery, left carotid artery, and left subclavian artery (*arrows*). (*B*) In addition there is stenosis of right pulmonary artery (*arrow*). (*C*) Wall thickening in the aorta.

throughout all layers of the artery consistent with GCA. Alternatively, patients with GCA may present with ischemic symptoms in the upper extremities. Angiography of such patients shows multifocal often bilaterally symmetric areas of proximal artery (subclavian/axillary/brachial artery) narrowing.

The American College of Rheumatology Classification Criteria are largely related to symptoms and biopsy results,[11] yet imaging can be used in equivocal cases to ascertain the extent of disease, for biopsy planning, or in lieu of biopsy. Ultrasound scan has been found to show a dark halo around the lumen of the artery, a specific sign for GCA[7] attributed to arterial wall edema. Inflamed arteries may also have wall thickening and enhancement on MRI[12] (**Fig. 2**). PET/CT provides greater sensitivity and specificity for vasculitis involvement in patients with GCA than that seen with Takayasu arteritis and can be used to ascertain extent of disease.[9]

Medical therapy with steroids and other immune-modulating drugs remains the mainstay of treatment of GCA. Given that the upper extremity stenoses are asymptomatic, endovascular therapy is rarely applied.

MEDIUM-VESSEL VASCULITIS
Polyarteritis Nodosa

Polyarteritis nodosa (PAN), first described by Kussmaul and Maier in 1866, is histologically characterized by a necrotizing vasculitis affecting small- to medium-sized vessels, eventually resulting in necrosis and vessel wall destruction. The prevalence of PAN ranges from 2 to 33 per million with an annual incidence in Europe of 4.4 to 9.7 per million with the variation likely secondary to differences in diagnostic criteria.[13,14] The peak incidence is in the sixth decade, and there is a slight (1.5:1) male predominance. Most PAN is idiopathic, but there is a known association with hepatitis B, hepatitis C, and hairy cell leukemia.

The clinical signs and symptoms of PAN are varied and are the result of organ-specific inflammation or ischemia secondary to arteritis. There are no specific antibodies or serologic markers; laboratory findings (leukocytosis, thrombocytosis, elevated ESR/CRP) are often nonspecific. The American College of Rheumatology has established 10 criteria to classify polyarteritis nodosa: (1) weight loss greater than 4 kg, (2) livedo reticularis, (3) testicular pain or tenderness, (4) myalgias, (5) mono/polyneuropathy, (6) new-onset diastolic blood pressure greater than 90, (7) elevated blood urea nitrogen and creatinine levels, (8) hepatitis B infection, (9) characteristic angiographic findings, and (10) biopsy of a small to medium artery containing polymorphonuclear cells.[15]

Because PAN typically involves small- to medium-sized arteries, angiographic findings are often observed in the branches of the abdominal aorta including the renal arteries (70%–80%), mesenteric arteries (50%), skeletal muscle (30%), and central nervous system (10%) (5). The most suggestive finding is 1- to 5-mm arterial aneurysms/ectasia (61%); other findings including luminal irregularity, wall thickening, stenosis, or occlusion may be seen on CT angiography, MR angiography, or catheter angiography[16,17] (**Fig. 3**). Angiography remains the gold standard; however, complications including organ infarction are best visualized on CT or MR imaging. Other diseases including rheumatoid vasculitis, systemic lupus erythematosus, and Churg-Strauss syndrome may have a similar appearance. However, PAN is rarely associated with glomerulonephritis or pulmonary involvement differentiating it from Churg-Strauss syndrome and granulomatosis with polyangiitis. Medical therapy is through

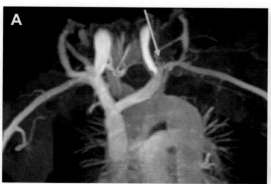
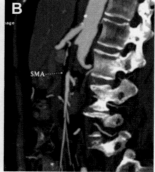

Fig. 2. (*A*) A 60-year-old woman with GCA. Contrast-enhanced MR angiogram shows high-grade stenosis (*arrow*) of left subclavian artery. (*B*) A 70-year-old woman with abdominal pain. There is wall thickening and occlusion of proximal SMA. Biopsy of the arterial wall confirmed GCA.

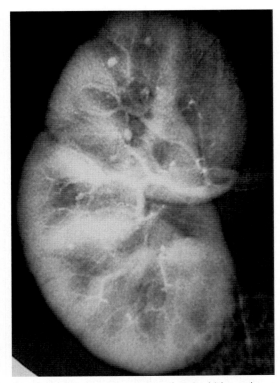

Fig. 3. Catheter angiography of right kidney shows multiple microaneurysms involving the small vessels in the kidney, consistent with PAN.

corticosteroids and immune-modulating drugs. Endovascular therapy is limited to treatment of large aneurysms with embolization using coils or n-acetyl cyanoacrylate.

Kawasaki Disease (Mucocutaneous Lymph Node Syndrome)

Kawasaki disease (mucocutaneous lymph node syndrome) is an acute, self-limited, febrile illness, which, if left untreated, can lead to a systemic vasculitis of medium-sized vessels in all organs but particularly the coronary arteries. The pathogenesis is incompletely understood but likely occurs secondary to an autoimmune reaction to an unknown infection.[18] Kawasaki disease typically affects children younger than 5 years and has a male to female ratio of 1.3 to 1.5. The clinical diagnostic criteria of Kawasaki disease involves fever lasting at least 5 days without other explanation combined with 4 of 5 of the following: (1) bilateral bulbar conjunctival injection, (2) oral mucous membrane changes, (3) peripheral extremity changes (erythema of palms/soles, edema of hands/feet, periungual desquamation), (4) polymorphous rash, and (5) cervical lymphadenopathy.[19] If therapy (ie, intravenous immunoglobulin or aspirin) is not initiated during this acute phase, patients can have complications including coronary artery aneurysms, depressed myocardial contractility, arrhythmias, and peripheral artery occlusion.

The imaging findings may be seen 12 to 25 days from disease onset as perivasculitis and endarteritis progress to pan-vasculitis. CT angiography, MR angiography, echocardiography, or angiography may find saccular and fusiform aneurysms (Fig. 4), which typically occur at vessel bifurcating sites, during the pan-vasculitis stage. The pan-vasculitis eventually leads to granulation tissue formation causing vascular stenosis and occlusion.[20]

The first-line imaging technique remains echocardiography because of its reasonable sensitivity for detecting right and left coronary artery stenotic lesions (85% and 80%, respectively) and its concurrent ability to show cardiac function abnormalities.[21] CT angiography can provide clear visualization of the coronary artery aneurysms and has improved sensitivity and specificity for detection of

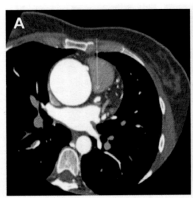
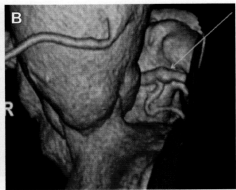

Fig. 4. Mild dilation of the left coronary artery consistent with left coronary aneurysm (arrow) in a patient with known Kawasaki's disease. (A) Axial CT angiography. (B) Three-dimensional reformation of CT angiography data set.

stenotic lesions relative to echocardiography. Myocardial perfusion single photon emission CT can be used to evaluate myocardial perfusion and ischemia. MR angiography is typically the second step in the algorithm after echocardiography, especially in adolescents in whom there is a poor acoustic window. The MR angiogram shows the aneurysms, occlusion, and stenosis.[22] However, the utility of cardiac MR imaging is its ability to show associated abnormalities including myocarditis (manifesting as patchy areas of increased T2 signal in the myocardium in 50% of patients), regional wall motion abnormalities (with measurement of end diastolic volumes, systolic ejection, and ejection fraction with steady-state cine images), and infarction as a results of the above processes (on delayed gadolinium enhanced images). Angiography best shows the size and extent of the aneurysms but because of its invasive nature is typically reserved for therapeutic interventions including embolization of the aneurysms or thrombolytic therapy.

SMALL-VESSEL VASCULITIS
Antineutrophil Cytoplasmic Antibody–Associated Vasculitis

Antineutrophil cytoplasmic antibody (ANCA)-associated vasculitis encompasses 3 distinct entities: granulomatosis with polyangiitis (GPA), microscopic polyangiitis (MPA), and eosinophilic granulomatosis with polyangiitis (EGPA). Both GPA and MPA are associated with 90% to 96% ANCA positivity, whereas EGPA has 60% ANCA positivity. GPA, previously known as Wegener's granulomatosis, results in small-vessel necrotizing vasculitis with involvement of the upper respiratory tract leading to necrosis of nasal septum, tracheal necrosis, lung nodules, and necrotizing glomerulonephritis. Imaging may show nasal blockade, loss of nasal septum, and lung nodules. No specific angiographic findings

are described (**Fig. 5**). Similar to GPA, MPA results in small-vessel necrotizing vasculitis with glomerulonephritis and pulmonary capillaritis. EGPA is associated with eosinophilia, asthma, upper respiratory tract granulomatous disease, and mono-neuritis multiplex. Treatment involves steroid therapy and other immune modulating drugs.[23]

VARIABLE-VESSEL VASCULITIS
Behçet Disease

Behçet disease is a chronic, relapsing inflammatory disorder caused by autoimmune vasculitis. It is a rare disease that presents with a wide array of clinical and radiographic abnormalities. The diagnosis is usually made clinically by recognizing the presence of relapsing oral ulcers, genital ulceration, and uveitis; however, symptoms may be less specific given that it can also commonly involve the nervous, gastrointestinal, and cardiovascular systems.[24]

Behçet disease can involve the entire spectrum of vessel sizes. Large vessel involvement is radiographically apparent as saccular pseudoaneurysms, which can involve large vessels such as the aorta, iliac, femoral, popliteal, subclavian, and pulmonary arteries. In many cases, these aneurysms may be multiple; rupture of such aneurysms is a leading cause of sudden death in patients with this disease.[25] If recognized early, such aneurysms can be treated by embolization or aneurysmal exclusion. Small vessel and capillary involvement, however, is not as readily imaged. Venous involvement is much more common than the arterial involvement. Patients may present with superficial thrombophlebitis with associated linear erythema or thrombosis of larger veins such as the hepatic veins and inferior vena cava resulting in Budd-Chiari syndrome and cerebral venous thrombosis leading to papilledema and optic atrophy (**Fig. 6**).

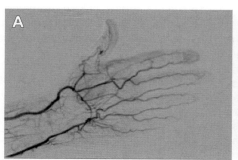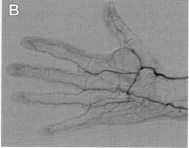

Fig. 5. Digital subtraction angiography in bilateral hands of a patient with an ANCA-positive vasculitis. The left image shows areas of occlusion and aneurysmal dilation (*A*) in the digital artery of right thumb. Contralateral hand (*B*) shows normal vasculature.

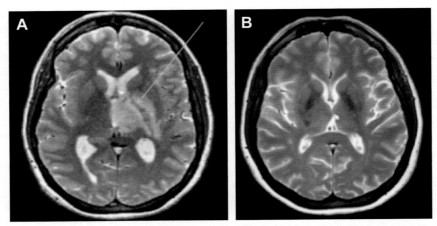

Fig. 6. A 48-year-old woman with a history of uveitis presented with right-sided weakness. MR imaging found left thalamic lesion (*arrow*) (*A*) (atypical parenchymal Behçet), biopsy showed inflammation, eventually resolved with steroids (*B*). Later, Behçet disease was diagnosed.

Largely because the underlying cause of Behçet disease is still unknown, treatment consists of a combination of steroids and cytotoxic/immunosuppressive drugs tailored to the organ system that is involved.[24]

VASCULITIS ASSOCIATED WITH SYSTEMIC DISEASE
Rheumatoid and Seronegative Arthritis–Associated Vasculitis

Although uncommon and poorly understood, vascular manifestations are also observed in patients with severe inflammatory arthritides, including seropositive (rheumatoid arthritis) and seronegative spondyloarthropathies.

The incidence of vasculitis related to rheumatoid disease seems to be decreasing worldwide, likely related to improved treatment and modification of environmental factors such as smoking.[26] Occurring in less than 5% of patients with rheumatoid arthritis, rheumatoid vasculitis remains, however, an important cause of morbidity and is one of the extra-articular manifestations of the disease that is associated with a significant increase in mortality.[27]

Rheumatoid vasculitis is thought to be mediated by immune complex deposition in the vessel wall, followed by a cellular response leading to presumed injury.[28] It generally appears late in the disease process and varies in its clinical presentation and imaging features, as it can affect nearly every organ system. Cardiac, pulmonary, gastrointestinal, and nervous system involvement have all been reported. Involvement of small- to medium-sized vessels predominate this process and can be seen radiographically as circumferential wall thickening and smoothly tapered luminal narrowing. This aspect of the disease process can lead to skin ulcers, which can often be the first clinical presentation of the disease.

In contrast, vasculitis associated with seronegative spondylo-arthropathies, such as ankylosing spondylitis and reactive arthritis, is a more common manifestation (**Fig. 7**). Also unlike rheumatoid vasculitis, there is preferential involvement of large vessels with intimal proliferation related to associated vasculopathy that can lead to aortic regurgitation and aortitis.[29] Interestingly, psoriatic arthritis, also an HLA-B27 associated spondyloarthropathy, has only rarely been reported to affect the aorta.[30] Small vessel involvement, particularly that which results in vasculitic skin lesions, is rarely described in seronegative spondylo-arthropathies.[31]

Consequently, the early imaging findings for these entities, particularly ankylosing spondylitis, include aortic valve regurgitation, heart failure, valvular thickening, and nodularity, which are most readily detected by echocardiogram or gated cardiac CT/MR imaging. Late but common findings of aortitis include dilatation of the aortic root and wall thickening with or without surrounding inflammatory changes that are best seen on CT or MR imaging.[32]

As with other inflammatory causes of vasculopathy, mainstay therapy includes steroids and aggressive management of the underlying cause.

Systemic Lupus Erythematosus

Systemic lupus erythematosus is an autoimmune, collagen vascular disease with multiple presentations (which are beyond the scope of this discussion) that may include vasculitis. When present,

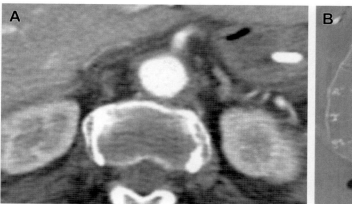
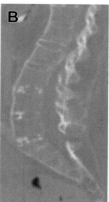

Fig. 7. A 66-year-old woman with ankylosing spondylitis. CT angiography (*A*) shows thickening of the abdominal aorta at the level of the celiac artery. Sagittal reconstruction of CT data shows spine findings consistent with ankylosing spondylitis (*B*).

lupus vasculitis often presents with ischemic symptoms involving the distal extremities but may rarely affect the viscera.[33] Care must be taken to evaluate for antiphospholipid syndrome as the associated microthrombi can present similarly.[34] Angiography can be used to evaluate a patient with symptoms of acute arterial ischemia for reversible causes, such as thrombus. Angiography is commonly used to assess retinal perfusion and detect retinal neovascularization. Peripheral angiography may show diffuse small-vessel involvement in the upper extremities with long tapered narrowing and occlusions of the digital arteries.

VASCULITIS ASSOCIATED WITH PROBABLE ETIOLOGY
Thromboangiitis Obliterans (Buerger's Disease)

Thromboangiitis obliterans is a nonatherosclerotic, segmental, inflammatory disease involving small- to medium-sized arteries and veins of the extremities, which may ultimately lead to vascular occlusion.[35] The typical patient is a young (20–40 years) male smoker. The average incidence is 4 to 5 patients in 100,000 with the incidence decreasing since the 1970s, likely secondary to a decrease in smoking rates.

The vascular involvement typically begins in the distal arteries and veins followed by more proximal involvement with 2 or more extremities typically involved.[36,37] The lower extremities are affected more than the upper extremities. The most common presentation is digital (toe, finger) ischemia with ulcers or gangrene. However, other symptoms include superficial thrombophlebitis, migratory phlebitis, Raynaud's phenomenon, and (as more proximal involvement occurs)

claudication. There are no specific antibodies or serologic markers; laboratory findings such as leukocytosis, thrombocytosis, and elevated ESR/CRP are often nonspecific.

Although CT angiography/MR angiography can be used, these modalities often do not provide sufficient spatial resolution, and an angiogram is typically performed. Angiographic findings consistent with thromboangiitis obliterans include absence of atherosclerotic disease or thromboembolism, segmental arterial occlusion with interspersed normal-appearing segments, and collateralization around the occluded areas resulting in a characteristic "corkscrew" morphology of the vessels.[38] The most common arteries involved include the posterior tibial artery (40.4%), anterior tibial artery (41.4%), and the ulnar artery (11.5%) (**Fig. 8**).[37] Treatment includes smoking cessation, prostaglandin analogs, calcium channel blockers, revascularization, and pain control.

Drug-Induced Vasculitis

Drug-induced vasculopathies are a rare entity and usually reserved as a diagnosis of exclusion. Although it can affect any size vessel, small and medium vessels are commonly affected. Usually, there is a temporal course between drug initiation and onset of symptoms with younger and middle-age patients more likely to be affected. A multitude of drugs have been associated with vasculitis, as described in **Box 1**.[1]

The exact pathogenesis of drug-induced vasculopathy is unknown and varies depending on the drug and its biochemical effects. Common pathways have demonstrated a correlation between perinuclear ANCA and activation of neutrophils and free radicals that result in a cascade of

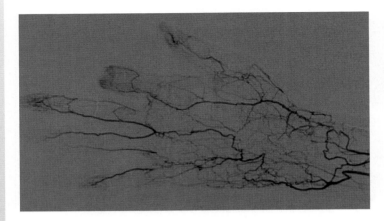

Fig. 8. Digital subtraction angiogram image in a patient with history of tobacco use after autoamputation of the index figure. Focal occlusions are noted with corkscrew collateral formation. Findings are consistent with Buerger's disease.

events that break up the endothelial barrier and induce focal edema and thrombosis.[39–41] Other drugs use a hypersensitivity response or neuroendocrine receptors to elicit responses of focal stenosis and narrowing.

Symptoms of drug-induced vasculopathies are difficult to discern from other etiologies and may have to be differentiated based on patient age and symptom onset after drug initiation. Most drugs have a cutaneous component that manifests as a rash or purpura in the hands, ears, nose or cheeks. Additional symptoms include strokes, arthralgias, renal failure, and peripheral ischemia.[1]

Imaging of these conditions usually begins with a screening MR angiography or CT angiography. Drug-induced vasculitis usually affects small- and medium-sized vessels, and imaging should be targeted to those regions. However, both of these modalities may be insensitive in detecting the vascular involvement, especially in the presence of small vessel disease. Digital subtraction angiography is the gold standard for imaging diagnosis. Affected organs show ischemic changes or patchy geographic enhancement on contrast-enhanced CT/MR imaging/angiography. Affected vessels show luminal irregularities, likely caused by focal areas of edema and thrombosis, areas of luminal stenosis, and occlusion and wall thickening (Figs. 9 and 10).[42,43] Treatment varies depending on the offending agent. It includes but is not limited to agent withdrawal, plasmapheresis, steroid use, and other supportive care.

VASCULOPATHY ASSOCIATED WITH CONNECTIVE TISSUE DISORDERS

Connective tissue disorders such Marfan syndrome, Ehlers-Danlos syndrome (EDS), and Loeys-Dietz syndrome (LDS) are a group of clinical syndromes in which genetic defects in the

formation of the extracellular matrix ECM result in weakened arterial walls and aneurysm formation as well a variety of nonvascular features related to weakened connective tissues.

Marfan Syndrome

Marfan syndrome is an autosomal-dominant connective tissue disorder caused by a defect in the FBN1 gene that encodes for the extracellular matrix protein, fibrillin-1.[44] The incidence is approximately 1 in 20,000 individuals.[45] The most associated vascular complications are aortic root dilation and thoracic aortic dissection (Fig. 11).[46]

Loeys-Dietz Syndrome

LDS is an autosomal-dominant connective tissue disorder caused by mutations in one of 2 genes encoding for the transforming growth factor–β (TGF-β) receptor, either TGFBR1 or TGFBR2 (causing LDS type 1 or 2).[47] First described in 2005, the prevalence ranges from 1 in 20,000 and 1 in 250,000. LDS is characterized by

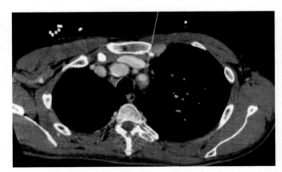

Fig. 9. Axial CT angiogram in a patient who took infliximab with wall thickening (arrow) of the subclavian artery consistent with chemotherapy-induced vasculitis.

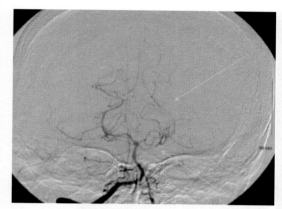

Fig. 10. Digital subtraction angiogram image of selective vertebral artery injection shows luminal irregularities (*arrows*) of the posterior circulation in a young patient abusing amphetamines.

craniofacial deformities and marked arterial tortuosity with a propensity for extracranial carotid and vertebral arteries.[45] Whereas dissection and aneurysm can involve the head and neck, abdominal, and coronary arteries, aortic root dilatation is nearly uniformly present. Thoracic aortic dissection is the most common cause of death, as in Marfan syndrome (**Fig. 12**).[46]

Ehlers-Danlos Syndrome

EDS is a heterogeneous group of syndromes united by defects in the production of collagen. Vascular EDS (type 4) is caused by a defect in the COL3A1 gene that encodes for the α chain of type III collagen 1.[48] The prevalence is approximately 1 in 250,000.[45] In EDS, aneurysm and dissection may occur throughout the arterial system, particularly in the abdominal aorta and its main branches (**Fig. 13**). Because of the fragile nature of the arterial wall in patients with type 4 EDS, dissections, ruptures, and arteriovenous fistulae can occur spontaneously or in response to minor trauma.[49]

All patients with connective disorders should be monitored with serial echocardiography to assess the heart and aortic root and with CT angiography/MR angiography of the chest and abdomen to assess aortic dissections and aneurysms. Patients with LDS should also undergo angiographic imaging of the head and neck. The mainstay of medical management has been β-blocker therapy. Recent and ongoing studies of Marfan syndrome have used the angiotensin II receptor antagonist, losartan, with promising results, thought to be related to decreased TGF-β pathway signaling.[50] When aneurysms or dissections occur and require intervention, surgical repair is preferred over endovascular stent-graft approaches because of underlying tissue fragility and increased incidence of endoleaks and disease progression.[51] Typically, aortic root repair is pursued when the aortic root diameter reaches 5 cm in Marfan syndrome and 4 cm in LDS or increases by 1 cm/year. EDS lesions are typically treated conservatively due to generally poor surgical outcomes.[46]

MISCELLANEOUS VASCULOPATHIES
Fibromuscular Dysplasia

Fibromuscular dysplasia (FMD) is a nonatherosclerotic, noninflammatory arteriopathy that causes narrowing of small- and medium-sized vessels. It is characterized by segmental areas of fibrotic tissue proliferation and smooth muscle overgrowth in the arterial wall.[52] Although a variety of mechanical, genetic, and hormonal factors have been proposed, the cause of FMD remains unknown. FMD predominantly affects younger women and children, with average ages of 15 to 50 years, and most often involves the renal arteries (60% to 75% of cases, of which 35% have bilateral renal artery involvement).[53,54] FMD has been described in almost every anatomic location but rarely involves other visceral and nonvisceral arteries, with the extracranial carotid and iliac arteries as the second and third most common sites, respectively.[54] Classic imaging findings include a string-of-beads appearance on

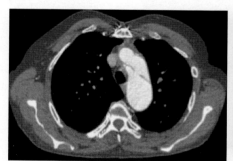
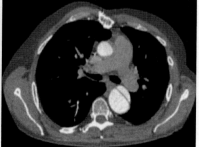

Fig. 11. Type B dissection in a 61-year-old man with Marfan syndrome.

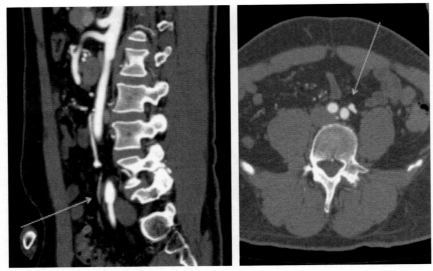

Fig. 12. A 35-year-old man with LDS with an inferior mesenteric artery aneurysm.

angiography involving the mid to distal portion of the artery, which typically presents as short segments of focal concentric stenoses alternating with aneurysms slightly larger than the normal caliber of the artery. Complications of FMD include arterial stenosis or occlusion with distal ischemia, dissection, rarely distal embolism, and, most commonly, hypertension in the setting of renal artery FMD.

Renal artery FMD is the second leading cause of renal artery stenosis after atherosclerosis and is the cause of 10% of cases of renovascular hypertension.[52,53] In contrast to atherosclerotic renal artery stenosis, which typically results is ostial narrowing, FMD affects the mid and distal renal artery. Another distinguishing feature of FMD

from other vasculitis syndromes is the lack of elevation of inflammatory markers typically seen in vasculitis.[53] Five histopathologic subtypes of FMD are described, including medial fibroplasia (75%–80%), perimedial fibroplasia (<10%), intimal fibroplasia (<10%), medial hyperplasia (<1%), and adventitial fibroplasia (<1%). Medial fibroplasia is characterized by the classic string-of-beads appearance of the mid to distal renal artery with the beads being larger than the normal vessel and pathologically proven to be true aneurysms **(Fig. 14)**.[52–54]

Duplex ultrasonography is the best initial screening examination, which has a high sensitivity and specificity for detecting main renal artery stenosis. CT angiography and MR angiography

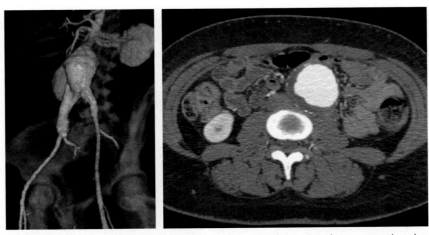

Fig. 13. A 26-year-old woman with EDS with a CT angiogram and 3-dimensional reconstruction shows an infrarenal aortic aneurysm.

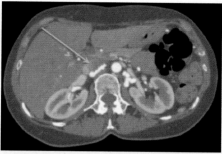
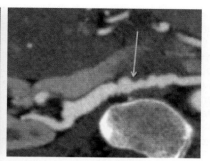
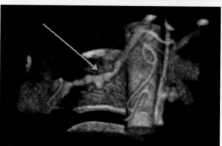

Fig. 14. CT angiogram shows a beaded (string of beads) appearance in the renal artery consistent with fibromuscular dysplasia. Bottom image is a 3-dimensional reconstruction of the renal artery.

are sometimes used to make the diagnosis but are limited by spatial resolution of the distal branch vessels affected by FMD. Therefore, catheter angiography remains the gold standard for diagnosis.[52–54] Pharmacologic management of hypertension is first-line therapy in patients with renal artery FMD. In the context of refractory hypertension with FMD, the treatment of choice for short-segment disease in the mid and distal renal arteries is percutaneous transluminal angioplasty, which is effective at disrupting fibrotic stenosis. Stenting should be reserved for stenosis greater than 30% after percutaneous transluminal angioplasty and for cases complicated by dissection or rupture after angioplasty. The definitive treatment of FMD involving long segments not amenable to angioplasty or stenting is surgical excision with bypass reconstruction to restore normal blood flow.[53,55] Asymptomatic FMD involving the carotid and vertebral arteries is often managed with antiplatelet drugs.

Segmental Arterial Mediolysis

Segmental arterial mediolysis (SAM) is a nonatherosclerotic, noninflammatory arteriopathy, which is characterized by dissecting aneurysms resulting from lysis of the outer media of the arterial wall. The most common presentation is abdominal pain and hemorrhage in the elderly.[56,57] Some literature describes SAM as a variant of FMD; however, a key distinguishing feature is the presence of dissections, the principle morphologic expression of SAM.[54,56,57]

SAM most commonly involves the abdominal aortic branches, especially the mesenteric arteries

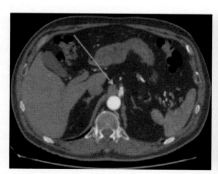
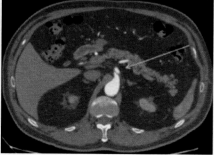

Fig. 15. A 45-year-old man with an isolated dissection of the celiac artery consistent with segmental arterial mediolysis.

(Fig. 15).[58] In addition, involvement of the carotid and vertebral arteries and iliac arteries is well described. On CT/MR/catheter angiography, fusiform aneurysms, stenosis, irregularity of the vessel wall, dissections, vessel wall thickening, and occlusions may be seen, often indistinguishable from other vasculitis.[56] Unlike FMD, SAM affects the middle and older age men, associated with sudden arterial dissection and rupture and involves the mesenteric arteries preferentially.[56,57,59]

The acute phase of SAM carries a 50% mortality rate most commonly owing to acute intra-abdominal hemorrhage.[56,60] Because of the rapid onset and progression of dissecting aneurysms, early detection with imaging is crucial. Complications of aneurysm rupture and mesenteric ischemia are often managed surgically; although, endovascular options are becoming more prevalent with each case managed uniquely.[56]

SUMMARY

Systemic vasculopathies represent a wide variety of heterogeneous vascular disorders characterized by vessel wall or luminal abnormalities. The imaging findings, in isolation, are rarely characteristic of any specific entity, but a combination of clinical and serologic findings and pattern of vessel involvement help differentiate various entities. Treatment depends on the underlying clinical entity. Endovascular and surgical options are used for treatment of ischemic symptoms and aneurysms at risk of rupture.

ACKNOWLEDGMENTS

The authors acknowledge the contributions of Jed Hummel, MD (UT Southwestern, Dallas).

REFERENCES

1. Wiik A. Clinical and laboratory characteristics of drug-induced vasculitic syndromes. Arthritis Res Ther 2005;7:191–2.
2. Jennette JC. Overview of the 2012 revised international chapel hill consensus conference nomenclature of vasculitides. Clin Exp Nephrol 2013;17:603–6.
3. Arend WP, Michel BA, Bloch DA, et al. The American college of rheumatology 1990 criteria for the classification of Takayasu arteritis. Arthritis Rheum 1990;33:1129–34.
4. Sharma BK, Jain S, Suri S, et al. Diagnostic criteria for Takayasu arteritis. Int J Cardiol 1996;54(Suppl):S141–7.
5. Tso E, Flamm SD, White RD, et al. Takayasu arteritis: utility and limitations of magnetic resonance imaging in diagnosis and treatment. Arthritis Rheum 2002;46:1634–42.
6. Eshet Y, Pauzner R, Goitein O, et al. The limited role of MRI in long-term follow-up of patients with Takayasu's arteritis. Autoimmun Rev 2011;11:132–6.
7. Schmidt WA. Role of ultrasound in the understanding and management of vasculitis. Ther Adv Musculoskelet Dis 2014;6:39–47.
8. Keo HH, Caliezi G, Baumgartner I, et al. Increasing echogenicity of diffuse circumferential thickening ("macaroni sign") of the carotid artery wall with decreasing inflammatory activity of takayasu arteritis. J Clin Ultrasound 2013;41:59–62.
9. Soussan M, Nicolas P, Schramm C, et al. Management of large-vessel vasculitis with FDG-PET: a systematic literature review and meta-analysis. Medicine 2015;94:e622.
10. Liang P, Hoffman GS. Advances in the medical and surgical treatment of Takayasu arteritis. Curr Opin Rheumatol 2005;17:16–24.
11. Hunder GG, Bloch DA, Michel BA, et al. The American college of rheumatology 1990 criteria for the classification of giant cell arteritis. Arthritis Rheum 1990;33:1122–8.
12. Bley TA, Uhl M, Carew J, et al. Diagnostic value of high-resolution MR imaging in giant cell arteritis. AJNR Am J Neuroradiol 2007;28:1722–7.
13. Mahr A, Guillevin L, Poissonnet M, et al. Prevalences of polyarteritis nodosa, microscopic polyangiitis, wegener's granulomatosis, and churg-strauss syndrome in a French urban multiethnic population in 2000: a capture-recapture estimate. Arthritis Rheum 2004;51:92–9.
14. Watts RA, Lane SE, Scott DG, et al. Epidemiology of vasculitis in Europe. Ann Rheum Dis 2001;60:1156–7.
15. Lightfoot RW Jr, Michel BA, Bloch DA, et al. The American college of rheumatology 1990 criteria for the classification of polyarteritis nodosa. Arthritis Rheum 1990;33:1088–93.
16. Hekali P, Kajander H, Pajari R, et al. Diagnostic significance of angiographically observed visceral aneurysms with regard to polyarteritis nodosa. Acta Radiol 1991;32:143–8.
17. Stanson AW, Friese JL, Johnson CM, et al. Polyarteritis nodosa: spectrum of angiographic findings. Radiographics 2001;21:151–9.
18. Rowley AH, Baker SC, Orenstein JM, et al. Searching for the cause of kawasaki disease [mdash] cytoplasmic inclusion bodies provide new insight. Nat Rev Microbiol 2008;6:394–401.
19. Ayusawa M, Sonobe T, Uemura S, et al. Revision of diagnostic guidelines for kawasaki disease (the 5th revised edition). Pediatr Int 2005;47:232–4.
20. Chung CJ, Stein L. Kawasaki disease: a review. Radiology 1998;208:25–33.
21. Mavrogeni S, Papadopoulos G, Karanasios E, et al. How to image kawasaki disease: a validation of

different imaging techniques. Int J Cardiol 2008;124: 27–31.

22. Greil GF, Stuber M, Botnar RM, et al. Coronary magnetic resonance angiography in adolescents and young adults with kawasaki disease. Circulation 2002;105:908–11.

23. Kallenberg CG. Key advances in the clinical approach to ANCA-associated vasculitis. Nat Rev Rheumatol 2014;10:484–93.

24. Davatchi F, Shahram F, Chams-Davatchi C, et al. Behcet's disease: from East to West. Clin Rheumatol 2010;29:823–33.

25. Chae EJ, Do KH, Seo JB, et al. Radiologic and clinical findings of Behcet disease: comprehensive review of multisystemic involvement. Radiographics 2008;28:e31.

26. Turesson C, O'Fallon WM, Crowson CS, et al. Extra-articular disease manifestations in rheumatoid arthritis: incidence trends and risk factors over 46 years. Ann Rheum Dis 2003;62:722–7.

27. Turesson C, O'Fallon WM, Crowson CS, et al. Occurrence of extraarticular disease manifestations is associated with excess mortality in a community based cohort of patients with rheumatoid arthritis. J Rheumatol 2002;29:62–7.

28. Bacons PA, Kitas GD. The significance of vascular inflammation in rheumatoid arthritis. Ann Rheum Dis 1994;53:621–3.

29. LaBresh KA, Lally EV, Sharma SC, et al. Two-dimensional echocardiographic detection of preclinical aortic root abnormalities in rheumatoid variant diseases. Am J Med 1985;78:908–12.

30. Slobodin GK, Khateeb A, Rimar D, et al. Aortitis in patients with psoriatic arthropathy: report of two cases and review of the literature. Rheumatol Rep 2014;6:6–9.

31. Kobak S, Yilmaz H, Karaarslan A, et al. Leukocytoclastic vasculitis in a patient with ankylosing spondylitis. Case Rep Rheumatol 2014;2014:653837.

32. Restrepo CS, Ocazionez D, Suri R, et al. Aortitis: imaging spectrum of the infectious and inflammatory conditions of the aorta. Radiographics 2011; 31:435–51.

33. Drenkard C, Villa AR, Reyes E, et al. Vasculitis in systemic lupus erythematosus. Lupus 1997;6:235–42.

34. Radic M, Martinovic Kaliterna D, Radic J. Vascular manifestations of systemic lupus erythematosis. Neth J Med 2013;71:10–6.

35. Buerger L. Landmark publication from the American journal of the medical sciences, 'thrombo-angiitis obliterans: a study of the vascular lesions leading to presenile spontaneous gangrene'. 1908. Am J Med Sci 2009;337:274–84.

36. Olin JW. Thromboangiitis obliterans (Buerger's disease). N Engl J Med 2000;343:864–9.

37. Sasaki S, Sakuma M, Kunihara T, et al. Distribution of arterial involvement in thromboangiitis obliterans

(Buerger's disease): results of a study conducted by the Intractable Vasculitis Syndromes Research Group in Japan. Surg Today 2000;30:600–5.

38. Lambeth JT, Yong NK. Arteriographic findings in thromboangiitis obliterans with emphasis on femoropopliteal involvement. Am J Roentgenol Radium Ther Nucl Med 1970;109:553–62.

39. Gan X, Zhang L, Berger O, et al. Cocaine enhances brain endothelial adhesion molecules and leukocyte migration. Clin Immunol 1999;91:68–76.

40. Gao Y, Zhao MH. Review article: drug-induced antineutrophil cytoplasmic antibody-associated vasculitis. Nephrology (Carlton) 2009;14:33–41.

41. Taborda L, Amaral B, Isenberg D. Drug-induced vasculitis. Adverse Drug React Bull 2013;279:1075–8.

42. Moritani T, Hiwatashi A, Shrier DA, et al. CNS vasculitis and vasculopathy: efficacy and usefulness of diffusion-weighted echoplanar MR imaging. Clin Imaging 2004;28:261–70.

43. Ha HK, Lee SH, Rha SE, et al. Radiologic features of vasculitis involving the gastrointestinal tract. Radiographics 2000;20:779–94.

44. Dietz HC, Cutting GR, Pyeritz RE, et al. Marfan syndrome caused by a recurrent de novo missense mutation in the fibrillin gene. Nature 1991;352:337–9.

45. Halushka MK. Single gene disorders of the aortic wall. Cardiovasc Pathol 2012;21:240–4.

46. Chu LC, Johnson PT, Dietz HC, et al. CT angiographic evaluation of genetic vascular disease: role in detection, staging, and management of complex vascular pathologic conditions. AJR Am J Roentgenol 2014;202:1120–9.

47. Loeys BL, Chen J, Neptune ER, et al. A syndrome of altered cardiovascular, craniofacial, neurocognitive and skeletal development caused by mutations in TGFBR1 or TGFBR2. Nat Genet 2005;37:275–81.

48. Pope FM, Martin GR, Lichtenstein JR, et al. Patients with ehlers-danlos syndrome type IV lack type III collagen. Proc Natl Acad Sci U S A 1975;72:1314–6.

49. Chu LC, Johnson PT, Dietz HC, et al. Vascular complications of ehlers-danlos syndrome: CT findings. AJR Am J Roentgenol 2012;198:482–7.

50. Bolar N, Van Laer L, Loeys BL. Marfan syndrome: from gene to therapy. Curr Opin Pediatr 2012;24:498–504.

51. Schepens MA. Re: "thoracic aortic endografting in patients with connective tissue disease". J Endovasc Ther 2008;15:626–7 [author reply: 7–8].

52. Hickey R, Nemcek A. Diagnosis and role of interventional techniques. In: Geschwind JH, Dake MD, editors. Abrams' angiography: interventional radiology. Philadelphia: Lippincott Williams & Wilkins; 2014. p. 621–2.

53. Slovut DP, Olin JW. Fibromuscular dysplasia. N Engl J Med 2004;350:1862–71.

54. Dahnert W. Radiology review manual. 7th, North American edition. Philadelphia: Lippincott Williams and Wilkins; 2011.

55. Begelman SM, Olin JW. Fibromuscular dysplasia. Curr Opin Rheumatol 2000;12:41–7.

56. Chao CP. Segmental arterial mediolysis. Semin Intervent Radiol 2009;26:224–32.

57. Lie JT. Segmental mediolytic arteritis. Not an arteritis but a variant of arterial fibromuscular dysplasia. Arch Pathol Lab Med 1992;116:238–41.

58. Hashimoto T, Deguchi J, Endo H, et al. Successful treatment tailored to each splanchnic arterial lesion due to segmental arterial mediolysis (SAM): report of a case. J Vasc Surg 2008;48:1338–41.

59. Armas OA, Donovan DC. Segmental mediolytic arteritis involving hepatic arteries. Arch Pathol Lab Med 1992;116:531–4.

60. Heritz DM, Butany J, Johnston KW, et al. Intraabdominal hemorrhage as a result of segmental mediolytic arteritis of an omental artery: case report. J Vasc Surg 1990;12:561–5.

Index

Note: Page numbers of article titles are in **boldface** type.